# About the au

## Michael A Crawford PhD, FRSB, FRCPath

Michael Crawford was born in Edinburgh and did national service with RCAF Winnipeg and RAF Oldenburg. In 1965 he obtained a doctorate at the Royal Post Graduate Medical School, Hammersmith, then established biochemical teaching at the Makerere College, Medical School in Kampala, Uganda. The UK had built a new teaching hospital in Mulago as a goodbye present for independence in 1962. With Sandy Rankin, he helped create the Muhimbili Medical School in Dar-es-Salam in 1963, returning to London in 1965. The experience in East Africa taught him the power of nutrition in health and non-communicable diseases which were in total contrast to those in the UK. At the Nuffield Institute of Comparative Medicine, he and Andrew Sinclair published the first evidence of the role

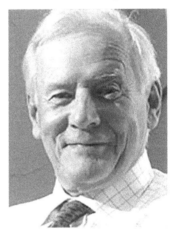

of DHA and arachidonic acid in the evolution of the brain in 1971. This was followed by the first evidence of an omega 3 deficiency causing severe behavioural disorders in a primate in 1973. He then turned his attention to maternal nutrition during pregnancy, when most of the human brain cells divide. On retiring in 2010 he was invited to work at Chelsea and Westminster Hospital campus of Imperial College, London, as a visiting professor. The prime interest of the team under Professor Mark Johnson, head of obstetrics and gynaecology, is in preventing preterm birth and the neurodevelopmental disorders which handicap a child for life. He has won many international awards and was elected as a Freeman of the City of London in 2017.

He has published 300 peer-reviewed scientific papgers and three books

web: www.imperial.ac.uk/people/michael.crawford
michael.crawford@imperial.ac.uk

## David E Marsh Dip Agric

D avid trained initially in agriculture (Shuttleworth College, Bedfordshire) with ten years experience farming in Bedfordshire. In the late 1970s and early 1980s David interviewed many medical doctors and scientists who had unusual ideas regarding the noncommunicable diseases (NCDs) and began writing the storyboard for a television series... thus meeting Michael Crawford in 1981 whilst he was director of Nutritional Biochemistry at the Nuffield Foundation Laboratories at London Zoo, (ZSL).

David then moved to human nutrition and co-authored The Driving Force; Food in Evolution & the Future (1989) – later Nutrition and Evolution (1995), with Professor Michael Crawford (Inst. Brain Chem. & Human Nutrition, Imperial College London). He has since written broadly (for Resurgence, Positive Health, Positive Health Online, Healthy Eating, Nutrition 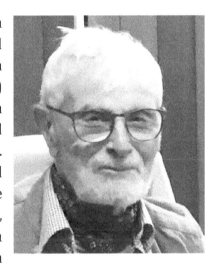 and Health amongst other publications) about nutrition, evolution, environment and integrated medicine, including a series in the Journal of Alternative & Complementary Medicine on energy or vibrational medicine.

This book is of particular interest to the author as it brings his special interests in nutrition and food production together in full circle. The Origins of Diversity: Darwin's Conditions and Epigenetic Variations, (Nutrition & Health 2008) won him the presitigious Cleave Award from the McCarrison Society for

Nutrition and Health in 2016.

David edited the McCarrison Society for Nutrition and Health Newsletter for ten years, together with many and various articles with it, and for the society's Journal Nutrition & Health; (see www. mccarrison.com). He lectures very occasionally on the history of evolution theories.

David can be reached at **davidmarsh.dip.ag@gmail.com**
www.davidmarsh.org.uk
**search <David Marsh Darwin>**

# In Memoriam

*To my late mother Joy (nee Thomas) – Marsh - Hilton whose tragically early death inspired me to attempt this and our previous books, The Driving Force: Food, Evolution and the Future (Heinemann, London) & Harper & Row (USA) 1989. Nutrition and Evolution, Keats 1995. Crawford M A & Marsh D E.*

# Dedication

To the recovery of the planet, now that epigenetics demonstrates the true role of environmental forces on our health and continued evolution.

To those dedicated people urging us to respect and re-build our environment.

To all young people and children of today, and those yet to be born.

# Acknowledgements

I firstly must thank David Marsh my co-author. Without his help and persuasion, this book might not have been written. His insights into Darwin's true story became an important motivation in the writing. We also wish to thank our publisher Chris Day whose encouragement has been of immense support. Then we must thank Alex Proud who bought my 1987 stretched version of the Citroen Prestige. It took only a matter of minutes for our chatting to reveal he shared the vision of the present crisis in humanity and offered to host the launch of the book at his gallery with support from one of his restaurants. A tower of strength and support!

I have a deep debt of gratitude to Uganda and its Makerere University Medical School. To witness and have the privilege of writing several research papers on the cause of non-communicable diseases (NCD) of East Africa which were in absolute contrast to the NCDs we encountered on return to the UK. That gave me an unshakable insight into the power of nutrition in human health. And for that insight I recall it was the late Professor Malcolm Milne, my PhD supervisor and Sir John McMichael then professor of medicine at the Royal Post Graduate Medical School, Hammersmith, who persuaded me of the wealth of opportunities for research in East Africa.

Then when we returned from Uganda, it was my much-loved wife Sheilagh who persuaded me to write a book "What We Eat Today" on our experience in East Africa and its health implications, As joint author, she put much of her own insight into the book. Having studied art at the then Ecole des Métiers et d'Art, in Paris she was asked to take over medical art at Makerere Medical School in Kampala. That was when the incumbent did not return from leave. It was a critical time as

Denis Burkitt needed her to draw his maps and figures for his seminal papers on the first evidence for a viral cause of cancer: Burkitt's Lymphoma. The experience with Denis, gave her a special insight to health in Uganda and the UK from a different perspective to mine. That was invaluable in the joint effort of the book which, published in 1972. We predicted the present rise in mental ill-health unless people included the nutrition of the brain in their food production and nutrition policies of which of course they did not.

On returning from Makerere in 1965 to head Biochemistry at the then Nuffield Institute of Comparative Medicine, I successfully managed to get a good grant from the Medical Research Council to work on lipid nutrition and the brain. With this grant, I was able to attract Andrew Sinclair to come to London and worked with us for 5 years. Together we uncovered new knowledge on arachidonic and docosahexaenoic acids with their selective incorporation into brain structures, and their role in evolution leading to the first evidence of an omega 3 deficiency inducing severe behavioural pathology in a primate in 1973. I thank Andrew and all the several good people who worked for us during those years of discoveries.

In the writing of this new follow on from the "Driving Force" I need to thank my family all of whom have been so encouraging, from time to time contributing with incisive thoughts. We sadly lost my wife Sheilagh to cancer. Later, I was gifted with Mandy my current wife whose help and attention to proper food and exercise. She has been a constant support and with an eye for the straight and narrow providing much needed guidance. Then I wish to thank Professor Mark Johnson and Dr Enitan Ogundipe who gave me a new lease of life by inviting me to join them at Chelsea and Westminster Campus of Imperial College, after retiring from London Metropolitan. The research work at Imperial College has opened the supreme importance of maternal health and nutrition before and around the time of conception. It also points the way to the prevention of developmental disorders of the brain, with their high prevalence in babies born preterm and at low birthweights. We need to thank the late Professor Letten F Saugstad for her sponsorship which helped fund the work through the Mother and Child Foundation. Exploring the relationship between nutrition and brain development with Mark and Enitan kept David and I up to date with the rapid developments in lipids and neuroscience where with Dr Yiqun Wang we also pushed back some boundaries in knowledge of maternal nutrition and health and the brain. David and I wish to thank Rachel Gow who throughout has been pushing us to get the book completed and advocating various organisations to help with its launch. There are so many people I wish to thank. But without taking up several more pages in an already long book, I know that they know – They are all over the world – So many in the USA, including my relations, Australia,Canada, Denmark, Dubai, France, Germany, India, Israel, Lebanon, Mexico, New Zealand, Oman, Pakistan, South Africa, the Sudan, Sweden and Norway: thank you truly for your science and support. A special thanks to Julian Simpole for his first edit of our writing and continued support. We also deeply thank the quiet, patient editing of Paul Sullivan. Paul has been remarkable for his generosity of effort, understanding of our frailties and mindful support of the principles echoed in the pages of this book.

**Michael A Crawford**

My thanks to Chandra Masoliver, without whose enthusiasm, hard work, encouragement, editing abilities and generosity over many years, this book would not have been written.

To both the late Simon House, MA Cantab (Nat Sci & Theol) and Professor Edward (Ted) Tuddenham MD, FRCP, FRCPath,

FacMed, Emeritus Professor of Haemophilia, University College London. For their advice in interpreting the human genome map and the role of epigenetics in our evolution.

Thanks to Positive Health Online for permission to re-publish Chapter 3 as they had previously published an earlier version.

**David E Marsh**

David was joint author with Michael of the Driving Force (Heinemann 1989) and Nutrition and Evolution (Keats, USA 1995).

We need to acknowledge Alex Proud and his gallery staff for holding the launch in his Proud Gallery with support from one of his restaurants. As Master of Ceremonies, Alex was a tower of strength and support for the theme of the book.

We absolutely wish to thank Rick Stein for launching our book on the 7th June 2023. His supreme skills in cooking fish and seafood added to the scientific needs of the brain, made a great combination of reason for protecting the oceans and enjoying much more of its wealth to save our brains. We also wish to thank his brother Professor Emeritus John Stein for his well-chosen words explaining why proper management of the ocean's wealth will stop the shrinking of our brains so enhancing the health and intelligence of future children.

Thanks are also due to Dr. Bill/William Spears for writing the foreword to show that David and Michael are not the only people concerned about the global crisis of brain health

# The Shrinking Brain

## The role of the environment in its evolution and future

Michael A Crawford

David E Marsh

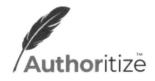

Published by
Authoritize Ltd
14, Croydon Road, Beddington
Surrey, CR0 4PA

+44(0) 20 8688 2598
www.authoritize.co.uk

ISBN 978-1-915465-12-2

Printed in the UK

# CONTENTS

# Foreword

My favourite "fish story" happened in 2012 when I personally met my omega-3 mentor, Dr. Michael Crawford. We were both speakers at the Global Organization for EPA and DHA (GOED) in Japan. Michael was the seafood scientist. I was the show-me-the-science pediatrician. We blended well then as speakers and now as authors who have a mission to make this world a smarter environment for human brains to thrive. I first met Michael at a conference on brain health in Japan. We were on the same platform. We listened to each other and after, sat together to talk about our common views on DHA, the brain, and the challenge of mental health. In so doing, we bonded our friendship and our mission.

During dinner we slowly savoured each bite of seafood and enjoyed the Japanese custom of *umami* (take time to dine and enjoy the good mouthfeel and gut-feel of the delicious seafood). Michael downloaded his decades of omega-3 research and imprinted his lessons into my seafood-enriched brain, and from that night on I upgraded my own eating habits and teachings to include his mantra: "Eat more seafood; grow a smarter and happier brain!" After that brainy night, I became a sea-foodie and had more fish stories to tell my children, grandchildren, and patients. You will enjoy these authors' fish stories throughout this book.

Meanwhile, back at my medical office. When expectant parents consult me for prenatal counselling, I get their attention by smiling and saying, "You're growing a little fathead inside!"

Naturally, they prod me to explain "fathead", as the authors explain so simply and scientifically in this book. I start by congratulating the mother, "You're doing the most important job in the world – growing a little human being." Continuing the consultation, "Your baby's brain is growing the fastest inside you than at any other time in his or her life. And the number one 'grow food' for your little fathead is the omega-3 in seafood, or seafood-based omega-3 supplements." I quickly add another motivator: "Your baby gets first dibs on the omega- 3s in your diet during pregnancy and breastfeeding when there isn't enough for two. Baby gets an omega-3-sufficiency, and you may suffer an omega-3-insufficiency, which is one of the top contributing factors to why some women suffer depression during and after their pregnancy. Your 'little sucker' literally milks the omega-3 DHA out of you - smart for Baby, but not so smart for Mommy since you also need enough omega-3s to meet the challenge of feeding and caring for your precious new baby."

In *The Shrinking Brain* parents will love reading about the importance of nutrition prenatally and postnatally, especially during the most critical period of brain development, before birth, when a baby's rapidly growing brain soaks up seventy percent of the total energy Baby receives from mother through the placenta. I love the authors' description when they write about baby-brain development in the womb: *Powered by maternal nutrition.*

At the six-month check-up I play the role of Dr. O. Mega III and continue the "fathead" talk by surprising parents with this advice: "Begin feeding salmon at seven months." I explain that the earlier parents can shape their baby's taste toward savoring seafood, the better for baby-brain development. Our greatest national treasure is our children, yet we do not treasure how we feed them. This one simple seafood start gets the child's brain into a growth path for life, in addition to supporting a healthier heart, gut, and nearly every other organ in a rapidly growing little body. DHA is the smartest nutrient our brains and bodies need, yet it is the nutrient that most of us eat less of and know little about. This book helps fix that.

After reading this book you will be convinced that seafood is the smartest food on planet Earth. Consider the brain- nutrient density of wild salmon. The smart nutrients that seafood provides, and that you will learn more about in this book, are omega-3 DHA/EPA, protein, astaxanthin (the powerful antioxidant that makes salmon pink), vitamins B6 and B12, vitamin D, choline, niacin, iodine, and tryptophan – all nutrients smart brains like. Seafood is smart see-food. That makes sense since the eyes are an extension of the brain. The top nutrient in the brain, DHA, is also the top nutrient in the retina of the eye.

When you read about the many nutrients in seafood, you will learn about an important nutritional principle called *synergy*, meaning that all these nutrients in seafood are partners in health. When you eat them together, they help each other exert more healthful effects. A great example is the partnership of vitamin D and omega-3 fats in seafood. Seafood is smart synergy food, a point the authors make throughout this book.

The title *The Shrinking Brain* says it all. At no time in our history has our knowledge of brain health been greater, yet the attack on our brains – and its smartest food – has never been more alarming. You will not only learn how to eat smarter but how to become a convincing voice in getting more and safer seafood from the sea into our brains. Our most precious organ, our brain (what makes us human and uniquely ourselves), is growing up in a polluted environment where it was never designed to thrive. The epidemic of mental unwellness is at the highest point in history, yet the most science-based and safest "medicine" is found in the sea.

So, my *Shrinking Brain* prescription for you: read it, eat it, do it, and teach it. You now have the tools to help yourself, your family, and our world live smarter and happier. And as a final note, this is a prescription for all ages. Not only is seafood the top grow-food for young brains, but it is also preventive medicine for maintaining senior brain health.

**William Sears, M.D., F.R.C.P.**
Author of *The Omega-3 Effect and The Healthy Brain Book*

# Preface

Since 1950, the prevalence of mental ill health has been escalating and measures of intelligence falling. In addition, brain size has been shrinking. This trend cannot be allowed to continue. Our book explains why and what can be done to reverse the trend, so as to ensure brighter children and progress for humanity.

We are concerned with the power of the environment in influencing evolution, our present and future. Hence we start with restoring Charles Darwin's importance of the environment. In 1859 and in his 5 further editions of Origin of Species he described Natural Selection being powered by 'the conditions of existence' (his term for the environment).

Ten years after his death in 1882, the creator of NeoDarwinism, August Weismann wrote two fatuously misleading and incorrect papers attempting to 'disprove' Darwin's theory, and succeeded by removing natural selection's powerpack: the environment, and opening the door for the gene-centric dominance..

From those late-19th-century days, thanks to Weismann, the environment became abused and treated as a dumping ground for mankind's waste. Weismann did the world a grave disservice from which we have not yet recovered.

A powerful example of Darwin's conditions of existence was the fact that during the first 3 billion years or so, of our planet's existence, life was photosynthetic and anaerobic. About 600 million years ago, enough oxygen accrued in the environment and seas for air-breathing life to evolve. All 32 phyla we have today evolved in the very short geological time frame, known as the Cambrian Explosion.

In the first, tiny single celled aerobic species like the dinoflagellates, sunlight was converted not into carbohydrates and proteins, as in the past, but into electricity. As multicellular species evolved, this sparked the evolution of the nervous system, and then the brain.

Also, the conversion of light to metabolic energy used omega 3 docosahexaenoic acid for its receptor structures. Amazingly, we still use the same for the structures and functions of our eyes, synapses, and neurons today. Obviously, the brain evolved in the sea but at first, it was very small, So what was the missing factor for its ultimate expansion?

When animals colonized the land, they reproduced by egg-laying. Then an asteroid, 7.5 miles wide struck the planet some 66 million years ago. The giant reptiles and the giant trees became extinct and were replaced by gentler flowering plants with protected seeds. The new environment provided the missing component for the brain's structures and is now essential for mammalian reproduction and brain size being several times bigger than before.

Our ancestors evolved a unique 1,600 cc brain from our ancestral, 350cc of the chimpanzee, despite our genomes differing by only 1.5%. This could only have happened with the provision of brain-specific building nutrients from both land and sea. Despite rising sea levels, there is incontrovertible evidence of early Homo exploiting both land and the marine food web in coastal Africa. This includes evidence of the controlled use of fire in cooking fish 780,000 years ago at Gesher Benot Ya'aqov, Israel.

Unfortunately, no government today has a food and agricultural policy that provides the special building blocks for the brain. In this book, we explain the rise and recent fall of the brain, exemplified by the rising prevalence of mental ill- health, and the declining measures of intelligence since 1950, due to Weismann's false science.

The change in the nutritional environment behind these adverse effects can be and must be reversed. The continued escalation of mental ill-health is logically a threat to the sustainability of humanity. https://www.ted.com/talks/josette_sheeran_ending_hunger_?

# CHAPTER 1
# An overview of the problem facing us

*"We celebrate the past to awaken the future"*
*John F Kennedy*

*"We cannot remain looking inwards at ourselves on a small and increasingly polluted and overcrowded planet"*
*Stephen Hawking*

This book is an attempt to retell the story of the planet and how we came to be here. Darwin is commonly associated with natural selection as a means for "the survival of the fittest" (an inexact phrase coined by philosopher and biologist Herbert Spencer in 1864). But he wrote more than that, and we shall discuss his concern over the impact of *environment* on evolution. This part of his writing has been ignored, but we shall re-visit it as it is relevant to our survival.

Humanity faces four crises: population growth with limited food and fresh water; pollution and climate change. The fourth is little recognised but of profound importance to our survival. It is the rise in mental ill-health and decline in measures of intelligence since 1950. The continuation of this trend is a greater threat to the survival of our children and theirs, than climate change, as serious as that is. It is only logical that the loss of intelligence leads to a poor ability to learn and make intelligent decisions. The greater the loss the greater the dehumanization. Inexorably, it is human evolution in reverse: it can only lead to the extinction of *Homo sapiens*.

Despite the fact that is the brain which makes us different

from animals, no Government has any recommendations for nutrition and brain health. There are recommendations for protein and body growth, but the brain is not made of protein it is made of lipid – i.e. highly specialised fats. The escalation of mental ill-health has been brushed under the carpet.

We like to get our messages from Nature. Take the composition of human milk for example. It contains the least protein compared to any of the large mammals. Yet it is rich in the essential fats needed to complete the building and function of the growing infant's brain.

In this book we explain how the brain evolved and what was required to make it. We illustrate the crucial importance of the environment in evolution. Indeed, we restore Darwin's interest in the environment as more powerful than natural selection. Indeed, it is obvious that natural selection can only move in directions permitted by the environment. This point is exemplified by the simple fact that air breathing animals could not evolve unless there was enough oxygen. For some 3 billion years life was basically anaerobic with not much happening evolution wise. Then when there was enough oxygen – big bang- all 32 phyla we have to day appear in the fossil record in what is called the *Cambrian Explosion*. Unfortunately. Darwin's interest in the environment was kicked out of touch by August Weissman's totally unscientific experiments leading to a gene centric philosophy. We will explain how this happened with its adverse consequences.

In so doing we hope to provide a solution to the crisis in mental ill health which has been highlighted with this new pandemic of Covid-19. With the decline in IQ since 1950 and the shrinking brain we are on a path of no return unless we sort the problem. .

The only real sense of urgency on all these issues comes from the young – campaigners like Greta Thunberg, inspiring 'climate crisis' demonstrations in London and cities worldwide. Their activity has at last won the attention of politicians – but for how long? The urgency does not just spring from rebellious youthful imaginations – it is very real. Each of these crises individually has the power to annihilate humanity. Their joint impact, to put it mildly, is bad news.

Following on discoveries we made in the 1970s and since, we offer a better evidence-based understanding of the origin of the brain, its nutritional needs and why we now face a mental health crisis. This leads to the last chapter in which we propose a solution to the decline in mental health and intelligence. It's a fascinating one, because it puts the priority of *human biology* with a focus on the supreme importance of the mother at the centre.

The development of a food system to reverse the decline, will simultaneously through carbon capture, take out much $CO_2$. We propose that the answer to arresting the rise in mental ill-health will lead to brighter children, enhance health in general and help address climate change.

## Covid-19 and the wake-up call

The image of a human mother with her child is one which underlines all our history and hopes for the future. She is pivotal to our story because most of the adult number of brain cells divide before birth. But timeless and enduring as this image may seem, the healthy continuity it represents is in grave danger. Covid-19 is a stark demonstration on the thinness of the thread that holds life. The Black Death, carried by flea-infested animals and textiles, reached its peak in Europe between 1347 and 1351. There were around 100 million deaths in Eurasia, which was about a fifth of the population. Whole communities were wiped out.

Bill Gates gave a TED lecture in 2015 in which he pointed out that 'Our society is woefully unprepared for a bad pandemic'. The kind of pandemic Gates was talking about is now among us, and it allegedly came from a mutated virus in a wild animal or escaped from a laboratory in Wuhan China, November 2019. In November 2020 Covid-19 spread to mink in Denmark, where there is a likelihood of another mutation. This new dimension raises the chilling possibility that a more lethal mutation of the virus could be even worse than the Black Death. It is important to note that males are more likely to be mentally affected and to die of Covid-19 than females. Apart from the elderly, the highest risk groups are amongst the ethnic minorities. Note that these are the same groups that are at the highest risk[2,3] of heart disease, diabetes and western cancers. They are also the groups at highest risk to low birthweights, moreover, males are more susceptible to the impact of dietary inadequacies of essential fatty acids, which are responsible for critical issues such as the integrity of the vascular cell membranes, the response to injury and immune function and are also responsible for the growth and function of the brain and its signalling systems. It is evident that some of the long-term impacts of Covid-19 infection involve impaired brain function [4,5,6,7]

There is good evidence that vitamin D has a protective effect. Bear in mind that dietary vitamin D co-exists with certain essential fatty acids important for the lipids (technical jargon for biological fats) needed to build cell membranes and the brain. It is a lipid- or fat-soluble vitamin, so it occurs in the liver of animals and is abundant in the lipids and oils of fish and sea foods of nearly all kinds. Corona-type viruses have a lipid membrane, and to infect you they have to penetrate the lipid membrane which surrounds our cells. They then remodel cellular membranes to form viral replication compartments (VRCs), which are the sites where viral RNA genome replication takes place. To induce VRC formation, these viruses 'extensively rewire lipid metabolism'. Recent research has provided evidence that 'membrane contact sites and lipid transfer proteins are hijacked by viruses and play pivotal roles in VRC formation'. [8]

That is, the health status of your lipids is likely to be a determinant of cell membrane integrity, immune system competence, brain defence systems and your ability not only to defend against infection but also to fight the worst it can throw at you. The sectors of the population which have the poorest nutrition regarding vascular, immune system and brain health are those at the highest risk.

The long-term adverse effects of Covid-19 and its variants on brain function is a worrying scenario, and It is clear that Covid-19 is a wake-up call for mental health. On 3 March 2022, the European Council opened negotiations for an international agreement on pandemic prevention, preparedness and response. The 194 members of the World Health Organization (WHO) agreed in December 2021 for pandemic prevention, preparedness and response. Very large sums of money have now been committed for a global research effort into preparedness and dealing with a future pandemic. Granted covid-19 has raised awareness of the global threat of extinction by a novel virus as infective as influenza but totally lethal. Here within we see again the opportunity to address the issue of mental health is missed.

This book is about the origin of the brain and the principles of nutrition which powered it from a 340 gram sized chimpanzee brain to the large brain of *Homo sapiens*. That incremental generation by generation of cerebral expansion could not have occurred without the special nutrients needed to build the brain and enable it to function.

No other land-based animal managed this feat. Indeed their brains shrank in relation to body size as they got bigger and bigger and grew faster and faster, We shall tell the simple story as to how *Homo sapiens* escaped that trap.

That story is of supreme importance to our survival. Since 1950, the prevalence of mental ill-health has been escalating and IQ has been diminishing.[9] Continuation of this trend logically leads to dehumanization and the end of our species. The evolution of our large brain depended on our ancestors finding the right nutrients to power its expansion. The present-day food system is failing to properly nourish the brain. In fact it is putting neural evolution into reverse with a shrinking of brain size and cognitive ability. Yet this threat is nowhere visible. We shall make a plea for its recognition and for a world-wide effort to stop the decline in mental health and restore the upward thrust of neural evolution to secure a future for our children and theirs. It is their future which is at stake.

## We need to sort the food system

The ancestors of *Homo sapiens* separated from the chimpanzees some 7 million years ago. Our genomes are only 1.5% different. This means our genome was adapted to wild foods. That is an obvious and undeniable fact. Now there are many ideas about how we evolved –We will present paleoanthropological evidence in support for our case describing the specifics of the wild food principle.

Sir Robert McCarrison, was a doctor major general in the British Army and served in the Indian Medical Service. He was impressed by the high prevalence of malnutrition in the cities compared to robust health he encountered when posted to Coonoor in 1927. Sir Robert was the first to demonstrate the power of malnutrition by feeding colonies of rats either on the diet of the country or city people! [10,11]. He founded the Medical Research Institute in Hyderabad which thrived and developed to become the prestigious, National Institute of Nutrition, in Hyderabad. Sir Robert's answer to nutrition, long life and health gained from his experience with the Hunza, is simple

*"The unsophisticated foods of Nature"*

Whatever you believe, it is unquestionable that the food we eat today bears little resemblance to the food and nutrition that powered our ascendency from the 350cc chimpanzee brain to *Homo sapiens* 160,000 to 200,000 years ago, with a 1,450 cc brain, a size that had been attained in the earliest known members of our species. The skulls of these earliest modern human fossils were found in Herto, Ethiopia by a team of Paleoanthropologists led by Tim White, professor at the University of California, Berkeley, in November 1997. Cro Magnon 1 lived closer to our time and skulls dating to about 30.000 years ago were even larger at over 1,600cc. It is now accepted in the topic that in recent times our brains have been shrinking. Based on the evidence of 8,000 autopsies, the average brain weight of the adult male is now 1,336g, and 1,198g for the adult female. With increasing age, brain weight decreases by 2.7g in males, and by 2.2g in females per year.

This reduction in the capacity of the brain is alarming. It is the brain which makes us human. If it is lost, all is lost. Covid-19 is a wake-up call on many fronts, but importantly, with mental ill-health on an escalating course to destroy humanity, it is a wake-up call for us to sort the food system. Moreover, the increasing prevalence in disorders of the brain threatens the very essence of who we are – what it is to be human. And at the root of the threat is the food we eat.

This book offers readers the opportunity to readjust their dietary perceptions – to liberate themselves from past dogmas and realise the beauty and power of food, of how our bodies can find a perfect balance with the nutritional environment, and how that simple fact has shaped our evolution. There's nothing stopping this equilibrium from being reached. We've been there before – for 90% of our existence as a species, in fact – and we can return via relatively simple measures. All most of us lack is information. The role of this book is to act as the missing instruction manual. We do not offer recipes or cooking instructions. Instead it is our hope that through an understanding of how things came to be people will be able to rationalize and make their own choices. This book we hope, will help people make an informed choice about the food they eat.

## The tasks ahead

It is our task, whether as parents, friends, guardians, or simply lovers of humanity, to leave a legacy for future generations by giving them the best possible nutritional start in life. We need to guide and educate politicians and thought leaders, informing them of the role that nutrition plays in the biochemistry of the brain and, critically, in preventing mental ill-health. Specifically, we need to highlight the vital role played by the omega-3 fats and brain-specific nutrients central to the evolution of the brain more than 500 million years ago. This evolution took place in the seas; hence the richest sources of brain-specific food are fish, other sea foods and certain algae.

This book provides a new look at evolution based on physics and chemistry and shaped by the nutrients available in the environment. Make no mistake, all the good work of evolution is in danger of being undone! In 2004 the EU decided to carry out an audit of the cost of health. When reported a year later, brain disorders carried the greatest cost at €386 billion.

The rise in mental ill-health has overtaken all other burdens of illness. It cost £105 billion in the UK in 2010, a sum greater than cancer and heart disease combined, and a rise from £77 billion in 2007. These are the Department of Health's own data; and yet the topic is below the radar of most politicians even though the media is beginning to pick up on the message.

## Brain food

We hope this book will draw attention to the supreme importance of the brain and indeed to 'brain food'. Just as our bones, skin and hearts have special but different nutrient requirements, the same is true for the brain. But its very special needs have, to our cost, been ignored. This nutritional information is particularly pertinent to anyone thinking of starting a family, and for all who wish to reach old age with their mental capacity intact. The following chapters are also required reading for the people responsible for policy regarding food, education and health. With an ever-expanding human population, the story we tell is supremely important for shaping the environmental, nutritional and agricultural polices needed to ensure the sustainability of humankind.

Although in a practical sense our story kick-starts at the next World Health Organisation gathering, EU food policy board meeting or International Food Policy Research Institute summit, the bigger picture starts way back with the origins of multi-cellular life. As John F Kennedy said, "We celebrate the past to awaken the future". The central focus of The Shrinking Brain is encompassed in that quotation. The message contained in our origins as a species holds the key to our current and future mental health and wellbeing and the challenges we now face.

## A new insight

We also hope to provide new insight into the past of our planet and its inhabitants, challenging the present self-view of our species. The astonishing fact is that the brain has been ignored in the fields of food policy and education. We have overlooked or simply ignored the importance of nutrition for the brain and the wild food which came from land lakes, rivers and seas.

Based on the current science, our book exposes stark choices for the future. The choice is on the one hand an increase in general human intelligence, prosperity and peace, and on the other a continued, diminishing IQ, and escalation of mental ill-health which threaten sustainability of humanity. In 1804 the world population stood at 1 billion. It took 127 years to add another billion. In 1966 when we first began to write on these matters the world population was 3 billion. In 2000 it reached the predicted 6 billion. In 2011 it reached 7 billion. It will hit 8 billion shortly, and 9 billion a little later.

Foresight Think Tank on "The Future of Food and Agriculture" reported to governments as far back as 2011 that there is not enough arable land on the planet to feed these numbers of people equably.

Note, however, there is another unmet concern. *"It is not just a full cup of food that matters, but what is in the cup"*, as Josette Sheeran, CEO UN World Food Programme, succinctly phrased it in June 2010. Foresight was repeating much of the same stuff as before, with little attention to what needs to be in the cup for the brain. There was little if any mention of sea foods, for example. And yet it is the sustenance of the brain that will determine our future. [12]

The truth is that we urgently need a revision of the food system. We need to sort out the food system whereby the intensification of food production has lost nutrient value which is replaced by fats and sugar. [13,14] We need foods essential to reverse escalating mental ill-health and replace it with a continued expansion of our intellect. Stupidity will exacerbate the several global crisis we presently have. We need better not poorer brains to deal with the world's growing social and political challenges and to bring into reality the dreams we have for a sustainable future. To achieve this we need to change the focus to serve the needs of the brain.

We need attention to the importance of the mother, even her health and nutrition before she conceives [15]. The importance of preconception nutrition has already been established by the folic acid story and neural tube defects. The majority of brain cells develop before birth and set the immutable stage for life. Poor parental health and nutrition before conception – in mother and father alike – along with maternal and infant malnutrition, sentence a child to a lifetime of physical and mental limitations. What happens before birth sets the stage for health and cognition.

The fertilised cell implants into the mother's tissue seven days after conception. That *milieu intérieur* environment is not created out of thin air. It is created by the health, nutrition and behaviour of the mother in the period covering the weeks, if not months, before conception. Indeed, even puberty may be relevant for the health of prospective offspring as this is the time when reproductive physiology is established. Nature prepares in advance for important matters, even storing fat during pregnancy to support lactation, which is the time of greatest energy challenge to the mother. But how many people, or even maternity units, act on this elementary issue?

This underlines why nutrition education in schools is of such crucial importance. And yet in the 1960s and 70s the UK government removed home economics from the curriculum, the original bread-and-butter subject in which food nutrition and cooking skills were taught. Today these skills are woefully lacking. Ready-meals and junk food takeaways are now commonplace.

## The United Nations World Food Programme 2020 Nobel Peace Prize

Last century we were engulfed in two world wars. This century has not started much better. The Russian invasion of the Ukraine with its bombardment of the homes of so many families, the destruction of their lifelong possessions and the deaths and wounding of men, women and children, is a stark example of failure of humanity being already with us. The failure of governments to create peace has given us the threat hung over our heads of a nuclear finale.

The rise in mental ill-health is the greatest threat humanity has ever faced. Alongside obesity and diabetes, according to a report from FAO in 2019, 821 million were afflicted with hunger in 2018. The United Nations reports that over 7.6 million people die annually because of hunger and hunger-related conditions or food insecurity. Inadequate nutrition in the early years of life stunts a child's brain development, resulting in a life of mental dysfunction. Mental dysfunction means failure to obtain good jobs and a descent into poverty, violence and crime. This brings us back to Josette Sheeran's assertion that it not just the full cup that matters, but the actual contents of the cup. To a large extent, that is what this book is about. To solve the escalation of mental ill-health, we need to fill the cup with the right stuff. With escalating populations and food insecurity escalating, this problem must be solved immediately, or it will be too late.

Peace and prosperity can only arrive through intelligent action and the elimination of hunger and the double edged scourge of malnutrition. In tackling these huge issues, priority must be given to the needs of the brain, as eliminating the mental ill-health associated with nutritional deficiencies would lead to a significant enhancement of intelligence and humanity.

At stake is the health and ability of future generations: our children and theirs. Strangely enough, the solutions to the food supply and mental ill-health crises also address climate change, as we shall explain later. But we need the brain power to steer the willpower that can fit all these pieces of the puzzle together.

There is hope. With the need for international solidarity and multilateral cooperation being more pressing than ever, the Norwegian Nobel Committee decided to award the 2020 Nobel Peace Prize to the World Food Programme (WFP) for its efforts to combat hunger, for its contribution to bettering conditions for peace in conflict-affected areas, and for its role in acting as a driving force in efforts to prevent the use of hunger as a weapon of war and conflict.

We are the only species that has a choice in shaping its future. We hope this book will help people make that choice an informed one. Too much is at stake to ignore the threat. Worryingly, time is running out.

# CHAPTER 2
# Biological philosophy.
# The history of the argument

## The Philosophers

If philosophy is the love or pursuit of wisdom, the study of phenomena, their cause and effect, it can be argued that the most important philosophers of the last two centuries have been the evolution theorists who devoted their lives to working out and explaining where life came from, and how we as human beings came to be on Earth. The cause or mechanics of how life began, and the mechanisms whereby simple life-forms turned into complicated ones, are questions which affect every one of us, for these laws concern not only our origins but the present and future conditions of life on Earth.

It is only in recent history that such speculation has been undertaken by scientists. Previously it was in the hands of theologians and classical philosophers. It was commonly assumed in many diverse cultures throughout history and the world that all matter and life emerged from an eternal mystical being, known by the many names of God.

According to such theistic thinking, this mystical power was the driving force which created all matter in the universe, and life; and to this divine force were attributed all things incomprehensible. So it can be said that such 'philosophical debate' has always been in existence. The pattern of the contemporary discussion has in fact been roughly similar for around the last 24 centuries; for the Greeks had pondered at length on the problem, and in their discussions can be seen the rudiments of the debate that exists today.

It is a complicated and triangular argument, centred as it is on whether life has purpose or is due to chance, and the nature of the force that drives the evolutionary process – whether this is some divine power, or natural selection propelling evolution in a continuous and progressive manner; or whether it is as the environmentalists have described, an organic unfolding of the environment driving the process in an upward direction.

Should the latter be the case, it would put all species at the mercy of the conditions of life, the medium within which all organic and inorganic life exists (and this includes food). This continues to be the burning issue, one that has a very real bearing on our future. It poses the rather delicate question: did those great characters of the last two centuries who might be described as the 'philosophers of science', actually get it right, or only partially right? Is it just conceivable there could be some additions?

Before looking at the contemporary debate, we will first look at the ideas on the subject included in some of the great cultures scattered around the world and through the centuries.

## Hinduism

While the Christian religion favoured a creationist origin – meaning that God, in a comparative flash, created the universe – some religions, such as Hinduism, contained a feeling of evolution within its philosophy of life. The Brahmins are the priestly caste of the Hindu religion. Theirs is probably the most ancient evolutionary theory in widespread use today; although it is just one form of a constantly recurring theme in Eastern cultures, and was around for thousands of years before the West's own 'ancient' civilisation of Greece had arisen.

This theme, which is indeed reflected in the Greek philosophies, is of the universe and life being a manifestation of sacred primordial matter, known usually by the local name of God for each of the cultures. In Hinduism this is Brahma, an eternal being of uncreated light out of which all things evolved, materially and spiritually. Such a process is seen as being metamorphic, of one form coming out of another, and of the original appearance of inert matter arising out of the unseen, omnipresent, infinite and eternal sacred source. It is transformation rather than creation.

Such ideas run through Egyptian, Chinese and Persian culture. They are picturesquely portrayed by the Sufi poet, Rumi, in the thirteenth century AD:

First he appeared in the realm inanimate: thence came into the world of plants and lived the plant- life many a year, nor called to mind what he had been: then took the onward way to animal existence, and once more remembers naught of that life vegetive. Save when he feels himself moved with desire towards it in the season of sweet flowers, as babes that seek the breast and know not why. Again the wise Creator whom thou knowest, uplifted him from animality to Man's estate; and so from realm to realm advancing, he became intelligent, cunning and keen of wit, as he is now... "Though he is fallen asleep, God will not leave him in this forgetfulness. Awakened, he will laugh to think what troublous dreams he had, and wonder how this happy state of being he could forget, and not perceive that all those pains and sorrows were the effect of sleep and guile and vain illusion. So this world seems lasting, though 'tis but a sleeper's dream; who when the appointed day shall dawn, escapes from dark imaginings that haunted him, and turns with laughter on his phantom griefs when he beholds his everlasting home.[1]

## Buddhism

The first "Buddha", Siddhartha, born approximately five hundred years before Christ to a princely Hindu family and

1    A.J. Arberry (ed) *Persian Poems*, an Anthology of verse translations, (Everyman's Library, London 1972)

educated by Brahmins, taught the oneness of life, emphasising the close connection between organisms and environment: a grand theory of relativity.

Life at each moment encompasses both body and spirit and both self and environment of all sentient beings in every condition of life, as well as insentient beings - plants, sky and earth, on down to the most minute particles of dust. Life at each moment permeates the universe and is revealed in all phenomena. One awakened to this truth himself embodies this relationship.

This poetry is attributed to the 13th century Buddha, Nichiren Daishonin, who also offered the following thoughts:

*"Man depends on food and clothing to survive in this world. For fish, water is the greatest treasure, for trees the soil in which they grow. Mans' life is sustained by what he eats. That is why food is his treasure."*

*"Life is like a lamp, and food like oil. When the oil is gone, the flame will die out, and without food, life will cease."* Buddhists have always considered the chain of being as results of cause and effect... *"Of all things that spring from a cause, the cause has been told by him "Thus come", and their suppression, too, The Great Pilgrim has declared."*

In this chain of causes, an understanding of which means that one has become Awake, it is emphasised that nothing whatsoever happens by chance, but only in a regular sequence... "THAT BEING PRESENT, THIS BECOMES; THAT NOT BEING PRESENT, THIS DOES NOT BECOME".[2] It is interesting that this view coincides with the idea we expressed earlier, of life depending on conditions.

## Taoism

The sacred book of the Taoists, the Tao Te Ching is attributed to Lao Tzu, an older contemporary of Confucius, (551-479 BC).

2     A. Coomaraswamy: *Hinduism & Buddhism*, (Philosophical Library, New York, 1950). First published 1943.

The opening of the Tao Te Ching portrays some of his ideas on our subject:

*'The way that can be spoken of is not the constant way; the name that can be named is not the constant name. The nameless was the beginning of heaven and earth; the named was the mother of the myriad creatures.'*

*'These two are the same, but diverge in name as they issue forth. Being the same they are called mysteries. Mystery upon mystery - the gateway of the manifold secrets.'*

This tract is also attributed to Lao Tzu:

*'In comparison with heaven and earth, man is but a mayfly. But compared to the Great Way (the Tao), heaven and earth too, are like a bubble and a shadow.*
*Only primal spirit and the true nature overcome time and space. The energy of the seed, like heaven and earth, is transitory, but the primal spirit is beyond the polar differences.*
*Here is the place whence heaven and earth derive their being.'*

## The Greeks

In early Europe, before the Judaeo-Christian creationist theory had taken hold, there were the Greek philosophers. These men, renowned for their zest in theorising about the reasons for life, had, generally speaking, a more mellow and organic view of the creation of the universe and life. Indeed, the word evolution itself comes from the Greek, and means literally 'unfolding'.

Before Socrates, the school of the Atomists worked out a Big-Bang theory of the creation of the universe, which tallies more with the findings of present day nuclear physicists and quantum mathematicians than with any of the philosophers of the intervening period. They saw the universe existing within an infinite ocean of atoms of invisible light. These had no beginning and no end. Vortices of streams of these atoms swirled and twirled through space, sometimes combining, and when their tails overlapped, the vast opposing electro- magnetic forces collided and clashed, releasing sufficient energy to create a new universe.

In terms of evolution theory, a similar argument was taking place amongst the Greeks – divine power and plan (of some sort) versus chance, and natural selection/survival of the fittest versus an organic unfolding; although in general there was rather more support for the organic approach, which had the environment pushing evolving life onward and upward, (an idea put forward by Aristotle). In the 6th century BC Anaximander wrote of indeterminate primordial matter being the basis of organic evolution. A hundred years later Anaxagoras adopted a widespread view that life arose from moisture, heat and earth; that air, mist and cloud made up plants, animals and inanimate objects; that seeds were carried down from the sky to Earth by the rain, and were germinated by heat.

But there were also those who championed the cause of the survival of the fittest. Empedocles (492-432 BC) thought that evolution was a series of attempts by nature to produce more perfect forms: "...And as they (the elements) mingled, a myriad kinds of mortal creatures were brought forth, endowed with all sorts of shapes, a wonder to behold". He was the first to argue the possibility of the origin of the best-fitted forms arising by chance rather through any sort of mystical design, to which of course the Greeks were notoriously attracted. Heraclitus in the 5th century introduced the concept of conflict and struggle for survival. Democritus (460-357), one of the best known of the Atomists, believed in adaptations of individual structures and organs.

Aristotle (4th century BC) saw a scale in nature, a progressive sequence of complexity culminating in man; that at primitive levels organisms arose by spontaneous generation, with organs being fashioned according to their necessity; thus the most universal being the most essential. He believed a relationship must exist between patterns of variation and evolution, and wrote of an internal perfecting principle impelling organisms to greater and greater perfection. Thus a complete gradation from mineral to plant, to plant/animal, animal with senses, to man. Henry Fairfield Osborn as one of the leaders of the Orthogenesis school in the first half of the twentieth century, wrote of him:

"Aristotle's argument for operation of natural law, rather than chance, in the lifeless and in the living world, is a perfectly logical one, and his consequent rejection of the hypothesis of the survival of the fittest, a sound induction from his own limited knowledge of nature. If he had accepted Empedocles' origin of the fittest through chance rather than through design, he would have been the literal prophet of Darwin."

In point of fact, Aristotle believed there were distinct reasons for evolution, of a mystical nature, thus bringing his theories under fire from those not liking the thought of anything teleological (doctrine or study of final causes). And in the evolution story there were a lot of those... the most notorious culprit being Darwin, perhaps with the exception of Professor Weismann from Freiburg University, whom we shall discuss later on in some detail. This real hatred of religious controls was initially a significant force in the evolution debate. So there is nothing very new in the theme of the argument which has taken place during the last two centuries; but a great deal of refinement.

## The Christians

For nearly two thousand years, the unquestioning Christian world had been happy to believe what the philosophy of the Church and the Old Testament had taught them; that the Earth had been made by the Creator in six 'days', that the different species had been created from the beginning in their original form, that they were immutable, and that the whole of life was planned and directed toward purposeful ends. These ends themselves were not very attractive to many – for those who had disobeyed the Creator's explicit instructions the future looked bleak indeed, with promises of holocaust and destruction, the final judgement of a vengeful Creator, and a fate worse than death for those who had not obeyed the commands of Holy Church. Those who supported such beliefs became known as Creationists.

The old Greek philosophy became the subject of a gigantic takeover bid, and was blended with the spiritual philosophy of the Church after the Roman Emperor Constantine (272-337 AD) converted to Christianity, with the result that the Greek-derived evolution theory was also converted to the account of creation in Genesis. In terms of the evolution of Europe, Constantine's conversion and his subsequent adoption of Christianity for the newly-holy Roman Empire, can be seen as a shrewd political move. For nearly four hundred years Christianity had been illegal, punishable by death, and astonishingly successful. It had spread like wildfire – underground, all over Europe, North Africa and the Near East. Making the movement legal had the effect of joining up many of those scattered secret groups into a semblance of unity.

Around this time there was a wide-scale persecution of the old mystery religions such as Druidism and Gnosticism. The Gnostics had been mystics within the Christian Church until outlawed in 367 AD, labelled heretics and excommunicated by Athanasius, then Bishop of Alexandria in Upper Egypt, (whose creed we still have today).

The Druids' sacred groves on the hills were felled, and the Gnostics' sacred texts were ordered to be burnt. Thus 'Orthodox' Christianity became the order of the day – a powerful political machine as well as a theological system, which ruled through a far-flung web of its own brand of mysticism. It was a curious mixture, portraying the elements of human weakness. While the central core was built on the purest form of selfless love, fear of denial of that love was used by the unscrupulous in their thirst for power; the fiery stake for heretics and the chill steel of the sword in its crusades and inquisitions were used to purify thought and destroy opposition in a ruthless drive for power and superiority, despite the exhortation to 'love thine enemy'.

Thus for a thousand and a half years the belief remained that life was not a random process, but directed towards purposeful ends by a divine Creator. The eighteenth century saw a re-awakening of reason, the so-called age of enlightenment with the re-emergence of science, which was to rediscover much of what the Ancient Greeks and Egyptians had known and develop it to our present state of knowledge. From several different geographical parts of Europe came the first publications of alternative theories of the origin of life. It is not surprising that the first few efforts had a distinctly Greek flavour. This can perhaps be attributed to the influence of St Thomas Aquinas, who was a staunch Aristotelian. This might explain how the work of both Dr Erasmus Darwin and Lamarck could be seen as a refinement of Aristotle's own theory.

## The retribution clause

These brief historical details portray how, throughout recorded history, practically every evolution theory of the 'organic - environmental - unfolding' type, be it Aristotelian, Sufi, Hindu, Jewish, Christian-Roman, French-Gnostic or English, all had their essential mystical backcloth, indeed driving force, which not only managed to answer otherwise unanswerable questions but also provided an ensuing retribution clause for those who broke the rules. In the East such a mechanism is known as 'Karma', or the Law of Consequence.

Most Eastern religions included reincarnation. It was believed that there was a gradual evolution of consciousness up the evolutionary scale, so that life through many lifetimes was seen as a pathway of spiritual evolution, with the end point being the emergence into an 'Ultimate Reality,' or God. Some even held that this process was the evolution of the 'Ultimate' itself, ever striving for greater heights of consciousness, stature and glory.

The Hindus commonly believed in an average of 8,600,000 incarnations, from inert matter to man, with a considerable number of these in human form. The purpose   of life was held to be growth in spiritual stature, culminating in fulfilment, enlightenment or 'bliss-consciousness', and release from the wheel of birth and rebirth. With the addition of reincarnation, it is not difficult to see the similarities with Christianity. In point of fact, early Christianity included belief in reincarnation, ("In my father's house are many mansions"), but it was dropped because the seers among the followers, who allegedly 'saw' other peoples' previous lives, were drawing attention and authority away from the priests.

The retribution clauses were for those who broke the moral code. Dis-encouragements usually included further lifetimes, in which one could "work out one's karma", until eventually all the lessons were learned. Negative aspects of an incarnation would be faced as problems or difficulties in further lifetimes, which would have to be overcome by selfless actions and deeds. In European culture we have the equivalents: "As you sow, so you reap", "Those who live by the sword shall die by the sword", and the once widely-feared threats of hell and eternal damnation. These systems represented a form of 'cosmic policing', which in Europe toward the end of the eighteenth century had become increasingly unpopular. For at their most subtle, they had a very real hold on peoples' consciences. At their most blatant, the principles were misused in, for example, the burning of heretics, as a mechanism for maintaining human, not spiritual power. The widespread and passionate dislike for such controls could have indirectly assisted the rejection not only of the mysticism, but also the unfolding-environmental evolution theory which so often accompanied the religious philosophies. Charles Darwin's own view of the Christian religion was probably shared by many others:

"I can indeed hardly see how anyone ought to wish Christianity to be true; for if so, the plain language of the text seems to show that the men who do not believe, and this would include my Father, Brother and almost all my best friends will be everlastingly punished. And this is a damnable doctrine." (From Darwin's Autobiography, 1876.)

Until recently then, environmental forces have always been explained in mystical, and therefore teleological terms. The environment's most considered aspect was always a theistic one; matter was a secondary consideration which emerged from a mystical essence. Modern evolution theory moved into a non-theistic explanation which looked at the other end of the problem, from the end product, thus avoiding the problem of mysticism but at the same time missing out on the meaning of the environment, and of food.

At first sight this new atheistic approach seemed to contradict the dogmas associated with the mysteries of religion. We are now proposing that evolution can be explained in terms of the principles of physics, mathematics and chemistry. When the chemical complexity of biology is reached, we   need different simplifications to come to terms with it, or to understand it, which results in a view of chemistry and food operating alongside the genetic mechanism and the 'truism' of natural selection.

While undoubtedly the most fascinating aspect of the whole process remains obscure – namely the actual mechanism whereby useful mutations are produced by nature in the first place – we can make the connections between hints which are only now appearing in scientific papers, and the 'biological law' on which the current theory of the Modern Synthesis is based, within which 'chance' still plays a prominent role.

In this book we will demonstrate how the physics and chemistry of food and environment is most probably connected to what hitherto has been explained as 'fortuitous' or 'positive' mutation. We will see how previously unknown factors in nature operating within food and environment could relate to that unknown aspect of evolution which up to now has been put down to chance.

## Awareness of environment in the first half of the nineteenth century

The air of thought in Europe concerning evolution during the first 50 years of the nineteenth century had been created initially by the Greeks, and later by the thoughts of Rousseau, Erasmus Darwin and Jean-Baptiste Lamarck, amongst others, in whose thinking the role of the environment and 'external conditions' had been very much to the fore. Although it was largely through the work of Lamarck that environmental considerations had become so widely accepted, the ideas of Robert Malthus had an important impact on evolution, through supplying Darwin with one of his most important clues. While Malthus did not make evolution his subject, but wrote on demography, his views emphasised the ultimate importance of what we know as the environment, and Darwin referred to as "external conditions" or "conditions of existence".

## Robert Malthus

A year after returning home from his historic voyage around the world aboard HMS Beagle (1831-1836), Darwin had come across Malthus' "Essay on the Principle of Population, as it affects the Future Improvement of Society". Having been impressed and influenced by the work of Sir Charles Lyell – whose book The Principles of Geology he read while on board, on the movements of continents and the evolution of geology – he had been primed for this extraordinary work, which was to give him the final clue to his own conundrum.

"October 1838, read Malthus' 'Essay on the Principle of Population'[3], being well prepared to appreciate the struggle for existence... it at once struck me that under these circumstances favourable variations would tend to be preserved, and unfavourable ones to be destroyed. The result of this would be the formation of a new species. Here then I had at last a theory by which to work."[4]

Darwin read Malthus "for amusement"; but the effect was considerable. The simple point argued in Malthus' Essay is that all organic species multiply in a geometric ratio, 3, 9, 27, etc., and the food on which they totally depend for their existence can only, in the most optimistic terms increase in a mathematical ratio, 2, 4, 16, etc. Darwin, having become used to the idea of the movement within geology through absorbing Lyell's work, was now able to see the progression of movement within the environment itself, and the growth of populations of organic beings living within them. He saw how all living systems have mechanisms whereby they produce vast numbers of seeds or eggs which far exceed the survival rate.

He saw the squeeze that nature puts on life, and how there was a constant struggle for available resources.

From this vital clue he began to see how any species with even the slightest adaptive advantage over competing neighbours would be the ones which survived. He termed this phenomenon "natural selection", meaning that the whole process appeared to have no observable causative mechanism, working in association with external conditions, a progression which nature threw up from time to time. Thus it was natural, by "chance" and fortuitous – fortuitous in positive change, called

---

3     T. R. Malthus: *An essay on the principle of population; or A view of its past and present effects on human happiness; with an inquiry into our prospects respecting the future removal or mitigation of the evils which it occasions*, 6th edition (John Murray, London, 1826) (First edition 1798).

4     C.R. Darwin *The Life and Letters of Charles Darwin, including an autobiographical chapter*, ed. Francis Darwin, (John Murray, London, 1887)

evolution; but disastrous in negative change, called extinction. Darwin explained that he did not actually mean by blind "chance" – by this expression he meant a mechanism caused by something of which people at that time were ignorant.

This mechanism was an entirely new concept to science. Although, as Darwin himself pointed out in his 'historical sketch'[5], he was not alone in feeling there was some such mechanism, and he lists over 30 other naturalists, biologists and observers who had by the late 1850s begun to think in the same terms. Darwin sat on his new idea for nearly 20 years before letting it become public knowledge, feeling it too revolutionary for the general good. His hand was forced by Alfred Russel Wallace who had come to similar conclusions through his work in the East Indies. Wallace sent Darwin his own ideas on Selection in 1858, and in that same year the joint papers were presented to the Linnaean Society; immediately after which Darwin hastily produced an abstract of the plot he had been hatching over the previous two decades, and published the following year. Malthus therefore can be seen to have lain the groundwork for natural selection. There are similarities between Darwin and Malthus insofar as they both observed what seemed to them to be hidden facts of nature, which today might not seem so far removed from common sense. Malthus argued the ultimate control of all populations by the food and space factor (Darwin's 'conditions'); Darwin argued natural selection. They both collected huge amounts of evidence from around the world. In Malthus' case, the question was of the nature of populations in relation to the perfectibility of society.

He first published anonymously in 1797, around which time the French Revolution had rather woken people up and given cause for consideration of demographic patterns. He was not the first. William Godwin and the Marquis de Condorcet had

---

5    "An Historical Sketch of the Recent Progress of Opinion on the Origin of Species", in the introduction to the third edition of *On The Origin of Species*, (John Murray, London, 1861)

worked on the problem earlier. But Malthus was the first to gather evidence from all over the world. What he did was to collect the writings of the very earliest European explorers. The book therefore held great fascination, for it was an anthology of such men as Cook, Vancouver and the earliest missionaries – the impressions of Europe's first intrepid adventurers into the unknown world. And most of these pieces of evidence supported Malthus' theory: that the ultimate controlling factor of the populations of all organic species was the food and space factor on which they totally depended.

Malthus was fascinating in that he was absolutely right and absolutely wrong (a recurring theme in this story). That he was wrong in so many matters is probably the reason why so little is heard of him today, when perhaps his greatest claims to fame are that he influenced Darwin and the economist Ricardo. In fact Malthus, who gained a first in mathematics at Cambridge in 1788 and became a clergyman in the Church of England, was not only a demographer but spoke and wrote authoritatively on politics, economics and sociology (his life spanned the first Industrial Revolution 1766-1834). As a priest he was a great moralist. He saw all populations as being held in check by their environments.

There were, according to Malthus, two types of limitations to the growth of populations. He divided these into 'positive checks', which were famines, epidemics and wars; and 'preventive checks' - vice and moral restraint. Being a clergyman he came down heavily in favour of moral restraint, (and to practice what he preached he put off marriage until he was 38). Never holding political power himself, he realised his theories would be of little value unless he was capable of influencing those who did. So he entered into contemporary debate on his many subjects of interest and became an extraordinarily controversial character, remaining so to this day.

In fact Malthus gained a more loyal following on the Continent than in Britain, for by using his theories on moral restraint he provided an explanation as to how Europe had gained its superiority. Other empires, such as China, might have greater wealth, but they depended on cruelty and dictatorship, whereas in Europe success was due to moral restraint, late marriage and controlled childbirth.

Thus Europeans were able to hold their heads high in any part of the world.

## Malthus relevant today

Malthus' ideas on the limiting factors of populations are of greater relevance today than they have ever been, especially when we begin to consider the driving force of evolution to be the power of chemistry in food and environment. Famines are obviously connected with food and space, and occur when a given area doesn't produce enough food for the population living on it.

Epidemics are less obviously connected, in that they are encouraged by widespread poor eating habits; if an area is not producing enough good quality food, or its quantity is restricted, then those people are going to have less resistance to disease through a lowered efficiency of the auto-immune system, be it infectious or deficiency disease. This is of particular relevance in the light of the degenerative diseases in the northern hemisphere today, which are widely regarded as having reached epidemic proportions, and in the rate of child-mortality in the southern hemisphere. Wars are connected too, as vividly illustrated by history, in that scarcity encourages plunder.

If Malthus were around today he would no doubt continue to argue, but with even greater passion, for moral restraint on behalf of the environment, on which the health and wealth of the world community depends. It could further be argued that if there is truth in the environment being so crucial a factor in size and survival aspects of populations (a fact that Darwin readily accepted from Malthus), then it is highly unlikely that the same factor would play an insignificant part in their creation. This is something Darwin understood, and which the neo-Darwinists did not.

## Malthus mistakes

This leads us to two obvious mistakes that Malthus made, which one rarely hears mentioned (even Darwin was uncritical and took Malthus 'as read'). One error was that he didn't think mature populations would stabilise, which in many cultures they have done. The fact that he didn't believe in birth control rather lets him off the hook; but a far more important error was that he considered (and advocated) the best way of producing maximum food from any given area on the globe was through deforestation and cash-cropping, which meant getting rid of the trees.

These ideas were typical of the times, with Europe colonising the Third World, taking its ideas on agriculture with them. This was a type of farming that was successful in the temperate climates of northern Europe, but in the arid, semi- arid and tropical areas to which it was introduced it was often, in the long run, disastrous. Desertification on the world map measures such disasters, which still increase annually. For these climates, so very different from those in Europe, were often unsympathetic to deforestation. What wasn't realised in those days, and is still not always taken on board today, is that in dry climates trees are an integral part of the irrigation system, and that such vital aspects as atmosphere and rainfall, soil-structure, water retention and drainage are directly linked to tree-cover, without which we get increasingly crippling periods of drought and flooding, followed by soil erosion and the sort of abject human misery that is regularly reported in our newspapers; typical of which is this:

"An Ethiopian peasant, remarking that a decade ago his harvest was good but since then the topsoil had been washed away, spoke for millions when he said: 'Now, all I have is a harvest of dust.'" (Alan McGregor, The Times, 2nd July, 1984.)

The tragedy was no doubt increased by the slow speed whereby land, which at first had seemed promising for grazing or cash-cropping, gradually deteriorated. Often there would be enough time for a number of harvests to be taken, not only to cover the cost of reclaiming from bush, scrub or forest, but to show a handsome profit. But then a gradual loss of soil-structure, erosion or blowing of topsoil, left vast and increasing acreages of desert. The process continues, constantly proving Malthus' hypothesis correct, with famines checking populations in the most dramatic and devastating way. Indeed, it has been estimated by Population Concern, a body headed by scientists, that more people have died in the last 100 years from hunger and malnutrition than in all the wars, murders and accidents in the same period. If genetic engineering could do anything to isolate the growth factor for increasing the speed of growth of (food-producing) trees for such arid climates, then this dreadful tide might at last turn, and investors given some realistic alternative to the disastrous cash-cropping policies which sadly they continue to perpetrate.

So while Malthus was to give Darwin one of his most important clues, he did not manage sufficiently to strengthen Darwin's own appreciation of the crucial role that the food and space factor played in driving evolution. Darwin saw the struggle for survival and the process of evolution which he termed natural selection, but he did not find a sufficiently scientific mechanism to explain the mighty push, the great upward surge which was giving the process momentum. In this respect he failed to see the true relevance of Malthus' food and space factor. He failed to see that within this geometric theorem actually lay the answer which he and many other students of evolution were looking for.

## The message

For the ultimate controlling factor argued by Malthus is itself a mirror-image of the role of food as the driving force of evolution, which is the message of this book. Evolution could not have happened had the basic raw materials not been there for evolution to come out of! Malthus' 'struggle for survival', yes; Darwin's (and others) natural selection and 'survival of the best-fitted,' yes; Mendel's 'law', also yes. But the message is this: it was the environment, or food, that supplied the builder's materials, the nutrition, water and atmosphere, the chemical building blocks which enabled evolution to happen initially, and afterwards to bear it along. Evolution was carried in great waves, by countless oceans of constantly moving atoms in relentless surges of rise and fall by the seemingly inexhaustible stores of bio-chemical energies of nature, which suddenly *do* become exhausted simply because animals grow faster than plants: the plants came first and they provided the food for animals. This is the simple secret contained within the food and space factor, otherwise known as the environment.

This, then, was the power of which Malthus spoke, the power that ultimately controls all species living in it, man being no exception. The major difference between humans and other species is that with our extraordinary (though not corporately wise) intelligence, we are now in the position whereby we could, if we were to gather the collective will of the policy-makers of the planet, create a future environment that is positive and nurturing for us rather than one which is negative and detrimental, for this is the factor that will exercise control over humans as a species in due course.

One factor which of course wasn't obvious in the first half of the 1800s was that the food and space resource was about to become extremely stretched. In those days European expansion was continuing, colonisation going full steam ahead; there appeared to be more land rather than less, and the thought of natural resources running short simply didn't enter peoples' consciousness then. Indeed, if land *did* become scarce, or useless through bad farming or exhaustion, there were plenty of other areas which could be opened up. Such thinking has been dominant ever since, and still is, as can be witnessed by the current desecration of the jungles of the Amazon Basin, with absolute disregard for ecological balance, or even for the fate of those people who are encouraged to carry out the work.

And so it is that Malthus remains a controversial character in history. But perhaps the time is ripe for a further review of his writings. For the world as it is today sadly shows the horrible truth in his ideas. The lesson should be taken further. For in Malthus' mistakes lies a lesson we would do well to learn – that environments, on which huge populations are entirely dependent, can be planned, landscaped and laid down by the foresight of those populations that will later be controlled by them. As the dominant species armed with an intelligence and foresight never before seen in the evolutionary tree, we have the priceless gift of being able to see and plan ahead.

When we can see the link more clearly between the environment and our own evolution, when it is more widely understood that there are factors outside the genetic structure of the nucleus which have a bearing on the future course of evolution, we will see that it is in our interests – and within our capabilities – to landscape that very factor which will later come to control our destiny. The question of renewable resources is even more pertinent now than in Malthus' own time.

## Lamarck

We will now examine the environment of thinking prevalent around the first half of the nineteenth century and take a look at the original evolutionist, Jean-Baptiste Lamarck of France, a man even more controversial than Malthus.

The philosopher Jean-Jacques Rousseau (1712- 1778) had been Lamarck's mentor in the early years of his career in France, introducing him to the study of botany. (It is an interesting coincidence that Darwin and Lamarck had both been students of theology and of medicine, which they both rejected before delving into the subject of evolution). Rousseau has been attributed with one of the first published theories, in recent centuries, of the effects of the environment in powering and steering evolution, and the consequent inheritance of acquired characteristics, which very broadly outlines Lamarck's own theories. Published in 1754, in his Discourse on the Origin and Foundations of Inequality among Men, Rousseau was discussing conditions of life in Sparta:

"Accustomed from infancy to the severity of the weather and the rigours of the seasons, trained to undergo fatigue, and obliged to defend naked and without arms, their life and their prey against ferocious wild beasts, or to escape them by flight, the men acquired an almost invariably robust temperament: the infants bringing into the world the strong constitution of their fathers, and strengthening themselves by the same kind of exercise as produced it, have thus acquired all the vigour of which the human species is capable. Nature used them precisely as did the law of Sparta the children of her citizens. She rendered strong and robust those with a good constitution and destroyed all the others."

Over the following ten or 12 years Lamarck compiled his Flora of France, which he published in 1778.[6] This won him acclaim, on the strength of which he was elected to the French Academy. He was granted a commission as Royal Botanist, and as a result of his recommendations for the reorganisation of the Royal Garden the Museum of Natural History was established. Having spent a considerable amount of his working life in

6    J-B. Lamarck: *Flore française, ou, Description succincte de toutes les plantes qui croissent naturellement en France (Flora of France)*, (1st edition Paris, 1778)

botany, Lamarck was made Professorship of Invertebrate Zoology. He published his first work on evolution in 1801, followed by a much fuller account in his Philosophie Zoologique in 1809; and between 1815 and 1822 he published his children, most of whom predeceased him.

He suffered a lifetime of poverty, was blind for the last ten yearsof his life and was buried in a pauper's grave. The sad story of Lamarck is not without humour, and is also one that arouses feelingsof humility when viewed from the present, looking back on the tragi-comedy of such eminent thinkers of recent history. It is understandable too, knowing what we do of human nature, and perhaps even more humbling when we realise how little even now is known about the 'mystery of mysteries' which makes up life.

The important connection between Lamarck and Malthus was that they both regarded the environment as strategically crucial. Publishing initially only four years after Malthus, Lamarck, while he managed to confuse everyone with his rather complicated laws, basically saw evolution emerging from the simplest life-forms, then being carried and transformed by the environment. Likewise, he saw species remaining stable and unchanging only while their environment remained stable. The essence of what Lamarck was saying was contained in his two basic 'laws', the first being the most important and the second following logically.

Lamarck's First law, in what we trust and believe is    an accurate interpretation (in English) is "...that organs, thus species, change in response to a need created by a changing environment". The Second Law, the one most people are familiar with is "...that such change was passed on through the genetic mechanism to the offspring", or "...the inheritance of acquired characteristics." It is ironic indeed that the law that this great man is remembered by is the second and that the first was not only misinterpreted, but lost among labyrinths of library shelves. But to have this latter law without the former is akin to having a cart without a horse.

Lamarck is often referred to as "the great tragic hero of science"; but he held high office, and commanded respect in France, until his death in 1829 at the age of 85. In fact Lamarck was the founder of evolution as we know it today. Despite his name having been repeatedly rolled in the mud, it was he who opened up the great debate nearly two hundred years ago, and despite the ferocity of Darwin's and others' attacks, to Lamarck must be attributed some of the most commonly accepted parts of contemporary theory. It was largely through the work of Lamarck that ideas concerning the effects of the environment had generally been taken seriously for long into the nineteenth century. Similarly, it was through his downfall that environmental and ecological considerations were thereafter not included in our culture's thinking. This was the great tragedy of Jean-Baptiste Pierre de Monet de Lamarck, shared by all those who have had the misfortune to be caught in the quicksand of a deteriorating environment.

Lamarck was also something of a poet and a considerable mystic. Small wonder then that he came in for some heavy-handed treatment from a large part of the scientific community, which at the time was looking for the same sort of precision and 'fixed laws' in biology as those seen at that time in physics and chemistry. The mood of the times was toward 'hard science', and away, rather than toward, religious feelings about life. Even though Lamarck's theories were attractive in a logical and common sense way, they were persistently difficult to prove in scientific research. Whether this was because he was so difficult to interpret, or that it has taken all this time for science to discover previously unknown cellular activities, is only being discovered with time: namely the science of epigenetics. But it is equally true that he has been as difficult to disprove. There is also the possibility that the political implications of his ideas were distasteful to those then holding power.

Perhaps the greatest tragedies of Lamarck's life were that he spent most of his life in the shadow of zoologist and palaeontologist Cuvier, and then had someone play the ultimate dirty trick on him by twisting his words after he died. The emotive air between the Creationists, who thought species were created according to a divine plan and were immutable, and the Transformists, who thought otherwise, can perhaps be likened to the unhappy relationship between Protestants and Catholics. Persecution, ruined careers and untimely death have littered both fields. The politics of theology and evolution share notoriously dangerous ground.

## Lamarck nobbled... By Cuvier?

In France, when a public figure dies, it is the custom for another prominent person to write and deliver a paper known as a eulogy. Not dissimilar to the English practice of writing an obituary, except the eulogy tends to be rather more lengthy and delivered in the form of a lecture. Now it so happened, unfortunately for Lamarck, that the man chosen to write this appraisal of the recently departed man's achievements just happened to be the leader of the opposition party of French evolutionary theory, M le Baron Georges Cuvier (1769-1832). He was an eminent man of science and culture, looked up to by the majority of France as a figurehead of learning and virtue, and a staunch upholder of conservative values. In eighteenth century Catholic France the belief was strong that species did not go through change, but had been made as they were by the creator for a specific purpose.

Cuvier was not only a creationist but a 'catastrophist', someone who believed that God made one set of species and every so often wiped them out, as in the Flood, and started over again with another set. Lamarck's ideas then must haveseemed extremely left wing and 'alternative' in the face of such sturdy opposition. What happened was that Cuvier inserted one or two slightly different keywords in his eulogy. Thus "le besoin" became, instead of "the need", "the wish or desire".

Therefore instead of an organ changing in response to a need created by changing conditions, it was, according to the eulogy, simply wishful thinking. But to be charitable, Lamarck's language was so poetic, flowery and filled with "vital force" and "willing", that the subtlety Cuvier's blistering put down was disguised to some extent by Lamarck's own lack of sharp, clear-cut definition. It has been said of Cuvier that this was "... the only stain on Cuvier's life, and it was unworthy of the great man."[7] But we cannot be sure that he was actually the culprit. Cuvier died only a year after Lamarck, and the eulogy, although originally written by Cuvier, was read in 1832 by M le Baron Silvestre. The Academy did not allow the text of the eulogy to be printed in the form originally delivered by Cuvier.

One can only imagine that the temptation must have been very great indeed for anyone put in that position. But the stunning effect it had was to reduce the reputation of Lamarck, especially in the English-speaking world, to a laughing stock. The trend of mockery was to be continued by Darwin who, while describing him as "...this justly celebrated naturalist" (in On the Origin of Species) and "...a source of inspiration endowed with the prophetic spirit in science, the highest endowment of lofty genius" (in an early notebook), had also condemned his "... views and erroneous grounds of opinion" (in a footnote of the Origin) as "veritable rubbish" (in letters). Indeed the farce was to be taken even further when Darwin's chief disciple delivered, in a series of lectures which were subsequently published, that according to poor old Lamarck, long-legged wading birds, such as spend hours on river banks or lakes' shallow edges, "... developed their long legs by wanting to keep their feet dry." It was to be Darwin's own daughter Henrietta who eventually sent a pert little note to the subscriber of such misinformation, suggesting that surely it should have been the birds' bodies that wanted to be kept dry!

---

7    A.S. Packard *Lamarck: The Founder of Evolution - His Life and Work* (Longmans, Green, and Co, New York, 1901

# Mistake perpetuated

The misreading, however, had been firmly planted, nor was it allowed to lose itself in the quiet obscurity of an unhappy grave. In 1936, an English translation appeared from the press of a university situated in the northern parts of Britain, of Cuvier's dastardly mal-interpretation. The mistake has been perpetuated ever since.

Darwin had also denounced his grandfather Erasmus Darwin's ideas, published in the 1794 book Zoonomia.[8] It will always remain an enigma as to whether Lamarck had read the elder Darwin's work, which had been published some six or seven years before Lamarck's, for their ideas were similar, sharing the thoughts of the formulating power of the environment. If, as is generally thought, he had not, then it seems possible that he had read the work of someone who had, for there is some similarity in style as well as content. But as both scholars' ideas concerning evolution were an extension of Aristotle's thoughts, this could well have been the connecting link.

The two ways of approaching such colourful and combative history seem to be, on the one hand, an intricate and maybe laborious discussion on what was or wasn't said; and the other, perhaps more refreshing and inspiring, to avoid too much raking of coals and rekindling of old fires of discontent, by making fresh appraisal and more accurate definitions. We shall do a little of the former, and rather more of the latter. It might also be suggested that an acquired and inherited, or at least perpetuated characteristic of the English is that they cannot, or will not, understand French. The more so when that particular piece of writing is more than a little obscure in its own language, a fact which is bolstered by what many regard as a glaring mal-interpretation in the first instance by a fellow Frenchman, who was trying (not unsuccessfully as it turned out) to protect his own position.

---

8    Dr Erasmus Darwin: *Zoonomia; or the Laws of Organic Life* (London, 1794)

## Lamarck's philosophy

Before we comment on the argument which was to follow, let us first look at the theories and style of the 'Father of Evolution.' The following extracts are from his *Philosophie Zoologique* published in 1809, and translated by Hugh Elliot. We shall see how the purpose of life for Lamarck was an unfolding of divine will on Earth, which he described as follows:

"Nature- that immense assemblage of various existences and bodies, in all who's parts proceeds an eternal cycle of movements and changes controlled by laws- an assemblage that is only immutable as long as it pleases her Sublime Author to continue her existence, should be regarded as a whole made up of parts, with a purpose that is known to her Author alone, but at any rate not for the sole benefit of any single part. Since each part must necessarily change and cease to exist to make way for the formation of another, each part has an interest which is contrary to the whole; and if it reasons, it finds that the whole is badly made. In reality however, the whole is perfect, and completely fulfils the purpose for which it is destined."

## Laws 1809

For Lamarck the environment was the greater power, and one which was always changing, forcing organisms living in it to change; thus evolution. His two main laws describing the mechanism of change are:

"Firstly, a number of known facts proves that continued use of any organ leads to development, strengthens it and even enlarges it, while permanent disuse of any organ is injurious to its development, causes it to deteriorate and ultimately disappear if the disuse continues for a long period through successive generations. Hence we may infer, that when some change of habit in some race of animals, the organs that are less used die away little by little, while those which are more used develop better, and acquire a vigour and size proportional to their use. Secondly, when reflecting upon the power of the movement of the fluids in the very supple parts that contain them, I soon became convinced that, according as this movement is accelerated, the fluids modify the cellular tissue in which they move, open passages in them, form various canals, and finally create different organs, according to the state of the organisation in which they are placed... Everything acquired or changed during an individual's lifetime is preserved by heredity and transmitted to that individual's progeny."

## Laws 1815

These two 'laws' were stated by Lamarck in 1809, and two more were added in 1815, contained in his massive *Histoire Naturelle des Animaux sans Vertèbres*. It is confusing that his two laws of 1809 became in 1815 laws 3 and 4. The new law 1 of 1815 proposed that :"Life by its own force tends to continuously increase the volume of every living body and to extend its parts, up to a limit which it imparts."

The new law 2 of 1815 was:

"The production of a new organ in an animal body results from a new need which continues to make itself felt, and from a new movement that this need brings about and maintains."

## The Vital Force

There is indeed a sense of poetry about Lamarck's writing which is attractive if one is not being too critical of its scientific reasoning, as can be seen in the next example, a description of the act of fertilisation:

"You may then conceive that an invisible flame or subtle and expansive vapour (aura vitalis) which emanates from the fertilising material, and which penetrates a gelatinous or mucilaginous embryo, that is, enters its mass and spreads throughout its supple parts, does nothing more than establish in these parts a disposition which did not previously exist there, break up the cohesion at the proper places, separate the solids from the fluids in the way required by the organisation, and dispose the two kinds of parts in this embryo for the reception of the organic movement."

## The Supreme Author of All Things

A little more can be seen of the beliefs of Lamarck when he comments on "...some existing prejudices", notably of the Creationists:"It has indeed been long observed that collections of individuals exist which resemble one another in their organisation and in the sum total of their parts, and which have kept in the same condition from generation to generation, ever since they had been known. So much so that there seemed to be a justification for regarding any collection of like individuals as constituting so many invariable species. Now attention was not paid to the fact that the individuals of the species perpetuate themselves without variation only so long as the conditions of their existence do not vary in essential particulars.

"Some existing prejudices harmonise well with these successive regenerations of like individuals, it has been imagined that every species is invariable and as old as nature, and that it was specially created by the Supreme Author of all existing things. Doubtless, nothing exists but by the will of the Sublime Author of all things, but can we set rules for him in the execution of his will, or fix the routine for him to observe? Could not his infinite power create an order of things which gave existence successively to all that we see as well as to all that exists but that we do not see? Assuredly, whatever his will may have been, the immensity of his power is always the same, and in whatever manner that supreme will may have asserted itself, nothing can diminish its grandeur."

So we can see Lamarck's belief in an unfolding evolution, but designed by God. But neither did he agree with the evolution theories of the atheists...

"Will anyone, it may be asked, venture to carry his love of system so far as to be able to say that nature has created single handed that astonishing diversity of powers, artifice, cunning, foresight, patience and skill, of which we find so many examples among animals? Is not what we see in a single class of insects far more than enough to convince us that nature cannot herself produce so many wonders; and to compel the most obstinate philosopher to recognise that the will of the Supreme Author of all things must be here invoked, and could alone suffice for bringing into existence so many wonderful things?"

The scope of Lamarck's work as one of the great naturalists cannot, of course, be fully grasped by these fragmentary examples, but what can be seen clearly coming through the quotations above is his own brand of religion, mixed with a highly imaginative viewpoint on biology. It may have been because of the political implications of his theory, which would of necessity have to be faced were he discovered to be right, involving environmental, ecological and sociological issues, as well as the 'theological' content of his ideas, that his biology was the more severely criticised, and then rejected. The same emotions would probably be experienced today. For the philosophy which emerges from Lamarckism is toward a more 'holistic' and ecological wisdom; in contrast, the philosophy which emerged from the unfortunate misappropriation of Darwin's original thought tends to support the old attitude of the right of might.

As we have seen, Lamarck's initiation and training were in botany, and the continental attitudes to plant physiology contained some advanced thinking which was not shared (it still isn't!) by zoologists, particularly in England. Botanists generally have had a greater awareness of the formative power of the environment; naturally perhaps, since plants are rooted to the spot and cannot move to pastures greener when the going gets tough. The effects therefore of changed environmental stimuli can be more easily examined. Examples of such views can be seen for example in Eduard Strasburger's Textbook of Botany (1894), now in its thirtieth edition.

Broadly speaking, then, we can see Lamarck's view, of an evolution emerging from a nurturing environment, related to some form of consciousness of the evolving organisms; but the overall view tended to be lost once his obtuse laws had been untangled. Add to this the fact that the mechanism which engineered the change was not isolated, and there appears a promising platform for another theory altogether. The story of Lamarck is indeed sad when one considers that many people regarded him as one of the greatest biologists who ever existed. His misfortune was that he came into the crossfire initially of the Creationists, and latterly the Atheists. But the interests of the environment and of ecological balance were furthered more by Lamarck than anyone else in the evolution saga... until now. In fact ecological consideration is only just getting recognition these days, drawn only recently into the limelight by economists and heads of state as it gradually dawns on the world of business that a sick environment means unhealthy balance sheets.

## Darwin and the scientific debate

From the end of the eighteenth century up to the present day, there have been recurring arguments concerning the mechanics of evolution. But for well over a century the two main protagonists have again been those who support the organic, environmental unfolding theory, and those who support the theory of natural selection. (It is confusing that both became known as Evolutionists, due to the initial battle being against the Creationists.) Nearly two hundred years of debate have accompanied the enormous progress, triumphs, and diversification of science. That the intricacies of the debate have become more complicated through reflection of the growing diversification of scientific specialty, there can be little doubt. Such specialisation has become so great that it has had the effect of making the original argument almost impenetrable to the untrained observer. Yet despite the progress and the euphoria there remains considerable dissatisfaction within the ranks of orthodox science itself, as well as amongst laymen, that current evolution theory is still incomplete, and that because of this we have inherited problems of magnitude which have become incorporated in our daily lives, concerning which there is an increasing sense of urgency.

The position from which we debate in this book is not one of condemnation but one of combination towards a more complete synthesis. The argument is not against the action of the genetic mechanism, nor does it deny the role of natural selection, but they are seen as *a posteriori*, that which takes place after the process of the creation of diversity, which itself is seen as *a priori*. This in no way denies the great service to science that earlier arduous and meticulous work has achieved, but we are saying that there is simply more to it: that the driving force acts initially on its own, propelled by the energy and laws of physics and chemistry, and that selection comes into play at a later stage (as indeed explained by Malthus). This can be clearly seen by looking at the Four Phases within each evolutionary epoch, which will be explored below.

## Pictorial sketch

We will now look at the course taken by the progression of Darwin's thinking, and it will be seen how, as his thoughts evolved, he methodically considered the factors we now explore. Not only did he consider the subject of environmental conditions but he vacillated greatly as to their importance,at first largely rejecting, then later including them within his theory. It then appears that the excitement of an entirely new scientific concept carried not only Darwin, but many others after him, on a safari which was to pay less attention to these earlier considerations. Amongst his followers were individuals who were even more Darwinian than Darwin, who were to cut out environmental consideration altogether while the great man himself could be seen in his later years embracing those factors he had earlier toyed with, to the alarm of certain ardent supporters who took successful steps to stem such 'heretical' reversion.

## Conditions of life

Darwin considered what he called "conditions of life" very seriously indeed. These conditions or external factors constantly appeared in his early notes and writings, being weighed carefully in the balance of his judgement, and, as can be seen from the first few pages of The Origin of Species, largely left unexplained. This 'cop-out' in his theory of any explanation of the food and space factor is, we believe, the main reason for the broad blank band of ignorance and lack of awareness surrounding nutrition, ecology and environment within the spectrum of Western culture today.

But from his early sketch of The Origin of Species, the first draft of which he completed in 1842, we can see to what extent Darwin himself had been impressed by the fashion of thought, created largely by Lamarck, which was in the air back in the 1840s, and which remained undisputed for some time afterwards.[9]

9    F. Darwin (ed.) *The Foundations of The Origin of Species: Two essays written in 1842 and 1844 by Charles Darwin*, (Cambridge University Press, 1909) http:// darwin-online.org.uk/content/frameset?itemID=F1556&viewtype=text&pageseq=1

## Anticipation of new evolution theory

So the picture emerging during the first half of the nineteenth century was one of quiet but growing excitement concerning the possibilities which lay within new evolutionary theory. It offered an alternative theory to that provided by the book of Genesis, and which would indeed be as remarkable as the discovery that the world was not flat, or Newton's discovery of the laws of gravity. Through the collective work of Lamarck and Erasmus Darwin, who carried on the tradition of the 'organic unfolding theory' of the (majority of) Greek evolutionists, the general attitude of thinking people was that environmental conditions were of great importance, but there was little rational reasoning and no scientific evidence to back up the theories. However, awareness of the formulating power of the environment, or the 'medium' as it was sometimes called, remained strong: until the scientific community became so carried away by the new concept of 'selection', which seemed to cover all the difficult problems with one gigantic and convenient blanket, that environment and conditions of life were relegated to disgracefully backward seats. Darwin himself protested vigorously:

"I have now recapitulated the facts and considerations which have thoroughly convinced me that species have been modified, during a long course of descent. This has been effected chiefly through the natural selection of numerous successive, slight, favourable variations; aided in an important manner by the inherited effects of the use and disuse of parts; and in an unimportant manner, that is in relation to adaptive structures, whether past or present, by the direct action of external conditions, and by variations which seem to us in our ignorance to arise spontaneously. It appears that I formerly underrated the frequency and value of these latter forms of variation, as leading to permanent modifications of structure independently of natural selection. But as my conclusions have lately been much misrepresented, and it has been stated that I attribute the modification of species exclusively to natural selection, I may be permitted to remark that in the first edition of this work, and subsequently, I placed in a most conspicuous position - namely, at the close of the Introduction - the following words: 'I am convinced that natural selection has been the main but not the exclusive means of modification.' This has been of no avail. Great is the power of steady misrepresentation; but the history of science shows that fortunately this power does not long endure."[10]

## The voyage of Darwin's thought

We can see, through looking at some of these early writings, the changing course of Darwin's own thinking, how seriously he considered environment, or 'external factors', when he returned from his voyage around the world, was perusing his notes, and making a rough sketch of the book that was to project him into prominence. The manuscript later published as The Foundations of the Origin of Species was written in 1842. It was discovered in a cupboard beneath the stairs at Down, Darwin's old home in Kent, when the family were moving out around the turn of the century. It was edited by his son Francis, and makes fascinating reading. For it shows how those very subjects which concern us now were close to his early thinking, subjects that had concerned such men as Lamarck and Erasmus Darwin, and later Herbert Spencer – who coined the phrase "Survival of the Fittest" – and indeed many other students of evolution. The pattern of Darwin's thought then undergoes considerable swings after his realisation that species were not immutable. By the time of his Foundations sketch in 1842, he was giving considerable space in his calculations to external factors, or those factors that we collectively call food. If Lamarck's definitions had been less fuzzy, Darwin at that stage could be seen to be leaning distinctly toward that same direction. He had

---

10    From the Conclusion in *On the Origin of Species*, 6th Edition, 1872

already taken Lamarck's ideas of the effects of use and disuse, or habit. He gave a significant place to environmental factors, but he was unable to offer a mechanical description. He channelled the issue into his latest thinking on the subject and created a new driving force, natural selection.

## Herbert Spencer

After 1859 and the publication of the first edition of On the Origin of Species[11], Darwin became more and more excited and convinced of the greater power of selection. But years later, toward the end of his life, with the sixth edition in circulation, he seemed to be coming back to the point at which he had started, and looking for other factors which might possibly be involved that he could have overlooked. Indeed, his hypothesis of 'pangenesis' was a pointer to what he was looking for: a clear indication that all along he could have made the most serious over-estimation. Not that the theory of natural selection is wrong, but that there are other factors crucial to enabling selection to operate at all. But here he was on difficult ground, having so damningly put down Lamarck and his grandfather. It was left to Herbert Spencer to suggest other factors upon which selection could rely: "Has the natural selection of favourable variations been the sole factor? On critically examining the evidence, we shall find reason to think that it by no means explains all that has to be explained." (Principles of Biology, 1864)

## The foundations of the Origin

Darwin wrote: "In June 1842 I allowed myself the satisfaction of writing a very brief abstract of my theory, in pencil in 35 pages; this was enlarged during the summer of 1844 into one of 230 pages which I had fairly copied out."

11    C.R. Darwin: *On the Origin of Species by Means of Natural Selection, or The Preservation of Favoured Races in the Struggle for Life*, (John Murray, London, 1859)

Here then are a few extracts from that first rough draft of The Origin of Species.

"According to nature of new conditions, so we might expect all or majority of organisms born under them to vary in some definite way. Further we might expect that the mould in which they are cast would likewise vary in some small degree...the (former) variation as the direct and necessary effects of causes, which we can see act on them, as size of body from amount of food, effect of certain kinds of food on certain parts of bodies etc etc; such new varieties may then become adapted to those external (natural) agencies which act on them."

"Introduce here contrast with Lamarck,- absurdity of habit, or chance -?? or external conditions, making a woodpecker adapted to a tree."

There follows a footnote here by the editor, who says..."It is not obvious why the author objects "chance" or external conditions making a woodpecker... He allows that variation is ultimately referable to conditions, and that the nature of the connection is unknown, i.e. that the result is fortuitous."

It should be made clear that this MS is difficult to read for several reasons. Charles Darwin's own hand was sometimes illegible, and there were often words missing, erasures, etc. What is particularly fascinating here is the double question mark, which could signify that he may have been asking himself, "is this absurd, or is there a clue hidden away in there somewhere?"

"Variation depends on change of condition and selection, as far as mans' systemmatic or unsystemmatic selection has gone; he takes external form, has little power from ignorance over internal invisible constitutional differences. Nature changes slowly and by degrees. There is no variety which [illegible] has been [illegible] adapted to peculiar soil or situation for a thousand years and another rigourously adapted to another; til such can be produced, the question is not tried. Man in past ages, could transport into different climates, animals and plants which would freely propagate in such new climates. Nature could effect, with selection, such changes slowly, so that precisely those animals which are adapted to submit to great changes have given rise to diverse races,- and indeed great doubt on this head." (Editors note "In the Origin ed i, p 141, vi, p176, the author gives his opinion that the power of resisting diverse conditions, seen in man and his domestic animals, is an example 'of a very common flexibility of constitution'.")

"Before leaving this subject well to observe that it was shown that a certain amount of variation is consequent on mere act of reproduction, both by buds and sexually,- is vastly increased when parents exposed for some generations to new conditions... These facts throw light on each other and support the truth of each other, we see throughout a connection between the reproductive faculties and exposure to changed conditions of life whether by crossing or exposure of individuals."

"It must I think be admitted that habits, whether congenital or acquired by practice [sometimes] often become inherited*; instincts, influence, equally with structure, the preservation of animals; therefore selection must, with changing conditions, tend to modify the inherited habits of animals.".... (Editor's note... "At this date and for long afterwards, the inheritance of acquired characters was assumed to occur.")

"Last case, of parent feeding young with different food (take case of Galapagos birds, gradation from Hawfinch to Sylvia) selection and habit might lead old birds to vary taste [illegible] and form, leaving their instinct of feeding their young with same food,- or I see no difficulty in parents being forced or induced to vary the food brought, and selection adapting the young ones to it, and thus by degree any amount of diversity might be arrived at." *(Note – could the illegible word have been "texture"?)* This is the nearest Darwin gets to seeing how food might precede selection, and is a tempting example of the driving force of selection itself.

"With the amount of food man can produce he may have

arrived at a limit of fatness of size, or thickness of wool [-], but these are the most trivial of points, but even in these I conclude it is impossible to say we know the limit of variation. And therefore with the (adapting) selecting power of nature, infinitely wise compared to those of man, (I conclude) that it is impossible to say we know the limit of races, which would be true [to their] kind; if of different constitutions would probably be infertile one with another, and which might be adapted in the most singular and admirable manner, according to their wants, to external nature and to other surrounding organisms,- such races would be species. But is there any evidence [that] species [have] been thus produced, this is a question wholly independent of all previous points, and on which examination of the kingdom of nature [we] ought to answer one way or another."

(All above quotations from The Foundations of The Origin of Species, 1909, edited by Darwin's son Francis).

Thus we can see that this was a period in which Darwin himself was most carefully considering (Malthus') food and space factor, weighing in the balance precisely the same factors that we are attempting to explain and evaluate in this book. As Francis Darwin has already explained, the general attitude and way of thought of the majority of people of that time was that characteristics were acquired from the environment, and that they were passed on through the hereditary mechanism. Maybe it was the extreme force of enthusiasm for natural selection which carried peoples' minds away from these delicate points, Darwin's included, as can be seen from the first few pages of the first edition of the Origin.

Another contributing factor could also be the cruelly damning attitude he took towards the ideas of Lamarck, who, though unscientific and rather woolly in his style, was often not so very far from those points Darwin himself was trying to reach. This becomes particularly clear when we look at Darwin's ideas concerning pangenesis, when he had been given time to thoroughly reconsider his views after more than a decade of public debate.

Before leaving Darwin's thoughts on the effects of environment in steering evolution, we will briefly look at his ideas on the apparent plasticity of species, which he reflects upon in the first edition of the Origin:

"The result of the various, quite unknown, or dimly seen laws of variation is infinitely complex and diversified. It is well worthwhile carefully to study the several treatises published on some of our old cultivated plants, as on the hyacinth, potato, even the dahlia, etc., and it is really surprising to note the endless points in structure and constitution in which the varieties and subvarieties differ slightly from each other. The whole organisation seems to have become plastic, and tends to depart in some small degree from that of the parent type."

The idea of plasticity is of particular interest to us in our study, as will become apparent later. For those interested in the progression of thought on the above topics, the version from the 6th edition of Origin appears in Appendix Two; there we can see how Darwin differentiates between definite and indefinite variation, having already noted this "plasticity" of species. The 6th edition was written in 1872, some 12 years or so after the first, 30 years after what became known as The Foundations, and obviously a reflection and refinement of this most crucial of issues.

This really covers the period of contemplation in Darwin's mind over a consideration of what gets changed, and what does the changing.

## The predominant power

Finally we can look at Darwin's conclusions, as portrayed in On the Origin of Species, where it can be clearly seen how important the environment was to him.

"To sum up on the origin of our domestic races of animals

and plants. Changed conditions of life are of the HIGHEST IMPORTANCE in causing variability, both by acting directly on the organisation, and indirectly by affecting the reproductive system. It is not probable that variability is an inherent and necessary contingent, under all circumstances. Variability is governed by many unknown laws, of which correlated growth is probably the most important. Something, but how much we do not know, may be attributed to the definite action of the conditions of life. Some, perhaps a great, effect may be attributed to the increased use or disuse of parts. The final result is thus rendered infinitely complex... Crossing appears to have played an important role... Over all these causes of change, the accumulative action of Selection, whether applied methodically and quickly, or unconsciously and slowly but more efficiently, seems to have been the predominant Power." (6th edition, end of chapter of 1.)

This final conclusion sees selection proceeding in a tempo related to the environment; there is an awareness that conditions play an important part; but here he is cautious... he is on Lamarck's own ground... ground where Lamarck came unstuck. Apart from paying homage to "external conditions" he offers no mechanical explanations, apart from the short-lived pangenesis theory, (which we will come to shortly). He shifts the whole focus onto selection, explaining and describing it as "natural".

We have now seen the gradual unfolding of Darwin's own thoughts, from initial belief in the then commonly accepted case of immutability; his appreciation of movement within geology, and the movement within the environment, the struggle for existence of all organic beings, the upward pushing of life; and his realisation that species do in fact change, slowly, imperceptibly. He was, after all, one of the greatest observers of nature, meticulously cataloguing what he saw, and one of the hardest workers, with a fabulous eye for detail. His production in terms of work was phenomenal (he wrote 20 books and 150 papers). He was also a great theorist. He simply couldn't help formulating theories around his many observations.

We have seen how carefully he weighed up the possibilities, considering most of the factors which could possibly have caused the upward unfolding of life-forms. And while being so inclusive in his deliberations, he finally came down in favour of the change being caused by natural selection, which was related to, and dependent on the environment, but in a way he could not explain. He considered the greatest factor to be the struggle for existence and natural selection producing the most refined forms, these being the survivors through being best adapted to cope with the struggle, best adapted to win the battle of insufficient resources, surviving because they were the most improved species arriving from the squeeze, pushed by nature into a state of superiority. But we can also see a certain degree of doubt popping up between the lines. Thus we are at the philosophy of the "survival of those best-fitted to the environment".

We can also sympathise considerably with the emotion of the final result being rendered infinitely complex! Through all this meticulous observation and evaluation Darwin had failed to explain the machinery of the initial diversity – that elusive factor which has ever since remained elusive, hidden as it is behind the veils of higher mathematics, population genetics and the largely unknown qualities of external conditions and the cytoplasm. But for 50 years the complexity of the argument, and the brilliant rhetoric with which it was argued, managed to mask the fact that selection on its own was an insufficient explanation for the causal mechanism of variation.

## Summary of Lamarck/Darwin differences

To sum up the original differences between the attitudes of Lamarck and Darwin, we could suggest that Lamarck saw the environment forcing change through the consciousness of the organism. Darwin saw the change happening, and realised that there was a relationship with the environment, but one he could not explain. He gave the resulting change a name, and convincingly argued it as a driving force. But both missed the essential driving force of *food*. They were of course both aware of nutrition, but neither made it a subject of primary focus.

## Natural selection takes shape

We can now jump ahead to the next part of the story, which first came to a head in 1868, nine years after the publication of Darwin's Origin of Species. The theory had attracted a great deal of attention, a lot of support from scientists, and much criticism. There had been time for some of the defects of the theory to be discussed. The significance of the new ideas had rocked the very foundations of the structure of society. There had been highly emotional scenes between the 'evolutionists' as they were now called, and the religious leaders of the day, whose authority was being openly challenged. For Darwin had now provided an alternative theory of evolution, based not on Vital Force or First Cause of any kind, nor on any theistic system. He had for many disproved the old myths in Genesis, although religious leaders were much later able to accept that his ideas had little to do with Genesis. He was about to start pulling the carpet from under the feet of the instigators of our moral code. He was taking thinking men and women away from the power of the Church; taking them away from any idea of mystical purpose, such as had originally formed the roots of European culture. There was jubilation in many quarters, hostility in others.

Darwin had reconfigured life from being a matter of purposeful design to a phenomenon based entirely on chance events. Other great thinkers of the period such as Marx and Nietzsche were co-authors of the cultural change. In the British Isles the full effects of this change on group-psychology would not be felt for a much longer period of time. Indeed, in many ways we are only seeing the widespread effects of the new philosophy now, more than a century after the death of Darwin himself.

## Pangenesis

But, back to 1868, in the face of criticism (which has never been entirely out of the picture since) centred mainly on whether natural selection was the actual driving force, or whether there were other factors not generally recognised, Darwin appears to have been aware of the shortcomings of his theory, searching for other mechanisms which would give a more plausible method of variation. He produced his hypothesis of pangenesis, published in a new, two-volume work, The Variation of Animals and Plants.[12] In this book Darwin was moving back towards the viewpoint from which he first argued, (as we saw in The Foundations of The Origin of Species), and supplies a series of alleged examples of Lamarckian inheritance of acquired characteristics. Pangenesis was an effort at floating a hypothesis which would have made such a theory scientifically acceptable – something which Lamarck before him had not managed to do. Pan ("including or relating to all parts or members") was also a rural Greek deity, one of his attributes being the instigation of panic...

Darwin, in his own panic, created the hypothesis of pangenesis. Briefly recounted, the theory was that every cell of every tissue and organ of the entire body had minute particles called gemmules. When any cell or organ changed, in response to a change in the environment, the gemmules would register the change also. The gemmules, or Darwin's Gene's as they became known, would then circulate in the bloodstream, eventually reaching the gonads, where the change of the organ

12    C.R. Darwin: *The Variation of Animals and Plants under Domestication.* (John Murray, London, 1868)

would be registered, thus enabling the organism to pass on such change to the offspring. It was indeed the sort of mechanism that has been sought ever since: something within the power of nature which can change the genetic mechanism, and thus pass the change hereditarily to the offspring.

Pangenes did not last long before they became extinct, there being no experimental evidence available to back up the theory. In fact it was Darwin's cousin Francis Galton[44] who was partially responsible, through his research on blood when he discovered nothing resembling gemmules. Had there been positive findings, such evidence would of course have proved Lamarck's earlier ideas correct, and re-instated the crucial status in evolution of environment, ecology and food.

Pangenes live on in certain dictionaries. Hugo de Vries (1848-1935), creator of the mutation theory, had his own theory of intracellular pangenesis at one stage. But Darwin realised within a few years that the hypothesis looked hopelessly unscientific, and pangenesis was allowed to drift quietly away. Mention is made of equal and opposite hypothesis, part of which became dogma and has persisted to the present day; and in a way, Darwin was getting very close with his 'invention' of pangenes to the mechanism of induced change, whereby something from the environment causes organs to change, with that change registering in the germplasm.

What Darwin had actually hypothesised with his pangenes was the first glimmering of understanding of what was to become known as epigenetics, a subject not fully described until 2010 with the publication of The Handbook of Epigenetics (in which the work of both authors of this present book is commented on).[13]

---

13    Francis Galton (1822-1911) was an English explorer, anthropologist and eugenicist noted for his pioneering studies of human intelligence. Knighted in 1909.

## Weismann's theory of the continuity of the germplasm

It was Professor August Weismann, from the University of Freiburg, who played the next opposing move. In 1885 – Charles Darwin having died in 1882 – he published his theory of the continuity of the germplasm. It was an equal and opposite idea to pangenesis, insisting on the absolute isolation of the germplasm – the reproductive cells – from 'somatoplasm' or other parts of the body. Weismann argued this absolute gulf with splendidly convincing rhetoric. While the body gave of itself, and actually created the germplasm, fed it, nurtured it and acted as its vehicle, it could never affect the germplasm itself. Thus, in its splendid isolation, there could be nothing which could affect the structure of the genetic mechanism via the body tissue. Some think this argument was motivated by the desire to bring an end to the line of thought Darwin himself was moving towards in his later years, veering uncomfortably close to the ideas of Lamarck.

It was indeed the case that Darwin, having been so utterly condemning of Lamarck initially, had taken his ideas on the effects of habit, or use and disuse (without giving any credit) and was now seen to be playing into the hands of the opposing camp of the old school naturalists and organic evolutionists... possibly posing political, even theological threats. But Weismann's insistence on the insulation of the genetic mechanism from any actions of the body put an end, for the time being, to this drift. His erudite argument, which was for his time scientifically remarkable, strongly reinforced the focus of attention on the internal, into the heart of the hereditary mechanism. Darwin had first taken the focus of attention into the organism, lessening respect for the food and space factor.

Weismann strongly reinforced those ideas, and was also responsible for the creation of neo-Darwinism. Like Lamarck, he was blind in later life, turning from experimental work to theory, and formulating his theory of germinal selection.[14] According to this, variation was "...directed by competition for nourishment among 'character-units' of the germplasm." (Genes had not then been discovered.) The theory was that by this mechanism, it was possible for any change to move in the direction favoured by selection! This early suggestion of evolution's involvement with food and nutrition is quite stunning in view of contemporary research work on heart disease and mental ill-health, which makes it look very much as if the very opposite could be happening.

Weismann's theories were founded on the idea that changes to 'germ plasm' – reproductive cells – could be inherited, whereas changes to other cells in the body – that is, changes to the physical health of the organism – could not. Later theories of heredity took this as an immutable truth, and the notion that environmentally-inflicted changes to the body could not be passed to the next generation was called the Weismann Barrier. Through his advanced thinking, Weismann removed that aspect of the original Darwinism which brought environment into consideration. He made a powerful case for the "All-sufficiency of natural selection".[15] His new theory should of course have been called Weismannism (a term which was, indeed, briefly coined).

In her 5th edition of A Short History of Natural Science, Arabella B Buckley[16] delightfully suggests:

"Professor Weissmann of Freyburg (sic) ... (has) brought forward of late theories which are a great help in forming a conception of the starting point of the embryo in plants and

---

14    Tollesfbol (ed.) *The Handbook of Epigenetics; the New Molecular and Medical Genetics.* (Academic Press/Elsevier, Cambridge, Mass., 2010)

15    *Über Germinal-Selection: eine Quelle bestimmt gerichteter Variation* (On Germinal Selection as a Source of Definite Variation) (first published 1896)

16    A.B. Buckley: *A Short History of Natural Science and of the Progress of Discovery from the Time of the Greeks to the Present Day. For the use of schools and young persons* (5th edition published by Edward Stanton, London, 1894)

animals, and the relations between growth, reproduction and heredity; but these theories are too new and too difficult to discuss here".[17]

Mendel's observations gave biologists the ammunition they needed to take this inward focus even further, and later the molecular biologists would invert this gaze even more. While most of the Darwin/Lamarck argument hung on the inability of research to isolate the suspected or expected 'Lamarckian Factor', another part of the thinking may have been centred, subconsciously or otherwise, on the implications of Lamarck's 'holistic' philosophy, which might have reanimated the spectre of religious domination that the evolutionists had been striving so hard, and so successfully, to avoid. Furthermore, there would have been unpopular political implications which would have to be faced should the environment be discovered to be a formulating factor in evolutionary direction. These would have included more socialistic attitudes than were favoured in the eyes of those who supported the 'fittest' theory, which became an extension and refinement of the 'right of might' argument. In recent heated rows in England, there have been allegations of Marxist leanings. But as this argument goes back at least half a century before Marx published, and as the state of consciousness coming from a social Lamarckism would be very different indeed to that we know of as Marxism today, they can be seen to be largely irrelevant.

But what undoubtedly was lost through all this passionate and learned debate was an understanding of the vital role in the evolutionary process of the Food and Space factor, the medium within which, and on which all living organisms totally depend. Thus it can be seen how this crucial omission could be at the roots of many of the more tragic and urgent problems we as a species face today.

17    This was the title of an article Weismann wrote in 1893 in reply to Herbert Spencer's defence of Lamarckism (published in Contemporary Review, 64 (1893) p.309

## The five phases

Students of evolution rarely fail to be impressed when, examining each evolutionary epoch and its various phases, they find again and again that in all cases when a new, more highly evolved lifeform becomes established, gathering itself for its future of dominance, the supporting 'conditions of existence' (to borrow Darwin's phrase for the environment) had to be in place and functioning first: preparing for the dance of the DNA with the environment.

To see this more clearly we'll look at a few epochs of evolution. An epoch can be divided into five parts.

- Phase One sees a rich nurturing environment supplying the right temperature, light, food and other basic living materials to small populations, which under such protective and stimulating conditions reproduce rapturously; populations thrive and grow successfully.
- Phase Two is more of the same, but population numbers have increased. In Phase Three populations have increased considerably, to the point where there is a dwindling of food and resources per capita - any species or type which has extra abilities in capturing their necessities will succeed over less efficient types. (This is where competition comes into play for the first time: not in phases One or Two.)
- This carries on through Phase Four, until its end, when an exhausted environment fails to supply the needs of hugely increased populations and even the best-fitted cannot survive.
- Phase Five is Phase One of the new epoch, when different species, better-fitted to the new environmental matrix become dominant (and the new chemistry involved in that matrix is often brought about by the activities of the sheer numbers of the previously dominant species).

One of the earliest life-forms, the blue-green algae, were dominant for over two and half billion years. They produced oxygen as a by-product of photosynthesis, and over this time slowly oxygenated the planet. Equally importantly they produced proteins, carbohydrates and essential fatty acids – or lipids – which were rich in omega-3 including docosahexaenoic acid – DHA. The Blue-Greens laid down the basic building blocks of life which we rely on, now and for the foreseeable future.

So DHA played a huge role in the 2.5 billion years of early blue-green life. In their teeming zillions the Blue- Greens (some divide into four every 28 hours) gradually oxygenated the planet which had previously been without oxygen (anaerobic). When the oxygen content of the air rose from 0% to the 3% of today's levels, and oxygen began to be used to provide superior fuelling, animal life fairly whooshed into being in top gear. Within 500 million years all the phyla – or branches of the animal family tree – were laid down, and evolution took off, with the creatures getting larger and larger until the age of the great reptiles, and of course the dear old dinosaurs.

Their 'conditions of life', or their environment, was a *sine qua non* of their success. A vitally important part of these conditions was an environment rich in DHA: a nutrient the landlocked food chain gives only limited access to.

Over thousands of millions of years' 'blue-green' activity, the environment of all living things was spectacularly rich in DHA. Fish and reptiles need omega-3 lipids for reproduction: they prospered for hundreds of millions of years, cashing in on the billions of years of the Blue-Greens' exertions.

Now we take a great leap to the end of the Cretaceous period, roughly 70 million years ago, when the dinosaurs disappeared, after which the mammals rose to dominance.

Here we can see a further example of the environmental mix coming first, before the evolutionary change actually happened – in the evolution of the placental mammals. For their evolution to be possible there had to be a widely available source of arachidonic acid (ARA, sometimes written AA) the long-chain omega-6 linoleic acid (see below) which became widely available only after the demise of the dinosaurs. Then a strange thing happened which no-one has yet managed to explain entirely.

In the terrible obliteration of most terrestrial animal life, when the dinos met their pitiful end and some creatures retreated to flourish in the sea, most plant life changed from ferns and ginkgoes to flowering and seed-bearing plants and trees.

We have the giant meteorite theory, the 100,000 year period of intense volcanic activity theory, and rare metal theories; but speculation also points to a giant sun-flare dowsing the planet with solar storms and unusual clouds of radio or quantum activity, which effected a genetic mutation - or was it a modification? - that suddenly produced seeds, a rich source of linoleic acid from which ArA is made, biosynthetically by the animals that eat the seeds. ArA is a vitally important part of the vascular system: the mammalian placenta is basically a new vascular system specially created to support the nutritional and other needs of the growing foetus. As we shall se later the mammalian explosion couldn't have happened without the ArA from omega-6 linoleic acid: which, it's worth repeating, only became widely available when the flowering and seed-bearing plants took centre stage.

# CHAPTER 3
# Origins of diversity:
# Darwin's conditions and epigenetic variations

To understand current progress in epigenetics we need briefly to visit 5th century BCE Greek thought onwards to our own 19th century CE. Empedocles, Heraclitus, Democritus, Hippocrates and Aristotle among others all had various views on environmental determinism, well described by Rebecca Stott in her excellent book "Darwin's Ghosts: In search of the first evolutionists." [1]

## Historical perspective

It is only within the last 120 years that the environment has taken a back seat behind the genetic determinism of the Neo-Darwinism created by Weismann, his Primacy of the DNA theory and later 20th-century Neo-Darwinist thought which remains the orthodox evolutionary model to this today. (And no doubt well beyond; although this old model is being challenged with our ever-growing understanding of epigenetics.[2])

Before this time, and for preceding millennia the nurturing and supportive qualities of the environment were considered crucial. In the 18th century, the work of Goethe, Rousseau and Lamarck stressed the important roles played by the environment in what was to become known as evolution, or *transformisme* in 18th and 19th century France.

Two decisive events during the 19th century collectively

denigrated the importance of the environment. These were Darwin's (and others') ideas regarding natural selection (1859 onwards), but particularly Weismann's 1890s papers Isolation of the Germ Plasm Theory and The All Sufficiency of Natural Selection.[3]

For although Darwin had stated that within his theory of evolution by means of natural selection "there were two great engines" driving evolution, "natural selection" itself, and "conditions of existence", he wavered over which was the most important.

In Chapter 5 of On the Origin of Species Darwin says:

*I am convinced that Natural Selection has been the most important, but not the exclusive, means of modification ... But the fact of variations... occurring much more frequently under domestication than under nature... lead to the conclusion that variability is generally related to the conditions of life to which each species has been exposed during successive generations.*

But he also stated, in the last paragraph of Chapter 6 (all 6 editions), that "of the two forces, conditions were the most important".[4]

This led to confusion, and to the fear that Darwin might be seen as straying into the ways of the discredited Lamarck, whose theories he had struggled so hard to distance himself from. It also made it easy for him to be misinterpreted: as indeed he was, only a few years after his death, by the German evolutionary biologist August Weismann.

## Handbook of Epigenetics

Weismann insisted on the "isolation of the germ plasm theory", in which he argued that no influences from somatic cells could affect the germ plasm, which existed in complete isolation. This is something we now know to be incorrect. Sadly, Weismann was blind by the time he published his ideas in this area: the 'isolation theory' was purely hypothetical. But acceptance of it led to the Primacy of the DNA theory leading to the genetic determinism we have known throughout the previous century until today. It is extraordinary to look back on it now to see how it all came about.[5]

However, the conventional viewpoint is now being challenged by scientists following completion of the human genome map and the growing understanding of epigenetics: the science of how environmental factors such as chemistry, nutrition, substrate, and stress and emotions can have a direct effect on the genome, making the same genotype behave or express itself in variable ways. These can lead to generational change in shape, form, function and behaviour; a growing number of scientists consider these impact energies play a more important part in the evolutionary process than had previously been realised.

The argument has flourished amongst evolutionists around the environmental theories of Jean-Baptiste Lamarck and Charles Darwin,[6] the genetic determinism of August Weismann the creator of Neo-Darwinism, and more recently the adherents of epigenetics and environmental evolutionists. A loose definition of the term epigenetic used to be covered by the phrase 'environmentally induced modification' (EIM). Until the beginning of the last century it was generally accepted that changes in the environment could result in reproducible change in the shape, form, function or behaviour of life forms. Such change was not the fixed type as occurs with mutations, but reversible. It was not therefore considered important in evolutionary terms. However, since the human genome map was completed in the early 21st century, such reversible change is at last being considered important: this is now known as epigenetic change. Debate continues amongst geneticists around this controversial subject to this day.

The late Simon House of the McCarrison Society says:

"Epigenetics is more than a fascinating and fast burgeoning field of biological research: it is of vital consequence to the human race, as we have come into arguably the worst crises in new forms of disease the human race has encountered.[7,8] These include the 'non-communicable' diseases related to the metabolic syndrome. Obesity, diabetes, cardiovascular and mental health disorders are increasingly recognised as connected with epigenetic changes of early origin."

House describes epigenetics as "the process of a gene being switched off (silenced), or conversely being switched on (activated) by removal of the methyl group". He goes on:

"Such changes reversibly modify the development of the organism without changing the basic gene-sequence (Epi- indicates 'on' the gene). Although the change is reversible, it can be passed on to subsequent generations.

"Epigenetic change can affect a cell's genome (genetic material) any time in the lifecycle, though the earlier in life the more potential. Reproduction involves major epigenetic changes in the genome of the developing oocyte (fertilised egg) and the genome from the sperm on fertilisation. These changes allow some fine-tuning of the new organism to parental environment yet can also give rise to problems. The grandmother is 'reading' the environment for her grandchild – and to a lesser extent the grandfather too.

Research articles are coming out fast on the relevance of epigenetic settings to many disorders, including: autism, psychosis, schizophrenia, Alzheimer's disease and cancer; the process of ageing; and trans-generational effects. Environmental factors shown to be changing settings include nutrition, medicines, toxins and metals. Surprisingly epigenetics studies in human vaccination against infectious diseases are not apparent. [9]

"There are two possible forms of environment- driven changes in organisms. One involves "switches" on the genes being turned on or off, in a process potentially reversible if and when the environmental conditions change." This is epigenetics. The other is a permanent change, where gene expression "sticks", freeing up the organism's limited resources for other purposes. This is the pathway to new species."

"The Human Genome Project completed in 2003 met with general surprise. Instead of the 150,000 genes expected, to account for wide human variation, there was a mere quarter the number. This highlighted epigenetics to explain the wide variation. A few pioneers, however, were not surprised, notably the authors of The Driving Force (1989) and Nutrition and Evolution (1995), Michael A. Crawford and David E. Marsh, who describe how evolution has been driven by nutrition, as powerfully as by any condition of existence. Contrary to the Neo-Darwinists they point out that Darwin himself, in On the Origin of Species, relates the theory of natural selection to 'the two great laws - Unity of Type and Conditions of Existence' (consistency of a species and environmental conditions). Of these two great laws, he declares (concluding Chapter 6): '... the law of the Conditions of Existence is the higher law; as it includes, through the inheritance of former variations and adaptations, that of Unity of Type'. Epigenetics is part of this law." [10]

Interestingly Darwin himself had proposed a mechanism for environmentally induced change, giving it the name pangenesis. This he published in his 1868 book The Variation of Plants and Animals under Domestication' (see Chapter 2). He maintained that all cells contain tiny granules he called gemmules, which register any environmental change. "They are collected from all parts of the system to constitute the sexual elements", he wrote, "and their development in the next generation forms the new being; but they are likewise capable of transmission in a dormant state to future generations and may then be developed".[11]

This was inspired guesswork, for although epigenetic change works with a different mechanism, it produces similar results. It took scientists another 140 years to work out precise mechanisms - collectively first published in the Handbook of Epigenetics in 2010.[12] Inspired prophecy might be a better term, seeing as genes had not been discovered in Darwin's time. Unfortunately Darwin was not that good at explaining himself. He had said in different parts of the Origin that 'natural selection' was the most important of the two mighty forces that he suggested were driving evolution – i.e. natural selection and conditions of existence – then in another place that conditions were the most important.

Dwelling on his various utterances, it seems clear that what he meant – and he says this elsewhere, "natural selection comprises of two great forces driving the upward thrust of evolution – natural selection, leading to "the survival of those species best-fitted to their environment" (later abbreviated to 'survival of the fittest' by Herbert Spencer); and "the conditions of life... meaning the total impact energies of the environment." It is unfortunate that he contradicted himself, so making it easier for successors to twist or misinterpret his message.


## August Weismann


After Darwin's death in 1882, the creator of Neo- Darwinism, August Weismann from Freiburg University in Germany (who we talked about in Chapter 2), argued in his paper The All-Sufficiency of Natural Selection that considerations of the environment - Darwin's Conditions – were not necessary, as natural selection was "a force sufficient unto itself". This he argued so convincingly all over Europe - including his lectures in Oxford, Cambridge and London – that for over a century scientists, medics, philosophers, etc., all fell hook line and sinker for his inexactitudes.[13]

Weismann should have called his theory Weismannism, rather than Neo-Darwinism, for he literally tore Darwin's original thesis in half, cutting out arguably the most important part – the environmental driving force which produced those species 'best-fitted' to their environment, enabling them to become, often over countless generations, the dominant species in their epoch of evolution – or in the not entirely precise terminology of Herbert Spencer, "the fittest".[14] Specialists regularly repeat this today, often calling themselves Darwinian when in fact they are neo-Darwinian, or rather Weismannian.

Because of Weismann's blindness, generations of our top brains have failed to realise the real power of the environment in almost every sphere of our lives. It explains why we do not appreciate or value it; why we do not understand the importance of, nor appreciate the quality of the foods we eat, the quality of the soils on which our food is grown, the quality of water in our streams, lakes, rivers and oceans, or the quality of the air we breathe... etc., etc. & etc.

Let us now jump to the current debate being played out on the world stage, by looking at Bill Sardi's "Let's Let Charles Darwin Sort-Out A Modern Debate In Biology".[15] This describes a US federal project that involved 440 scientists from 32 laboratories from around the world in a project known as ENCODE (Encyclopedia Of DNA Elements). This concluded that 80% of the library of human genes (known as the human genome) is biologically functional. The results of ENCODE were reported in September 2012; strong criticism of its "extremely loose definition of 'biologically functional' soon followed."[16]

ENCODE stunned the world of human genetics at that time as it was believed that only a small fraction (~3%) of genes actually produce proteins.

Sardi reports a further scientific reversal, 22-months later: scientists at Oxford University claimed that only 8.2% of our DNA is biologically active, with the rest of the genome being leftover evolutionary material that has undergone mutational losses or gains in the DNA code.[17] Moreover, these researchers claim only a little more than 1% of human DNA accounts for the proteins that carry out most biological processes in the body.

Sardi suggests this is seemingly good news, describing how the human genome is comprised of about 21,000 genes, meaning only a couple hundred genes need to be influenced to produce a beneficial effect. Researchers, he suggests, have found that "only 295 genes are robustly associated with human ageing.[18] There are natural or synthetic molecules known to activate or deactivate hundreds of genes at a time.[19] This suggests an anti-ageing pill is within reach."

Sardi goes on to describe how non-functional or "junk DNA develops from DNA mutations. Over time mutations arise in DNA. Mutations occur on the DNA ladder. The steps of the DNA ladder called nucleotides (adenine, guanine, cytosine, thymine) may be substituted or be out of sequence, producing a mutation."[20]

## Cytosine IN and OUT

Various studies estimate that humans sustain 2.1-10.0 deleterious mutations per generation. This suggests that, over time, 90% of the human genome has mutated and is non-functional.[21] Oxford University researchers say these mutations have rendered most of the human library of genes, a copy which is stored in the nucleus of every living cell in the human body, as non-functional.

But let's not overlook a convincing experiment where a segment of so-called junk DNA was deleted from laboratory mice. These animals experienced increased weight gain and mortality on a high-fat diet.[22]

## Sir Robert McCarrison – Genetic versus Epigenetic

"Inherited gene mutations represent only about 2% of all human disease.[23] Inherited diseases involve changes in the steps (nucleotides) of the DNA ladder. Gene mutations involves DNA structure.

"However, genes are not static. Genes can make proteins, a process called gene expression (gene is switched 'on') or gene silencing (gene is switched 'off'). Modifications in protein making of genes that occur without changes in DNA sequence is called epigenetics. Most chronic disease is now believed to be epigenetic, that is, derived from gene protein making." [24]

Sardi suggests that *"In between the lines of print readers find the scientific community is attempting to make the science fit an evolutionary model that makes little or no sense."*

*"The Oxford University scientists write that most of the human genome has been 'purified' by a theoretical biological mechanism called natural selection. The unfit genes become mutated and the fit genes remain intact. The largest part of the genome "can be deleted without impacting fitness" of the species, they say."*

## Genetic purification questioned

"The proposed idea of genetic purification by natural selection is on very shaky ground. As researchers at the University of Washington note, mutations rarely turn out to be beneficial.[25] "Another long unexplained phenomenon is that the genome size of the most advanced species, Homo sapiens, is 40 times smaller than a lungfish. An onion has a genome that is 5 times larger than a human.[26] One would think greater complexity would require more genes, not less."

## Nature versus nurture

"The behind-the-scenes battle going on is whether evolutionary forces are at work (genetic mutations over a long time) or whether relatively rapid epigenetic changes control the functionality of genes. Can biological function be explained without the dogma of random natural selection?

"The debate here is nature versus nurture, inherited biological destiny versus environmentally/molecularly alterable biology. The evolutionists cannot tolerate a departure from the evolutionary model. Oxford University researchers say the 440 scientists who authored the $123 million ENCODE project are dead wrong! It just can't be.

"Yet we know that most human disease is not inherited and involves ageing, which can be slowed or even reversed via epigenetics.

"The epigenome is not only 'imprinted' in early human development but can be altered molecularly later in life."


### Let Charles Darwin sort it out

Bill Sardi continues:

"With arguments for mutational/random natural selection/ evolutionary biology on the one hand and epigenetic/ environmental/alterable epigenetics on the other, it may be time to let the words of Charles Darwin sort out this argument.

"David Marsh of the McCarrison Society For Nutrition & Health in London, UK notes that Darwin spent a great deal of his time on his trips around the Galapagos Islands searching for possible mechanisms which communicate information from the environment to the human body. Darwin's eloquent drawings showing changes in bird beaks over a short period of time (not millions of years as evolutionists claim) strongly points to environmental factors rather than inborn inherited. factors that drive biological adaptation.

"Marsh notes that 'in each of his (Darwin's) six editions of the Origin Of Species he stated there were two forces in evolution - 'natural selection' and 'conditions of existence'; Darwin claimed the latter is more powerful', says Marsh. He points out that natural selection has weak predictive power because of its dependence upon random events. Marsh says recent changes in human height and shape over the past century strongly point to Darwin's 'conditions of existence'. The same goes for the modern epidemic of diabetes.

"Discover Magazine said it in 2006: 'DNA is not our biological destiny'. In 2010 Time Magazine's headline cover story said: 'Why DNA Isn't Your Destiny'.

"Epigenetics explains more about our biological destiny than evolution. Humans don't need to be resigned to thinking the diseases that plagued their forefathers will inevitably affect them. Even existing diseases can be reversed mid-course. There is a lot researchers in biology aren't telling you about epigenetics."

It seems apposite to allow Charles Darwin the last word, by looking at his comments on chance:

"I have sometimes spoken as if variations were due to chance. This of course is a wholly incorrect expression, but it serves to acknowledge plainly our ignorance of the cause of each particular variation."

Poor Darwin, arguably the greatest environmentalist ever, would be turning in his grave if he could only see what Weismann, and many others since, have done to his beloved powerfully environmental theory.

In conclusion: there have been few comments on the ENCODE debate since the publications mentioned above, due no doubt to the increasingly complicated nature of the research. However, we will look at what conclusions have been reached in Appendix 1, from an excellent paper from Rio de Janeiro State University, Science and Biology Teaching Department – Biology Institute, Rio de Janeiro, Brazil, in which they conclude that: "A gene-centric conception of the organism has to be reviewed."

Finally, the HGP and ENCODE projects accomplished a great map of the human genome, but the big data generated remain to be carefully analysed. We've been endeavouring to catalogue a number of phenomena in order to understand the language of nature. But it is not so evident. The key for understanding the "secret of life" has not been revealed. (Readers interested in finding out more about Encode should refer to Appendix 1: The Human Genome Map and the Encyclopaedia of DNA elements).

# CHAPTER 4
# The Order In Life

## A problem with little by little and random mutation

So! Did we really arrive here by random mutation? Or was it more down to Darwin's 'conditions of existence'?

When one stops to think about it, for random mutation and natural selection to work requires conditions in which there is a struggle for survival. That means a lot has to happen first. Darwin was correct: the conditions of existence had to be right first. In the search for extraterrestrial life people are looking for planets circling a star that have conditions appropriate for carbon life as we know it. They know the conditions of existence have to be right.

The temperature of the universe ranges from close to absolute zero at -273.15°C to way above 1,000,000°C or more. We can see that our own conditions occupy a very small window at the bottom end of the range. In searching for potential water-based life on other planets astronomers refer to the 'Goldilocks Zone' – a sweet spot that is not too hot, not too cold, but just right! This concept is a version of Darwin's conditions of existence.

Darwin was right about conditions of existence in many ways he could not have envisaged. The laws of physics are precise. If the proton was as little as 1% heavier, then matter as we know it would not exist. The conditions of our existence are dependent on extremely precise dimensions of the subatomic particles that make everything.

Out of the various theories of evolution Darwin formed a synthesis that seems impregnable. And yet it has not been without critics, and criticism has not only come from people affronted by a doctrine of evolution that seems to contradict sacred writings.

His thesis however contains one important oversight. Darwin considers how species changed little by little to become what they are today. He does not discuss how it all happened in the first place. Ironically, he does not actually address the *origin*, even if that word is in the famous book title.

There is also a separate problem which is not of Darwin's making. As we discussed in the previous chapter, he rewrote his thesis several times and attempted to find the solution to a problem which worried him. How, exactly, did species interact with their environment? By asking that question he recognised that natural selection was not the only operational force in evolution.

Darwin claimed there were two factors of paramount importance in evolution: natural selection and 'conditions of existence' (see chapters 2 and 3). The latter equates to the environment, and, to be blunt, physics and chemistry.

The evolution of organisms requires a conducive environment. This is obvious when you think of it in terms of the familiar world around us. Flowers could not have evolved without soil, and bees could not have evolved without flowers. These "conditions of existence", in which environment and organism proceed hand in hand, are the springboard of all species.

He argued that as natural selection was dependent on 'conditions', then conditions were the more important of the two controlling factors. So (to recap points made in the previous chapter), original Darwinism perceived the environment to be a major directive force, although a precise mechanism of how environment interrelated with natural selection was not clear. It was this problem that Darwin spent the rest of his life trying to work out. He searched for what he called pangenes, which translated environmental conditions to the germplasm – what we know today as epigenetics.

Darwin realised that as natural selection was dependent on conditions of existence, the latter must be the more important of the two forces.

## Has there been enough time for life to emerge?

There are several recurring objections to the narrower 'post-Darwin' view of evolution, in which random mutation reigns supreme. One objection can be put in the form of a simple question:

*'Has there been enough time for life to arise in the first place?'*

It seemed to happen quite quickly once the temperature of the water was agreeable.

Many scientists have questioned Darwinian 'collection of small, random changes' as a mechanism for the origin of life, let alone new species. Indeed, Albert Szent-Gyorgyi, the scientist and Nobel Prize winner, has presented the case that the probability of life emerging by chance is zero.[1] The Cambridge astronomer Sir Fred Hoyle, like Szent-Gyorgyi, was so convinced by the mathematical implausibility that he abandoned the idea of evolution taking place on our own planet and proclaimed that it must have arrived from outer space.[2] He calculated that you have to go through $10^{18}$ combinations (as a number, that's 10 with 18 zeros after it) one by one before you assemble the complete code. And that is just for one tiny protein. The chances of this happening are remote. The idea that life evolved by chance alone just doesn't compute.

This is because it evolved by design – not a design of theological origin, even if He designed it, but through chemistry and physics. In this book we are simply suggesting that the principles of chemistry and nutrition remove the element of chance. They define the conditions and what will happen when chemicals get together. It has the simplicity of 1 + 2 = 3. No less – no more.

## Monkey business with typewriters

Another champion of randomness was T. H. Huxley, a leading figure in British science and a great supporter of Darwin. It is instructive to look at a well-known analogy, the 'Monkey Theorem', which Huxley supposedly used to justify the chance process suggested by Darwin. This analogy has six monkeys tapping unintelligently on typewriters for millions of millions of years. We should rightly regard a monkey's successful literary achievements as a remarkable accident, and it was claimed that if we looked through all the millions of pages the monkeys had typed over the millions of years, we would find a Shakespeare sonnet *"somewhere amongst them, the product of the blind play of chance"*.

Huxley was supposed to have invited his readers to imagine this group of monkeys, each at his own typewriter, hammering away at the keys in a totally random way. In time, it is said, they would type out the complete works of Shakespeare.

Mathematically, this is sort of true. In time they would, perhaps: but the question is, how much time? To test this, we wrote an Alpha-Micro computer programme to calculate how long it would indeed take for one of Huxley's monkeys to type out just the first line of a single Shakespeare sonnet. The program ran, and the computer informed us that the answer was too large a number for it to print (note: these were early days of computing when you had access to the object code, unlike today when it is deliberately hidden – back then you could make the computer do what you wanted, but now you have to buy a load of so-called software!)

After this frustrating answer from our computer, we realised that you do not actually need a computer at all, simply a table of logarithms. By converting the problem to logarithms we were able to get a result. And it was quite long. If a monkey went on untiringly hitting three or four keys every second – say two hundred a minute – the job would take just under 30 billion years. If it had started typing at the moment the universe began, it would still be nowhere near halfway to producing that first line of Shakespearian verse.

What we forgot was that a typewriter has at least 45 keys, not the 26 we had computed for – and that does not include upper and lower case. When we mentioned our problems with the computer to our friend and mentor Norman Pirie FRS, an eminent scientist working at Rothamstead agricultural research station, he remarked that when he was at school a master tried to use the same argument concerning monkeys. Pirie immediately pointed out that with 45 keys and (say) 30 letters in a line, guessing that the log of 45 was 1.7 you had a number 50 figures long for the possible permutations. A computer is not needed. [4]

[5] This, of course, no more proves Darwin wrong than Huxley's analogy could have proved him right. What it does show is that arguments about what will occur by random change are valueless if we do not consider the actual arithmetic and logistics compatible with the mechanism. Although science has yet to describe the full range of numbers and the chemical mechanisms involved in evolution, it is astonishing that so many have swallowed this random monkey business!

Hoyle is by no means the only critic to believe that, for a simple model of the evolution of life and natural selection, the numbers do not fit. Professor C. H. Waddington, a geneticist who did much experimental work with animals, has compared the theory of evolution through chance to a builder "throwing bricks together in heaps" in the hope that they would "arrange themselves into a habitable house". [6]

These simple demonstrations give some idea of the sizeable mathematical constraints which convinced Szent- Gyorgyi, Hoyle and Waddington, among others, that evolution could not have happened by chance alone.

Many 20th century scientists have highlighted the staggering improbability of life being able to evolve by random mutation in the relatively limited time available. And yet the idea of random changes spearheading evolution remains the accepted narrative. In the hypothesis put forward in this book, chemistry and nutrition remove the element of chance – the driving force is not random mutation, but environment-led change based on availability, economy, and a situation akin to shopping from a metaphorical supermarket shelf stripped of everything except the absolute essentials.

## Chemistry and physics remove the randomness

So how could it have worked? Chemical molecules are themselves built to specifications which depend on the nature of the chemicals reacting together.

For example, sodium plus chlorine = table salt.

This property of chemicals is not lost simply because the chemical is part of a living system. Hence the chemicals which interacted to produce what we now call the genetic code and the further interaction with proteins, RNA and other molecules, had to be arranged in response to the options set by the laws of chemistry and physics. It is just a bit more complicated than sodium + chlorine = salt.

Then there are electrons, and biologists by and large forget about them; but, as we will discuss in due course, electrons are vital for brain and nervous system function.

Certain molecules, and arrangements of them, send electrical messages around the brain that enable you to see, hear, touch, think and act. That is a very important consideration for *Homo sapiens* with such a big brain!

This targeting by the laws governing how one chemical reacts with another and how complex systems grow from the simpler ones takes 'the guesswork' out of the game.

However, those with faith in the lottery theory have fought back. A computer programme, if given rules, can readily assemble meaningful phrases out of a jumble. Richard Dawkins uses this technique in his book *The Blind Watchmaker*. To solve the

Huxley paradox he analyses the data on the basis of cumulative selection whereby the first selection restricts the possibilities for subsequent selections. That is, you go down one path, and in doing so the survivable options of the next accidental step are dramatically reduced to a point where it is all possible by chance alone. So he says.

And yet Dawkins is still entirely focused on the notion of a lottery. He ignores the fact that you must have conditions which will lead to such severe competition for limited or diminishing resources that only the fittest survive. Nothing can work unless the conditions allow it or even encourage it. His technique is about modified selection, and chance. He does not consider, for example, the vast numbers involved in arriving at the correct assembly to make a protein like haemoglobin or building a complex structure such as the mitochondria which provides the energy for the cell. His Watchmaker trick does not solve the real problem of randomness. [7]

What Hoyle and Szent-Gyorgyi were worried about in the first place was not selection but the origin of life itself: selection comes at a much, much later point – possibly 3.5 billion years later, with the evolution of animal life during the Cambrian Explosion. Selection is fine tuning. Origin is a massively different ball game.

The difference between one animal or plant species and the next is tiny in comparison with the difference between the presence and absence of life. If, however, the beginning of life was the dedicated work of chemistry and physics, then we need not consider chance. But we do need to consider the conditions of existence – the environment.

The rules of chemistry are not at all those of a blind watchmaker. The blind watchmaker model can only have been postulated by people who lacked a grounding in chemistry and physics. Darwin had an excuse because chemistry and physics were in their infancy when he was formulating his theories. But in the twenty-first century there is no such excuse.

The rules of chemistry and physics were in place long before life evolved. Perhaps a few moments after the big bang, if not before! It is not a question of a blind agency but one with its eyes wide open to specific laws. The important distinction between blindness/randomness and rules is that rules allow predictions to be made about associations and directions. In comparison, randomness offers little predictive value. Prediction is a basis of the scientific method and when scientists get it right, the predictions are proved correct. When wrong – they start again. Rules enable us to predict what happens when A meets B or when a sodium atom meets a chlorine atom. Hence chance can be replaced by the inevitability of chemistry and physics.

The mathematical numbers involved in the creation of life by random events are difficult to comprehend, and it is also difficult to ascribe to chance the simpler question of the evolution of the sophisticated hierarchy of living things.

This difficulty is illustrated by a consideration of what needs to happen for what appears to be a single new modification to succeed.

## The mythical story of the giraffe and its long neck

Let us consider the long neck of the giraffe, which has been used often in the debate on natural selection. Those animals with slightly longer necks than their friends survived because they could reach higher into the trees and so gain the advantage of reaching foods that others could not.

It's an appealing image, but not one that survives close examination. If, say, some forerunner of the giraffe was born with a slightly longer neck than its parent, the greater length would be valueless if the animal did not also modify its heart to pump enough blood to increase the blood pressure to 200 mm Hg, to send the blood up to the brain. Then its vascular system has to be strengthened to take the strain. Its nervous system must change, too. It must also alter its pattern of behaviour if it is to seek food amongst vegetation formerly out of reach.

If the food that is brought within the longer-necked giraffe's reach is different to that which its shorter-necked parents browsed on (and this is indeed the case, and an important piece of the puzzle), then its stomach and digestive system will also have to be modified. So it is not just the time needed to develop the gene for a long neck – the time taken for all these other essential changes to coincide also needs to be taken into account.

Anyway, if the mutation works like this:

1.  a gene for a 50cm neck
2.  a gene for a 100cm neck
3.  a gene for a 200 cm neck; etc.,

- then you also need to include the genes for all the other things. A gene for long, strong arteries; a gene for superior blood pressure control, for blood to reach the brain; and no doubt a gene for better kidneys to handle the blood pressure problem. Perhaps the giraffe has the answer to haemorrhagic stroke. If ever there was a propensity for such a stroke it results from living with a blood pressure of 200 mm Hg.

Perhaps, after sitting for a long time, and then bending down to tie your shoe laces, and suddenly leaping out of the chair, you may have felt giddy for a moment or two? Well, think how giddy a drinking giraffe should feel if it raises its head after drinking water! Perhaps it hears or smells an approaching lion, lifts its head in panic, ready to make off in fast loping strides. The blood should drain from the brain. It should black out. But it doesn't. And the reason it doesn't is down to a sophisticated arrangement of blood vessels and valves and baro-receptors (pressure receptors which respond to a pressure-induced stretching of the artery) in its head, keeping the blood pressure to the brain constant. This blood pressure remains the same no matter whether the head is up or down. Of course, people will still say this was all managed by selecting only those random changes that worked. But it does sound like a tall story.

Another issue is this: if the mutations are random then they could just as easily go in the wrong direction, or some go one way and others somewhere else, instead of harmonising all those things needed for a long neck. You cannot build a long stretch of arteries to reach the giraffe's brain without the specific chemicals to build those arteries. Perhaps there is some mechanism linking these changes. The chances against them all happening simultaneously are enormous. The truth is that the actual changes taking place are not just *cumulative* but *coordinated*.

And for a start, *very specific chemicals* are needed to build these arteries. When discussing nutrition, we will later discuss the fact that the food of the giraffe is different in a meaningful way to the food of short necked grazing animals.

Indeed, if we take a moment to glance at the different lines of evolution, they are so coordinated that it is far from likely that chance alone could have produced the great variety of living forms that have come into existence. For the first two to three billion years since life first began, not much happened. The planet was covered in water. The vast sea was inhabited by anaerobic prokaryotes – single-celled bacteria and algae, and probably other life forms such as viruses. The creation of the animal phyla with all their great diversity happened in a brief geological time-frame in the Vendian and Cambrian, starting around 600 million years ago.

The basic biochemical functioning of organisms has remained largely unchanged since the very beginnings of life. This is because evolutionary changes are not just cumulative but are also coordinated, obeying simple chemical laws. Life moves forward according to a program dictated by chemistry and environment, which limits the possibilities sufficiently to explain the pace and diversity of evolution. It is like providing a channel for water to flow through, rather than letting it make random progress across flat terrain.

## Breathing space: the story of oxygen

For the first 3 billion years or so, life was anaerobic – i.e. it did not breathe oxygen. Oxygen is a highly reactive element and will combine with anything it can get its hands on: and it did. It has a low atomic weight – a lot of it would have been produced by exploding supernovas. Much of it combined with hydrogen to produce water. The blue-green algae and other photosynthesising bacteria did what plants do today, absorbing carbon dioxide and excreting oxygen. For a long, long time, other chemicals absorbed spare oxygen (e.g. rusting iron). Initially there were so many elements with a love for oxygen that it was mostly taken out of circulation.

However, a time eventually came when oxygen-trapping chemicals were saturated. The concentration of oxygen in the sea was at an all-time low; but the blue-green algae and photosynthetic bacteria did a great job for climate change, mopping up the $CO^2$ and pumping out the $O^2$.

Slowly, the oxygen tension rose, reaching the point when air-breathing life became possible. Consequently, there was a proliferation of air-breathing life, a phenomenon referred to as the Cambrian Explosion, when all the animal phyla we know today came into existence. The Cambrian Period lasted from approximately 541 to 485.4 million years ago. Although there must have been an abundance of life before the Cambrian, the bulk of air-breathing animal evolution occurred in this geologically brief time period, when oxygen became available in sufficient concentration. This was not chance. This is *not* a tale of random variation. It is one of sheer chemistry and conditions of existence.

The rise in oxygen tension would not have been uniform. Hence hot spots would be expected. Indeed, volcanic vents and the huge variations in water depths would have created a great diversity of different chemical conditions, temperature and pressures, and with differences in in the UV-dense, solar radiation too, paving the way for the different life forms to evolve as they did. The creation of the animal phyla happened in a geological blink of an eye. It had nothing to do with chance.

Why was life limited to single-celled organisms for 3 billion years? Why is it that the 32 phyla in existence today first appeared with the "Cambrian Explosion", with no new phyla evolving since? The answer is the same in each case – conditions of existence. A tipping point arrives; and in the case of the first blossoming of complex, multi-cellular life, that tipping point was oxygen.

The earliest life on Earth lived in an oxygen-poor environment. Oxygen built up as a by-product of photosynthesis in single-celled organisms, and oxygen availability enabled the production of highly unsaturated fatty acids. Carbon based life is built with carbon atoms which have four hooks to combine with other carbons in a chain and with other chemicals such as nitrogen, phosphorous, sulphur and others. These were the building blocks of life. Saturated fatty acids are simply a chain of carbon, joined by single hooks or bonds with the spare hooks joined to hydrogen and a oxygen acid group at one end. When oxygen came to be present in enough concentration, it stole two hydrogens from adjacent carbons so it could exist happily as $H_2O$. That left two hooks which joined together to make a double link – what we call a double bond or unsaturated bond. Indeed, oxygen played this game with many molecules but importantly the unsaturated fatty acids so formed became the building material for cell membranes, enabling the organisatiion of cells and various specialized compartments like the nuclear envelope inside, a major start to cell specialisation and the evolution of multicellular life as we know it today.

The important question is: what are the rules for the success of selection? Let's consider large herbivores. The chemistry and hence the nutritional value of tree foliage is different to that of the grass eaten by bovids. For example, to return to our old friends the giraffes, their favourite food *Balanites aegyptiaca* has thick fleshy leaves. The fruit – called the desert date as it is also used for food by nomadic people – contains an oil-rich kernel. Moreover, more than 60% of this oil is linoleic acid. Eating a lot of linoleic acid could contribute to the building of the tough blood vessels needed to take the blood to the brain at high pressure. Linoleic acid is converted to arachidonic acid, which just happens to be quantitatively the most dominant essential fatty acid in the inner cell membrane of the endothelium which lines the arteries. It is also the precursor for prostacyclin, a hormone-like substance that stops platelets adhering to the vascular walls, thus preventing thrombosis and helping control blood pressure. With the giraffe's constant high blood pressure, they would certainly need that.

The leaves of *Balanites aegyptiaca* are a source of alpha-linolenic acid, the parent of the omega-3 essential fatty acid family including EPA and DHA. There are many Acacia tree varieties that produce a bean that is also rich in alpha-linolenic acid. Giraffes loves the big, tall Acacias, which their grazing shapes into the familiar umbrella trees of the African savannah.

In the 1970s at London Zoo we studied the effect of an alpha-linolenic acid or omega-3 deficient diet in Capuchin monkeys. Apart from demonstrating severe behavioural disorders and poor hair condition, the veterinary pathologist at London Zoo reported that the monkeys had fatty livers and a loss of elastic tissue in their blood vessels. [8]

The opposite side of the nutritional coin is demonstrated by the widespread use of linseed cake (rich in omega-3) to induce a lovely shiny coat in horses before a show. No one has studied the effect of alpha-linolenic acid on the horse's blood vessels. Nonetheless, here is another mechanism whereby the alpha-linolenic acid rich diet of the giraffe could have contributed to their evolving elasticity and strength. The diet of the grass-eating herbivores would be nowhere near as rich.

There may be many other hidden factors that we do not know about. No one has looked. People just take it for granted that random selection will explain everything, and look for more and more devious ways to explain inconsistencies such as those pointed out by Rattray Taylor and Stephen J. Gould in his theory of *punctuated evolution.* [9]

## Evolution did not happen by slow, gradual modifications: it went in leaps and bounds

If change did indeed occur randomly through the accumulation of many tiny modifications, then it would be likely to occur at a steady pace until the eureka moments. One of the most important objections to this random idea concerns the many examples of sudden branching or new development in evolution, referred to as discontinuities, of which the Cambrian Explosion is the most striking example. Suddenly, when oxygen arrives, the old collapses and the new appears. Stephen J. Gould drew attention to these discontinuities as recurrent themes punctuating evolution which are difficult to explain through chance.

There has to be some reason why the evolutionary forces for significant change did nothing for the so long 3 billion years, then leapt into top gear before suddenly coming to a stop. If random mutation was continuous, as the accepted thesis supposes, was its potential for innovation held at bay? If so, what held it at bay and, even more interestingly, what was it that suddenly released the mechanism for change? Indeed, what called the sudden excitement to a halt? The Cambrian Explosion is a massive testament against gradual modification and a validation of Darwin's 'conditions of existence', and the death knell to chance.

Later, the dinosaurs ruled the Earth for 160 million years, and then over a period of a million years or so they disappeared. There was an explosion of diversity amongst the mammals, which took the dinosaurs' place. Flies and bees emerge in the fossil record as if from nowhere. There are no intermediate forms found. Some genetic changes have occurred with time, but their form has been largely unchanged since then. Much the same is true for modern mammals.

To explain these discontinuities Fred Hoyle has resorted to implicating visits from outer space.[3] Others have suggested recurring catastrophes – the whole world darkened with the dust of enormous volcanic eruptions, or struck by some giant meteor or asteroid. This book, without dismissing the meteor idea entirely, will suggest a less dramatic agency for change.

## Evidence from chemistry

Another problem lies in the basic chemistry of all the life forms we know about. If changes had been truly random we would expect them to have affected a random biochemical level of organisation as well as others, but in fact they have not.

The way in which modern plants absorb sunlight, use its energy to promote chemical reactions, and excrete oxygen into their surroundings is the same, as far as we know, as that of the earliest forms of plant life (and indeed the very first photosynthetic prokaryotes 3 to 4 billion years ago).

Still more curiously, the chemistry that transports oxygen in the human bloodstream is the same in all mammalian species. Some oddballs use copper instead of iron – crabs for example. However, the basics of copper and iron for oxygen transport in the blood are biochemically similar.

Indeed, the key processing systems in our bodies are not radically different to those of the first microscopic creatures that drifted in the primeval oceans. In a world of chance events, such persistence over millions and even billions of years needs explaining. The chemistry of our photoreceptors and the brain's synapses and neurons are basically the same as in the cephalopods, which evolved about 400 million years ago.

This uniformity of structure and function may be explained

by many different lines of evolution converging on the same answer as to what is best fitted for the purpose. On the other hand, the reason for uniformity may simply be, as the late Norman W. Pire remarked in 1972, *'that in similar environments, only one form of biochemistry is possible'*. He argued that, while evolution involves selection, *'it is not always certain from which direction the selection comes. Chemical structures first appear and then uses or new uses are made of them later.'*

Indeed, he believed that ideas on evolutionary progress are basically an aesthetic appreciation of morphology, *'coloured by anthropomorphism'*. For example, we are so familiar with the hand and its function that it is difficult to imagine any better design existing either in the past or in the future. The design of the human hand seems to be so perfect that it becomes a perfect piece of evidence for natural selection. And yet mice, rats and squirrels have little hands which they use for holding food when eating, like a child holding an ice cream cone.

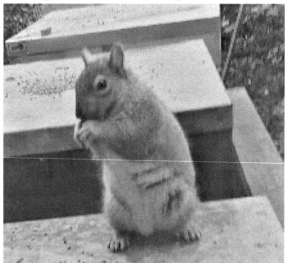

And then we have the dolphin, which has in its flipper all the bones found in the human hand. Now, if an engineer had to design two 'perfect' pieces of apparatus, one to propel a boat and the other to manipulate small objects, it is hardly likely that he would use the same structure of tiny rods for both mechanisms, simply varying their lengths and thicknesses. Yet that is what has happened with humans and dolphins. The changes to their forelimbs may have been selective, but they have not been random. The sizes of the individual bones have varied but, curiously, *their number and relative positions have not changed at all.* (We will offer an explanation in due course when we visit the shores of Lake Turkana in Kenya and the El Molo who thrive on its produce.)

Structure similar to the dolphin's flipper is seen in the limbs of other marine mammals. This may seem to suggest that there is some not-yet-understood restraint that makes certain kinds of change less or more likely to occur than others. Alternatively, there may be some biological mechanism which uses the same ground-plan and simply makes more or less of this or that. Did the dolphin evolve the bones of a hand inside its flipper? Or did the arm bones shrink into the body, and surplus skin join the fingertips to make flippers where a hand had once been?

In the light of this example, the design of the hand as evidence for natural selection is perhaps less convincing. We can ask: 'Is it more likely that the dolphin arrived at the shape and form of its arm and hand from a different and unknown starting point, or did it start from a similar plan to the human limb and was subsequently modified?' To us the former seems unlikely.

And if this is so, then evolution can be shown to work through changing shape and size but retaining the basic plan. One can then ask if the changes involved in becoming a dolphin, including a shrinkage of the bones and the covering of the hand with skin, were actually the consequence of epigenetic changes. That is, were they responding to the conditions of existence, with a high phosphorous and low calcium diet, and weightlessness (as with astronauts), shrinking the bones? In other words, did it have nothing to do with natural selection? We will ask later why on earth did a bunch of land mammals decide to make their life in the sea??

As in these details so in the broadest view, evolution displays certain curious streaks of conservatism on the one hand and astonishing diversity on the other. The most fundamental grouping of living things that biologists recognise is the phylum. There are about 32 phyla, although the exact number is still a matter of dispute. What defines a phylum is that its members share a certain overall plan or strategy of life. There are, for example, single-cell systems such as algae and protozoa, and multicellular systems such as trees and animals with backbones. Plants get their food from air, sun and soil, animals by eating plants or each other. Fungi, on the other hand, feed on organic matter as animals do, but stay rooted like plants. Again, there are different ways in which living systems are organised. The design that we humans have followed is based on the principle of two symmetrical halves - two eyes, two kidneys, two halves of the brain, each limb matching another on the opposite side. A starfish or a limpet is not like that: its design is radial rather than bilateral, and an oyster is different again.

## Evolution caught in a trap

Evolution, it seems, gets itself into certain grooves from which it finds it hard to escape. No new phyla seem to have emerged since the Cambrian Explosion. Again, that is not random. Many species, successful for long periods, have died out altogether. Natural selection presumably worked well for them for these periods, but ultimately the changes needed to adapt to a changing environment were simply not within the repertoire available to them. In fact, whole classes of animals get stuck in grooves. The buffalo, whatever the pressure on it, could never randomly change into a carnivore, nor can the lion learn to live on grass. If by random changes we mean that a change of any kind is as likely as a change of any other kind, then clearly this is not how evolution works.

Although the rules of chemistry and physics can be thought of as absolute, they do allow for the possibility of competition and we might envisage the element of chance taking the organism in one of a number of directions. The chemistry of the large molecules is complex and the number of letters in the genetic code so large that even obeying the rules of chemistry, the number of possible permutations is such that room for random variation would be expected alongside certain fundamental dictates.

One example is the favoured theory on immune system function, proposed by Australian virologist Sir Frank MacFarlane Burnett, which is decidedly dependent on chance. Lymphocytes (a subtype of white blood cell in the immune system) are generated with a vast repertoire of antibody variation. When an immune cell matches an invading antigen, it is stimulated to divide and so produces a clone of identical cells making an identical antibody. Further stimulation by the same antigen multiplies the rate of reproduction leading to a rapid expansion of the defence system. This mechanism is an elegant example of natural selection operating within our own bodies, relying specifically on the chance production of antibodies in the hope that one would provide a chemical match for the offensive agent. Or is it? Is there an interaction between the immune cell and the virus or bacterium which signals the identification of the pathogen to create an immune cell with a surface response to the unique pathogen? Is this an epigenetic type response, rather than the population of immune cells having a pre-existing responder facility in the outer membrane? Indeed, it could be viewed as an environmenal/epigenetic effect whereby the invader influencers the gene coding, which is of course what happens.

One oft-quoted example of natural selection occurred in the soot-laden atmosphere of the coal-burning industrial belt of England, on the bark of trees. Dark coloured Peppered moths (*Biston betularia*), successfully camouflaged against the pollution-blackened trees, survived, while lighter coloured ones were eaten by birds, providing a vivid example of Darwinian predation at work. That is the general view. However, if the moths are feeding on soot-laden vegetation then is it not likely that their bodies and wings would take on a darkened hue? Something similar is seen in city-dwelling pigeons, which are often much darker than the pigeons in farm land, or the rock doves (*Columba livia*) from which all feral pigeons are descended. Indeed, carrot juice fanatics take on a warm skin colour.

While we accept that natural selection is a factor here, we believe, as did Darwin, that it was not the only mechanism in evolution, and that chemistry operating through the environment is at least as important, if not more so.

The fundamental rule of chemistry is that those options which are thermodynamically most stable are the ones that persist. Chemistry will find a consistent direction, just as water will always run downhill. Rock is hard and stable on the surface of our planet only because the temperature makes it so. The fact that the molecules in an animal's body are more complicated than those in a rock does not mean that the laws of chemistry and physics are suspended.

If evolutionary change was obeying simple chemical laws, the persistence of traits, the problem of the evolutionary timescales and Stephen J. Gould's discontinuities and punctuated evolution - long periods when nothing happens, followed by sudden change – would all be explained. Instead of wasting time exploring innumerable dead ends, life would move forward according to a programme dictated by the nature of chemistry and the environment. The presence or absence of chemicals like oxygen, or nutrients like vitamin A, make certain directions possible or impossible. When chemical support systems (as in essential nutrients) for a particular line of species are exhausted, the biochemical system cannot cope, the line collapses and creates a new discontinuity. [10]

In a sense, the example of Burnett's theory of immune system function is not only an example of specific selection but also an example of the interaction of external influence as in the bunch of chemicals that constitute the virus..

The cells of the immune system are very different from the fertile egg, and this process of differentiation may offer insights into evolution. How does the combination of two single cells, the sperm and ovum, turn into an eye or a hand? This important question has been tackled Norman Maclean and Brian K Hall's book *Cell Commitment and Differentiation* . They start with the present understanding of cell differentiation which offers two alternatives. Cells become skin or muscle because certain genes are deleted or suppressed. [11]

Almost universally the latter strategy has been adopted so that the cell nucleus from any part of the body contains all the original DNA code and can be reused to produce a new animal. The authors comment that the recent rapid advance in knowledge of gene sequences might 'beguile' one into thinking this process of differentiation is well understood. '*That this is not so is simply because knowing the sequence of a particular gene, or even how it is regulated, does not itself provide an insight into how a cell becomes committed to a particular fate.*'

The remarkable similarity between different stages of embryonic development and the history of vertebrates  has raised the thought in the minds of many that embryonic development and cell differentiation emulate evolution. At about four weeks of age it is difficult to distinguish the human embryo from any other mammal; it has a long tail, a single-chambered heart like a fish, and a circulation with loops to four gill-arches, also like a fish. It seems as though it first organises itself in a manner similar to the fish and then develops this into the plan for a primate.

There is indeed an interesting similarity between cell differentiation and evolution. Cells differentiate and become committed. Animals evolved and became committed. The question that cell differentiation and evolution both ask is:

what is it that directs the paths they follow? The question that cell commitment and the rigidity of evolutionary lines – as in carnivores versus herbivores – also asks is: what holds them in place? That is, why is a limb a limb, and why does it stay as a limb? Why is a cow a cow, and why does it not turn into a lion, is basically the same question. Add to this the rigidity of genetic codes for certain key systems (e.g. oxidative enzymes) and the question becomes: *was evolution cell differentiation on a grand scale?*

## Chemistry at work in cell commitment

As Maclean and Hall point out in their splendid book, other than knowledge of anatomy, surprisingly little is known about cell commitment and differentiation. Similarly, little is known about regulation of shape and size. Although codes in the DNA may provide for much we need to know about the chemical reasons for change: why does this chemical increase and that one decrease in amount? If such matters can be controlled internally by chemical signals, can external chemicals also act as messengers?

Most gardeners will have used plant rooting compounds to encourage faster rooting of cuttings. These plant auxins are in fact messengers applied externally which stimulate DNA synthesis and so increase cell division and the elongation of the cell through making more cell wall materials. The effect is to encourage root formation where before there were apparently no root cells. The plant rooting hormone is indolylacetic acid and it also co-ordinates with gibberellic acid to act on undifferentiated plant cells. In plants which are capable of producing male and female flowers, a high proportion of indolylacetic acid will promote female blooms, while more gibberellins result in male flowers.

Tadpoles will metamorphose, lose their tails and develop legs when stimulated with thyroid hormone. If production of the hormone is prevented, they will not develop into frogs. The thyroid hormone is a simple 6 carbon, ring structure which contains iodine. The obvious conclusion is that if there were no iodine on the planet there would be no frogs.

The World Health Organisation's map of the incidence of goitre (iodine deficiency leading to mental retardation) shows that it is found mainly in mountainous and inland regions. These are areas where the soil has had its trace elements washed away by rain and melting snow. A low iodine content leads to inadequate thyroxine production. In humans this leads to physical changes most visible in the neck, face and eyes. In situations where the iodine content of the soil and food is very low, the deficiency results in impoverished brain development.

These simple examples suggest that the common view that 'food is just food', and that our primary concern should simply be whether there is enough of it, is inadequate. There is mounting evidence that it is not just the amount of food but its qualitative composition that matters. Indeed, the contemporary debate on diet and its relation to Western heart disease, mental ill-health and cancer is based on exactly that premise. It is not just a full cup that is needed, it is what is in the cup that matters. [12]

The question we are asking in this book is whether or not nutrition was a determinant in evolution which operated on – even directed – the basic plans of living systems. There is by no means enough evidence to spell out all the details, but such evidence as exists is compelling. It suggests that just as the beginning of life was determined by chemistry and conditions, so its later forms and expressions were also chemically shaped. Not exclusively – sometimes chemistry would operate independently, sometimes in tandem with selection, and sometimes selection would operate alone. But if the latter occurred, as Darwin recognised, it could only do so if the conditions allowed it. Hence we are back to chemistry and physics.

Our contention is that the origin of the planet and,

subsequently, the origin of life was determined by chemistry and physics operating within the conditions which prevailed at the time. Once the conditions of temperature and pressure had stabilised, life remained relatively stable. As with the Cambrian Explosion, there were crucially important changes in the conditions which brought about biological change.

## Our short lives obscure the big picture

Because the timescales involved in the life of the planet are so huge, it tends to be taken for granted that the conditions on the planet are stable. This is far from the truth: they are changing constantly and always have been. Since the terrestrial environment first emerged, rain has been washing salts, trace elements and waste products from the land into the sea and changing both as a consequence. If the North Sea and the Baltic can be affected in a few decades by fertilisers, think of the effect of rain and climate on land over million-year timespans. Although there may have been periods of relative stability in the physical conditions of the planet, chemical change has been constant - in part as a result of living systems, and partly through inexorable changes in the redistribution of the elements on the planet and variations in the behaviour of our sun. At first these changes were in simple chemicals coalescing into living systems; but as life became more complex, chemicals became food. Changes in the chemistry of food and differences in choice of foods are associated with different evolutionary paths. The implication is that *change in food or choice of food is an evolutionary instrument.*

For three-and-a-half billion years or so, blue-green algae dominated life on Earth. It produced oxygen, and what was ultimately a destructive pollutant to the algae was both a mutagen and essential nourishment for the animals that were to come. The evolution of air-breathing systems simply had to wait for the advent of oxygen. When it came it added the missing element to what was otherwise a rich niche for animal life 'waiting', as it were, for oxygen. The almost rapid coincident appearance of animal life is too much to ask of random chance.

The logic suggested by this example can be applied to us today in a manner that is vitally important for our future. The extension of the argument is that changes in chemistry or food can influence the expression of biological systems. This means that the food eaten by humans and lions throughout our separate evolution had some bearing on what we and the lion are today. And the story doesn't end in the past – nutrition will also play an important role in deciding our future. Bear in mind that our genome is only 1.5% different from that of the chimpanzee. *That means our genome is adapted to the wild foods we ate during our species' evolution.*

People need to think about the significance of that statement when visiting the supermarket. Apart from fish and seafood, there is barely anything on the shelves that fits the criteria of wild foods. Sir Robert McCarrison, a pioneer in developing an understanding of nutrition, health and disease commented that whenever a population departs from "*the unsophisticated foods of Nature*", ill-health of one form or another follows.

Once we understand the chemistry, we can understand how and why the first self-replicating molecules and then the first living things took the forms they did; and why, in time, they gave way to certain particular successors, from which all later forms of life descend. It was not a matter of chance: it was cause and effect. Given the nature of the environment and its chemistry, there was only a limited number of paths which chemistry, and hence evolution, could have followed. Perhaps as Norman Pirie said, there was only *one*.

# CHAPTER 5

# The chemicals of life

# Let there be light! Conditions in a star

# start it all

To understand what we are, where we came from and where we are going, it is a good idea to start at the beginning. Well, that means the Big Bang.

The energy of the Big Bang created matter. People are a bit vague about how this happened. Usually physics lectures inform the student that the first law of thermodynamics is the conservation of energy: "The law of conservation of energy states that the total energy of an isolated system is constant". However, those physics lecturers also say that at the Big Bang everything we know about was created out of nothing. This is in flat contradiction to that first law.

It all starts with a so-called quantum wall at the mind-bogglingly brief instant of $10^{-43}$ of a second. Prior to that moment, all rules and theories of physics and chemistry break down. Okay, so you don't like the rules, let's just suspend them! That sounds very unscientific; and yet people at the highest level of physics are happy to do just that. CERN with its big Hadron Collider which sends particles circling underneath Geneva and bits of France, to collide with each other to examine the bits and pieces, wants to develop a bigger and better particle accelerator to find an insight onto that very tiny time frame. That is, to see evidence of the breakdown of the laws of physics.

This whole topic is a lovely subject for ridicule but is very serious science. Indeed, the term 'Big Bang' was invented by Fred Hoyle, the Astronomer Royal, as a joke to ridicule the concept. But it is no joke! It is serious and, so far, convincing. At the same time, a key question few ask and no one answers is: what happened beforehand?

Some consider the Big Bang to have been the rebound after the collapse of a previous universe. Over time stars die forming black holes. Black holes absorb more and more stars until there are none left and the lights go out. Then, just as the first black hole exerted its gravitational influence to draw into it anything within range, so the immense gravity of the many black holes merge together until there is only one massive black hole left. Being so big this phenomenon becomes unstable and implodes into a singularity of nearly infinite mass and energy. The rebound explosion of the singularity kicks off a big bang with an unbelievable amount of energy at phenomenally high temperatures. So it is thought by some.

Einstein's great breakthrough was to define the relativity of energy and mass. They are one and the same under different guises. Hence as the phenomenal energy cools it becomes mass or matter. Tiny protons and electrons crystallize out of the energy. Our protons are positive, electrons negative. There should have been an equal number of positive electrons and negative protons, i.e. matter and anti-matter. So they should have cancelled each other out. But we live in a world with negative electrons and positive protons. Somehow, although much cancelled out there was somewhere a corner of only our stuff, odd as that seems. Anyway, cool it a bit further and positive and negative join, that is the electron joins up with the proton which is hydrogen.

This thing called gravity gets to work and brings the hydrogens together, more and more clumping into a swirling big, gigantic ball. If you scuba dive, you will know the deeper you go the greater the pressure which puts a limit on how deep you can go safely. So the bigger the ball gets the more intense the gravity and pressure in the middle of this ball. It gets so intense it fuses two hydrogen atoms together to make helium. The energy of the two hydrogens independently is greater than the one helium – economy of size! So a heap of energy is released which heats things up making it easier for more and more hydrogens to form helium. This is how our sun formed and the principle of the hydrogen bomb. There are now attempts to capture this fusion energy to provide a clean source of energy for the future.

In the beginning, this clumping is big and gets bigger. Soon the heat from the fusion of hydrogen atoms set off a chain reaction, it lights up and a star is born. Indeed, many clumps led to many stars then galaxies as we have today. This is how our sun formed. There are now attempts to capture this fusion energy to provide a clean source of energy for the future.

The life of a star is not plain sailing for it eventually must use up its hydrogen. As this disaster approaches it starts fusing helium and makes carbon and out of three helium atoms and then oxygen and even higher elements. When the hydrogen is used up making the heavier elements, the gravitational pull at the centre becomes so great that the dying star simply implodes creating a super-nova and throwing the debris out into space. Other stars pick up the debris and make heavier and heavier elements, and go *bang* again with bigger supernova. These have been seen with the naked eye at various times over the last 2,000 year, with a sighting in the year 185 AD in China possibly the first recorded. Modern astronomers are able to observe them, and the Hubble telescope has recorded some really beautiful and spectacular ones.[1] As you will know living systems are made up of carbon, hydrogen and oxygen in various combinations. Hence the carbon and oxygen used to make our bodies come from a dying star.

What came before the Big Bang? Where did all that matter come from? One theory suggests that big bangs are part of a vast cycle, fuelled by black holes. These eventually swallow everything in the universe, including each other. Eventually there is just one Mother of All Black Holes. Being unstable, it implodes. At the final moment of its implosion there is nothing in existence except a singularity of infinite mass and energy.

This bounces back, as it were, with a-rebound explosion – a 'big bang leaving a micro-wave radiation which enable physicists to discuss various happenings. This theory neatly explains the most recent of these bangs, and also accounts for an almost-but-not-quite- infinite number of previous big bangs. What it doesn't explain is the very first one. To crack this we need to discover what came before both the chicken and the egg!

But, fascinating as the discussion is, we have more mundane matters to discuss here, such as the beginning of life.

## The beginning of life – was it different in principle?

There is a belief that the creation of life was so complex it had to come from outer space. This idea is fuelled by evidence of amino acids and the like as we use in our metabolism to make proteins, in meteorites, or bits of rock from asteroids or comets. That just shifts the problem elsewhere. There is every good reason to accept that does not solve anything and is unnecessary: our life had its beginning here.

The elements ejected from a supernova are at first far too hot to touch anything else! When they start cooling many are of a positive nature and others negative so they join up. For example, oxygen is a really vicious element wanting to join up with anything going in the positive domain. At the still high temperature from a cooling region from a supernova it will burn silicon making the silicon oxides which form the rocks of our planet and elsewhere. Hydrogen is despite all that goes on in fusion, is the commonest element remaining from the Big Bang. Oxygen is doubly negative, and hydrogen is singly positive so we have H2O water - thankfully a lot of it.

The point here is that what happens in the creation of elements and compounds happen according to very fixed rules of chemistry and physics: there is no mystery here. Carbon is a very special atom as it has four hooks to join up with others. Oxygen has two so you have CO2!. With four hooks, carbon can connect with four different elements, it can connect with itself making chains or hydrocarbons. Its chains can connect with oxygen making fatty acids, or sugars, or with nitrogen making cyanide or amino acids and then proteins. Then sugars, other nitrogenous compounds and phosphates can join together to make nucleotides which can form strings and DNA!

## The chemicals of life can be made in the lab

The belief that there was some kind of life force making the chemicals of life, was destroyed in the 19th century by Friedrich Wöhler. Born July 1800 in Eschersheim, near Frankfurt, Germany, he studied and taught chemistry at the Polytechnic in Berlin. When he synthesised urea, an organic molecule, from simple laboratory chemicals, the gulf had been crossed. The gap between the living world and its environment was closed. Since then large numbers of biochemicals and all the vitamins have been synthesised. Swiss healthcare company Hoffman-La Roche began mass producing vitamin C in 1934 and sold it by the ton until it sold out its nutrition division to concentrate on pharmaceuticals. Indeed, there is no reason to suppose that we could not manufacture all the complex biochemicals that appear in living forms: if we were prepared to invest enough time and money. Craig Venter led the US team that decoded the human genome. May 21st 2010 at a press conference in Washington DC, he and his team announced they had made the first fully functioning, reproducing cell controlled by synthetic DNA: they had made synthetic life. [2]

There is nothing magical in any of the above. Once again it is a matter of conditions.

Water, chemicals, and the right temperature. That's the recipe for the cocktail of life. No magical "vital force" is required. Biochemistry simply boils down to chemistry and physics.

Carbon is the basis of life. The point is that building these and other substances is simply a matter of chemistry, and it can occur in the absence of life. The so-called 'molecules of life' are chemical certainties – they are to be expected and are indeed found in meteorites, and will be found on Mars or far away out there on the exoplanet Alpha Centauri Cb.

The union of elements is largely based on their number of bonds, and their ability to give or receive electrons. Carbon has four two-way bonds, making it a versatile giver and receiver that can bond with many other things, including itself. It is this versatility that gave rise to the possibilities of complex organisms.

So, with the versatility of carbon explained, we are approaching the boundaries of life, for it is the combination of different amino acids – built from carbon, hydrogen, oxygen and nitrogen – that form proteins, the building blocks of living tissue, where they are housed in membranes made by lipids made with fatty acids, phosphates and some carbon-nitrogen stuff and called phospho-lipids. These biological membranes are ultimately responsible for the organisation of compartments inside cells to do different things like energy production, signalling and even brain function, or supervise protein manufacture, and house the genome itself in the cell nucleus.

Question: What do you get when you take carbon, hydrogen, oxygen, nitrogen, phosphorous and sulphur, and add water? Answer: Pretty much everything that ever lived. But it requires specific conditions. This is why life doesn't spontaneously spring up in every corner of the Universe. It's also why evolution flows through narrow channels, where randomness is severely limited by environment.

Charged substances mix with water – whether positive

or negative, they are attracted to the opposite charge in the H2O molecule. This is how solids such as table salt dissolve. Dissolving can be understood as elements being 'trapped' by water molecules – they are not in suspension, but have become a solution – i.e. they cannot be filtered out.

Oil and water do not mix, as water carries an electrical charge and oil doesn't. So, water alone cannot wash oil from your hands; but if you add soap, it acts as a go-between, effectively merging the oil and water, and the gloop can then be washed away. Without the soap, the oil and the water will remain mutually exclusive. This principle is at work in cell membranes – a fatty acid water-insoluble barrier wraps around each cell like a protective wall.

## 4.5 billion years ago – wealth gifted from the stars

At the beginning of the life on the planet, there would of course be an extraordinary wealth of minerals and chemicals dusting the surface, if not knee deep. That is just the way it had to be in the aftermath of a star exploding, with a great amount of gold, silver, copper, iron, silicone, oxygen and carbon, with products of these forming with everything except gold, as things cooled off or heated up to the right temperature and pressure.

Such conditions would have formed the carbon-based, organic chemicals from the simplest as loosely described above, to those that were far more complex. It could not have been otherwise. The late N. W. Pirie commented that *"it would have been more surprising if it had proved impossible to make such 'biochemicals'"* Indeed, it is very likely that wherever in the universe there are appropriate conditions and raw materials, these types of biochemicals will be formed. So it is hardly surprising when NASA and others find the amino acids of life on a meteorite! These discoveries may get the media over-excited, but such discoveries are to be expected. *Not* finding them would be surprising. They may likely be found on Mars and get people unnecessarily very excited.

The possibility that the basic 'life chemicals' can arise spontaneously without life was tested experimentally by A. Oparin in Russia in 1949 and by S. L. Miller in the UK in 1953. A powerful electrical spark was repeatedly discharged through a sterile atmosphere of methane, ammonia, hydrogen and water vapour, and after running the apparatus for a week they were able to identify four simple amino acids in the water. Many other investigators have confirmed the results of this experiment and in addition have been able to observe a number of other organic compounds, including purines and pyrimidines – which are the building blocks of DNA. There would have been spectacular electrical storms after water had condensed on the surface of our planet.

In 1964, Professor Sydney Fox and Kaoru Harada of Los Angeles performed a similar experiment to Oparin's. Methane was mixed with a concentrated solution of ammonium hydroxide and put into a tube containing silica sand at about 1000°C. On analysing the residue they found 12 amino acids typical of those in proteins: alanine, aspartate, glutamate, glycine, isoleucine, leucine, phenylalanine, proline, serine, threonine, tyrosine, and valine. [3]

He was also able to show how mixtures of amino acids could, simply, be induced by heat to link together in long- chain molecules: a process known as co-polymerisation, the daisy-chaining of smaller molecules together in a line. The significance of Fox's observation is that it is by just such a process that amino acids joined to form proteins and eventually to form life.

These examples provide an insight into the question of chemical determinacy versus chance. Chemistry is actually based on the chance of collisions between atoms or molecules. However, the results of the collisions are not chance. The items either go their own way or they attract each other and form a new compound. That being the case then life cannot be based on chance. Chemistry is deterministic, and so life must be the same. Even if we do not understand some of its greater complexities, they will still be deterministic. 4.5 billion years ago at the beginning of the planet's formation, water started to condense on the planet and various comets would strike the earth with water as there was no protective atmosphere. It was bathed in ultraviolet light from the sun as there was no ozone layer. UV is a high energy form of sun-light and would have been a major factor alongside the electrical storms and volcanism which fuelled the chemical synthetic processes taking place in muddy pools and shallow waters, that led to self-replicating molecules and life.

There is a continuum from the creation of matter to the creation of the stars, the planet, and finally life. The formation of the chemicals of life were not random events. Like all other parts of that continuity, the origin of matter, stars, our planet and ourselves was governed by the laws of chemistry and physics: matter and chemicals from the simplest to the most complex in our living systems, simply responded logically to the different conditions of existence. That is why it is so important to get to grips with the present-day challenge of changing climate.

## INTRACELLULAR DETAIL AND THE ORIGIN OF ANIMALS

### The Cambrian Explosion

For the first 2.5 – 3.5 billion years of living systems on the planet, life was largely anaerobic converting sunlight into carbohydrates and proteins. Importantly for our story, there is no fossil evidence of intracellular detail in that period: blob like life. Although some aerobic life may have existed, it was minimal. Life was fuelled by photosynthesis which as in our plants of today, fixed $CO_2$ and excreted oxygen. The main products of photosynthesis were proteins, sugars and DNA. Change came when photosynthesis and the photolysis of water had excreted enough oxygen for air-breathing life to become thermodynamically possible. Astonishingly, when that happened about 600 million years ago, multi-cellular, air breathing systems evolved rapidly and all the 32 phyla we know today came into existence in a very short geological time span. In geological terms this was a sudden, almost instantaneous event. It is called the "Cambrian Explosion".

It is absolutely marvellous that at this time, intra- cellular detail appears in the fossil record. That detail was provided by cell membranes and cell membranes are built with phospholipids. Hence it is an undeniable fact that lipid biology came into the picture to provide for the compartmentalization within cells. This compart-mentalization is seen in every electron micrograph of a eukaryote cell as in Fig. 1.

## Lipids in the origin of multicellular life

Lipids formed bi-layers with water on either side creating specialised compartments inside the cells (e.g. nucleus and mitochondria).

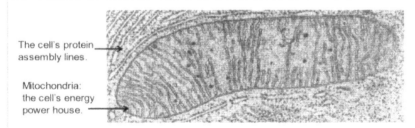

When oxygen became available in sufficient amount, complex molecules requiring high energy and oxygen were formed. Of these the polyunsatuated lipids played an important role forming the cell membranes which led to intracellular compartmentalisation .

The cell's protein assembly lines.

Mitochondria: the cell's energy power house.

Intracellular specialisation led to specialisation of the cell themselves. Lipid composition responds to temperature, pressure and chemistry. The intense, solar UV radiation, and varying conditions is a likely explanation of the speciation that led to the Cambrian Explosion of the phyla.

Lipids interacted with the proteins resulting in a range of special functions. We can see this today with different lipid and protein compositions in the eye, the neurons, the myelin, the heart, the liver and kidneys. The lipid membranes housed the transporters, ion channels, signaling and cell recognition systems. The absolutely new (but ancient) proposition is that it was the lipids rather than the proteins or DNA which was behind the intracellular specialisation, then cell specialisation leading to the cell cooperation which resulted in multicellular life.

You will not find this concept in any other book where the focus of attention will be on proteins and DNA. But for 2.5 - 3.5 billion years DNA and protein had their chance but did not do it. It had to wait for oxygen, its production of polyunsaturated molecules, the formation of lipids which naturally form micelles in water, leading to tiny life forms like the mitochondria in the picture above. As originally an independent life form it joined with the primitive cells in a symbiotic union making energy for the cell whilst the cell fed it with its needs. This explanation for an independent organism inside the cell with its own DNA was put forward by Lynn Margulis [4,5]. She received the National Science Award from U.S. President Bill Clinton in 1999.

The lipids, by forming membranes and playing host to certain proteins, made possible intracellular specialization. See the image of the powerhouse of the cell, mitochondria above. With the varying environments, temperatures, pressure and chemistry, the lipids would change in response to the different environments and chemistries. So different proteins would be favoured for incorporation, leading to different designs. And that leads logically to speciation and multi-cellular evolution into the phyla we have today.

For the first 2.5 billion years of life on the planet, DNA, RNA and protein had their day. We know lipids respond to temperature and pressure. We also know the fatty acid components influence the way the gene expresses its instructions and have a major role in epigenetics. The space filling electrical and liquidity characteristics of the membrane lipids enable a response to pressure from high mountains to the Mariana Trench 10,911 meters deep.

The Panathalassic Ocean of the late pre-Cambrian 600 million years ago had 85% more water than today and the land was barren because land plants had not evolved But there would have been fiords, shallows and very deep places with volcanism in land and in the ocean. The resulting diversity of conditions under the influence of strong solar UV radiation as the ozone layer as we have today had not been formed, could well have contributed to the development of the different phyla.

## EPIGENETICS

Dr David Barker of Southampton University, published evidence that poor maternal/fetal nutrition left life long marks, by generating risk of heart disease, stroke and diabetes in later life [9]. There is now extensive epidemiological support for his findings. The persistence of this effect of poor prenatal development can be explained by epigenetics whereby, environmental influences switch genes on and off resulting in an apparent genetic change without altering the genetic code. The unravelling of DNA as the genetic blueprint led to the Crick dogma that information flowed from the DNA but never backwards, a part of the scientific paradigm. Epigenetics falsifies this dogma. Dr, Bastiaan Heijmans and others, of the Department of Molecular Epidemiology, Medical Statistics, Gerontology and Geriatrics, Leiden University in Holland, studied the effect of the Dutch famine during WWII in the winter of 1944-45 [10]. They found DNA methylation to be altered 6 decades later in those born from mothers exposed to the famine. The females also had children born with a higher proportion of low-birth-weight infants than normal.

In 1900, the British Army had to lower its height of entry to 5 feet to get enough recruits for the Boer War (1899- 1902). Shortly after average height started to increase by 0.4 inch every decade. If you had a time-machine and stood the people of 1900 beside the people of today, you would be forgiven if you thought they were genetically different races. We changed in height, size, and health in a century and height is still increasing with people over 6 feet quite common. The late Simon House has an excellent U-Tube presentation on the topic 11. Whilst the effect is considered reversible, so far no one has considered the impact of long-term multigenerational persistence on the nature of a species. Perhaps epigenetics has been involved in the change in shape and size of the land animals which went into the sea and our now our marine mammals. In a marriage between a 6ft, 3inch male and a 6 ft 1 inch female today, we would not expect to see the children to grow up to be just 5 feet tall adults. People have been getting bigger but brains, smaller.

## A return from land to the sea

The history of the mammals following the collapse of the giant reptiles and the giant trees, is an example of long- term epigenetic influences. This evolutionary principle in the origin of mammals is discussed in our paper just published Crawford MA, and 11 others: (The imperative of arachidonic acid in early human development Prog Lipid Res. 2023 Feb 4:101222. doi: 10.1016/j.plipres.2023.101222. Epub ahead of print). Another but more visible example is the extraordinary business of land mammals returning to the sea! Shortly After the Cretaceous–Paleogene (K–Pg) mass extinction event of 66 million years ago at about 50 million years ago, certain land mammals started occupying the land-water interface before going back into the sea, species after species – Whales, dolphins and porpoises, manatees, seals, walrus, sea lions, sea otters and some might include polar bears. One after the other until about 7 million years ago. These species, which had once been land mammals, became marine mammals.

Why, one may ask, did animals take the trouble to colonise the land and then go back into the sea? No one seems to have answered that question. All groups exhibit aquatic adaptations directly related to feeding, particularly changes in the eyes, dentition and rostrum. Mark Uhen from Department of Paleobiology, National Museum of Natural History, Smithsonian Institution, Washington, DC wrote "The earliest representatives of each clade all show morphological features that indicate they were feeding while in the water, suggesting that feeding ecology is a key factor in the evolution of marine mammals"..[12]. What factor is different to land food?

It simply had to be the brain which drove them from land to sea. Umami! Nothing else would do it! We think is it was the marine nutrients which powered the evolution of the brain in the sea in the first place which would have influenced the brains of these migrating animals We know DHA encourages brain growth, is rich in sea foods and poorly available on land. There are also the trace elements on which the brain relies for protection against peroxidation. Dr Joe Hibbeln, a psychiatrist who recently retired from the NIH USA, considers EPA and DHA to be anti-depressant and a happiness factor [13]. Could the consumption of sea foods and fish have been a factor drawing the land animals deeper and deeper into the wonders of the marine food web and THE stunning beauty of marine life, to living in the sea full time? They certainly ended up with big brains, the adult dolphin brain weighs 1.7 Kg!. The sperm whale something like 8Kg. That is of course in a very large body. One wonders if the depletion of the soils by the dinosaurs, with the trace elements being washed into the sea, led to the enhancement of the oceans which is where you find the giant species of today?

The take home message here is that the brain evolved in the sea as everyone knows if they think about it. They would also know that to do so it would have had to use marine nutrients even if they knew nothing about DHA. No government has any recommendations which prioritize the nutrition of the brain in food policy. We are ignoring the dependence of our brain on sea foods at our peril.

The idea of the land mammals gradually changing shape to be better adapted to feeding in the marine habitat is intriguing. We know that diet can change shape, size and disease pattern so assumedly can work for both worse or better. Interestingly, unlike most evolutionary jumps, there is on this occasion fossil evidence of intermediates – the whale ancestors with one foot on the land, as it were, before full commitment to the sea. This went against the concept of punctuated evolution as put forward by palaeontologists Niles Eldredge and Stephen Jay Gould [14], who we have mentioned before. Given the evidence of the whale intermediates, Gould commented: "The embarrassment of past absence has been replaced by a bounty of new evidence - and by the sweetest series of transitional fossils an evolutionist could ever hope to find."

In 1992 a fossil had been excavated from sediments  of an ancient seabed in Pakistan by Dr. J. G. M. Thewissen, an anatomist and paleobiologist at North-eastern Ohio Universities College of Medicine in Rootstown, USA. It was about 10 feet long and named *Ambulocetus natans*, which means 'swimming walking-whale'.[15] It had short legs which were probably used for paddling more than walking, and a snout and mouth like a crocodile. Also found in Pakistan was a fossil named *Rodhocetus kasrani*. Two partial skeletons put together gave a reasonable idea of what the mammal looked like. It had short arms and legs and long fingers which were probably webbed. The evidence suggests these transitional mammals were feeding around the shorelines before their lineage became fully committed to life in the sea.

Modern dolphins have vestigial legs which shrank and disappear which means they once had legs as we know. This does not sound like a gene mutation but is more like epigenetics.

# Why did the leg bones shrink?

In the wild the dolphin eats fish, and fish do of course have small bones; but us much as 50 per cent of its diet can be made up of squid and similar species which have no bones. They use cartilage instead, and the squid flesh is rich in phosphorous.

The amount of calcium in squid and octopus is low. In the meat of salmon and cod there is 13.4 and 13.7 times more phosphorus than calcium and about the same ratio in whole squid. However, the fish also have bones, and seawater contains a significant amount of calcium (0.4g/100m1).

Muscle function and movement requires more phosphorus than calcium. In the beginning, animal biology was boneless and involved a high-phosphorus low-calcium ratio. Hence the low-calcium level in marine life would be a function of the biology at the start of the food chain and life. What is clear from present knowledge is that a high-phosphorus low-calcium ratio acts against the hormonal and metabolic mechanisms involved in bone growth. Is it just possible that weightlessness combined with a high-phosphorus low-calcium diet may have dictated an economy in bone formation in the transitional marine vertebrate species. Such an economy might explain the sacrifice of the dolphin's legs and its shrunken arms.

The effects of weightlessness have been demonstrated in space exploits. The Soviet cosmonauts, who hold the world record for living in outer space, had to be carried out of their ships in special chairs after prolonged exposure to weightlessness. Yuri Romanenko who in 1987 lived on the Mir space station for 326 days lost about 5 per cent of his bone calcium and had probably lost up to a third of his blood volume too.

The shrunken arms of the dolphin are even more interesting because inside the flipper there are all the bones of the human arm and hand.. The photo below was taken in the museum in Tromso, Northern Norway. The idea of gene mutations to produce hands as a paddle is bizarre. This is more like epigenetics (see chapter 6) whereby the environment changes the behaviour of the genes without altering the code. The genes for legs are present but supressed. The genes for arm bones and hands and fingers are still obviously there but their activity truncated to accommodate the poverty of bone building nutrients: as the bones shrank, the hands simply got covered in surplus skin. The day of the dolphins may be yet to come![18]

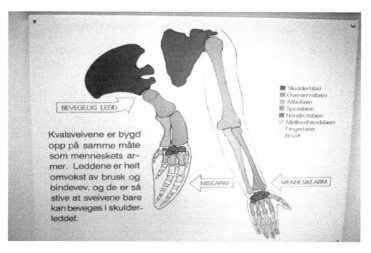

Image with thanks to the Museum of Tromsø, Norway.

## Michael and the El Molo – the near-aquatic human lifestyle

Michael writes about another piece of evidence regarding the nutritional involvement, and hence epigenetics was provided by a visit Michael made to the El Molo in Northwest Kenya. The El Molo are a tribe who relied almost entirely on fish from Lake

18    The dolphin embryo has vestigial legs. Once H. sapiens has gone, the coastal resources will flourish again. If some dolphins start to make use of it again and their legs re-appear, they would begin to make use of nearby land foods and with epigenetics at work its legs would extend and the skin from the flipper retract to reveal the bones of the hand. Once they learn to sleep on land instead of half the brain asleep at any one time, then the full power of the 1.7 Kg brain would be available. The planet then would have at last a hyper intelligent species hopefully to restore from our lost opportunity.

Turkana. Sir Vivian Fuchs first visited them in the 1930s, and he reported a curious fact: they all had bent legs.

In 1965 Michael decided to see if this was still true, and to establish whether the reason was a genetic abnormality. His late wife Sheilagh Crawford arranged a safari to the El Molo with Roy Brown, a paediatrician at Makerere Medical College, in Kampala, and Roy Shaffer, a flying doctor in Kenya. Roy Shaffer was familiar with similar people like the Samburu and Masai, and indeed had a Masai-speaking assistant. It was known that the El Molo language had a similar root to that of the Masai. We also took along with us Michael's Danish, biochemist colleague Inge Berg-Hansen and her sociologist husband. Sheilagh was the organiser, and supervisor of food and the two children Adam and Lyndsay, then aged 3 and 9.

Roy Brown roundly criticised the plan to take the children, saying that we were visiting dangerous territory. That was true. The Shifta would mount raids from Ethiopia, to kill and plunder. They liked to steal the women but take the men's testicles as trophies, turning their scrotums into purses. We felt reasonably confident, as we did have a comprehensive collection of firearms, although their role was to provide food en route rather than fend off bandits.

Sheilagh was not going without the children, so she put her foot down and told Roy, "Michael is paying for the safari and we are travelling in his Land Rovers, so the children are coming! They have done many safaris before; but we need you to assess the El Molo children, so I hope you will join us".

Swallowing his misgivings, Roy did indeed join us, and claimed the driver's seat in the long wheel-base Land Rover. He was a great companion and was a hit with the El Molo children and their mothers.

After three days of dust and dirt, we found ourselves in northern Kenya at the top of an escarpment of over 1,000 feet down to the Jade Sea, then called Lake Rudolf but renamed Lake Turkana in 1975. The view of the Jade Sea below was a sight never to be forgotten – stunning; it was called the Jade Sea for good reason. After two days of lava desert the sight of this great mass of sparkling, jade-coloured water stretching as far as the eye could see north and south was mesmerising. With not a habitation in sight, it was as though we had reached another planet. We all got out of the Land Rovers and just stood in silence for a long time.

However, the pitiful track we had followed seemed to end there as though whoever had made it only wanted to see the view! To contemplate the way down was a challenge to say the least. It was indeed the proverbial nightmare. The way was strewn with rocks. There was some semblance of a path, but it was difficult to know if it was real or imaginary. We had to make the road ourselves, shifting the larger rocks and gently easing the vehicles over the smaller ones.

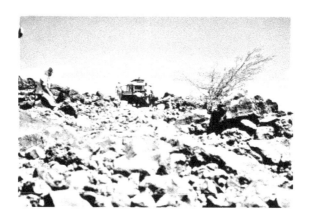

The road to the El Molo – climbing down the escarpment to Lake Turkana involved making the road. A rare bit of path can be seen.

When we reached the bottom of the escarpment, we were confronted with a lava beach at the lake shore. At one point there was a lava pile some 50 feet high, as though a mountain at Loiyangalani had funnelled its debris onto the beach to stop trespassers. The only way was up and over, which was a challenge for the Land Rovers. It was almost like trying to climb a sand dune, as the lava rubble just slipped under the tyres.

When we reached the top, we could at last see the El Molo huts in the distance. The plain between the escarpment and the lake became quite wide, so we were able to drive the Land Rovers side by side. The three were throwing up a lot of lava dust, creating a moving cloud which would have been visible from a considerable distance away. It might well have been an alarming sight for the El Molo. This suspicion was bolstered when we finally saw them. At the edge of the village stood a line of warriors, facing us, shoulder to shoulder and armed with spears and stamping on the ground.

Not encouraging. We stopped and began to discuss what we should do and how we could make friends!

While the adults were debating this pressing issue, our two children, obviously weary of being cooped up in a hot Land Rover, left the vehicle. Not registering the spears, which might as well have been walking sticks to them, they waved at the El Molo and half ran towards them. They had seen what we had not, four El Molo children. The four squeezed between the legs of the warriors and come forward to greet our two. They had never seen white people of the same size as them. It took very little time for all six children to be playing and talking together, blathering away in their own languages. It did not seem to matter that our children knew nothing of the El Molo language nor the El Molo children of English. In some strange way they seemed to understand each other. And so the ice was broken! We were welcomed and taken to the village.

Roy Shaffer's assistant was able to talk to them, as their language was close to the Masai tongue. When dusk fell, a fire was lit, and food cooked. The El Molo gave us fish they had caught and we gave them some of our food, which they eyed with great suspicion but none the less gave it a try. After the meal Roy Shaffer took out a tape recorder and put it on the top of his Land Rover. His assistant told the El Molo that we had brought a song from their cousins the Masai. There was at first great astonishment at the song coming out of the black box, but that vanished quickly, and they were soon jumping in the air and singing themselves. Quite a performance. Roy then got them to send a song back to the Masai. They danced and had us all dancing too under a bright, starlit sky.

We spent two weeks with the El Molo, carrying out health checks, giving aspirins, taking blood pressures and collecting blood. In relation to the issue of the locals' bent legs, it was soon noted that outsiders who joined the idyllic life by the lake produced children who started life with straight legs, but which bent when they learnt to walk. All the children were equally affected, so the reason for the weak leg bones was therefore unlikely to be genetic. Even the dogs seemed to have slightly bent hind legs. The photo below is of one of the oldest of the El Molo and is an extreme. None the less it makes the point. They all had sabre shaped shins to a greater or lesser extent.

As for the El Molo themselves, apart from their bendy legs they were truly healthy. Their blood pressures did not rise with age to any significant degree and their blood cholesterol levels were remarkably low, with little rise again with age. Moreover, their blood levels were lower in linoleic acid but richer in arachidonic acid and DHA in comparison with the Buganda and Europeans living in Kampala[16].

Claudio Galli, a professor at the Department of Pharmacology in Milan, Italy, carried out a similar study of people living in the fishing villages on the shore of Lake Nyasa. He compared their cholesterols and blood pressures and other heart disease risk factors with their more vegetarian compatriots living inland[17]. The results were essentially the same as the El Molo case study, only in greater detail for heart disease risk factors.[18]

El Molo Fish eaters: Bent tibia – photo from Dr Roy Shaffer

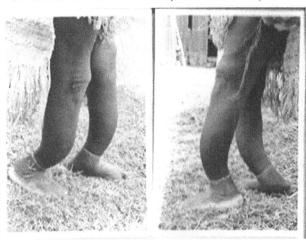

Our analysis showed that Lake Turkana had a very low-calcium content. The El Molo were restricted to a diet of lake fish and flora because of their otherwise barren surroundings; the lava desert which ran right down to the lake shore.

We had brought some grain and fresh game meat for them, which they enjoyed. Occasionally they would travel north to a place some distance away where there were hippos, and so they did occasionally have meat; but not often. They also ate fresh water plants but the lava desert stretched down to the lake so nothing of any merit grew on the land.

They invited us to join them on one of their fishing exploits. As fish were abundant in the lake, they had no difficulty in catching them. They used fishing nets made from the palms in a nearby little oasis where there was a freshwater spring and surrounding greenery. The net we used was several yards in diameter. We waded into the lake until the water was nearly up to our shoulders, each of us holding a part of the net perimeter. Then we let it sink.

The El Molo became excited and started singing to the Gods of the Lake. The singing reached a crescendo and at a sign from their leader we all pulled like mad, staggering backwards and raising the net to the surface. There were plenty of fish, and they were all big ones. The spaces in the net were quite large so they only caught large fish – very conservation-ecologically-minded, you might think; but the real reason was the scarcity of materials to build nets, making the gaps large.

By only catching large fish they were not eating edible bones from smaller ones. They would often suck a fish bone and crack their lips in so doing. The bones of smaller fish would have provided the El Molo with a valuable source of calcium, but by eating only the meat from the large fish, they had a diet that was low in calcium and high in phosphorus. Not unlike the would-be dolphins. All their weight-bearing leg bones were weak and bent as a result: the evidence incriminated their low calcium intake. To them, their sabre-shaped legs were natural.[19]

So here is more evidence of nutrition affecting shape and form in our own species. And there was another fascinating aspect to the story. The El Molo told us that they often had pain in their legs, but not when standing in water, assuredly because the buoyancy of water relieved the pressure on the legs. They spent quite a bit of time in the lake of course, with their fishing nets, or in their little boats made of palm logs, from which they would spear the plentiful fish or visit one of the islands. Perhaps the El Molo were on the way to becoming freshwater human dolphins.

Note: In this chapter, we have talked about the shrinking bone adaptation to a marine life by the mammals. It is important to note that this does not mean they had light bones. In fact, the remaining bones are actually heavier than otherwise expected. This is doubtless to aid deep diving. The sperm whale can dive to 2,000 meters in search of giant squid whilst Cuvier's beaked whale can dive to 3,000 meters and stay below the surface for up to two and a half hours. With the extraordinary pressures from the water column at these depths heavy, strong, and flexible bones would be an advantage.

At the same time, the shrinkage of the arms and loss of legs would doubtless have helped in calcium economy.
(Sulman J Rahmat, Madelyn G Crowell & Irina A Koretsky (2020) Correlation of Bone Density in Aquatic and Semiaquatic Animals to Ecological and Dietary Specializations. doi 10.31031/OARA.2020.02.000537).

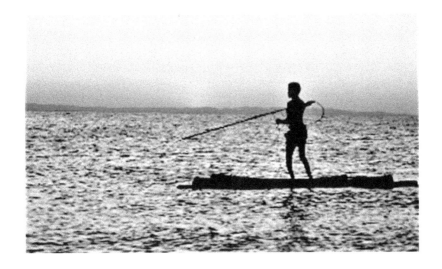

An El Molo spear-fishing. The photo was taken by David Coulson and sent to us by Patrick Holford. It illustrates the link with water, beauty and peace.

We have changed in height, shape, mental and physical health in one century. The question we are asking is where will this lead us? With the escalation of obesity, diabetes II and mental ill-health the answer does not look comfortable. Perhaps we will provide an answer.

# CHAPTER 6
# More on Epigenetics and the favoured predators

## THE EYES HAVE IT

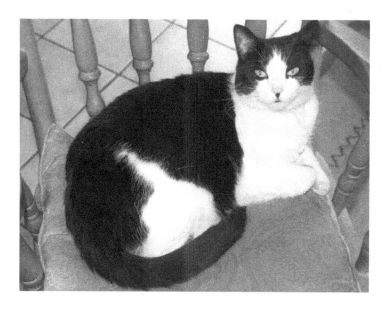

The basics of eye design, with a retina and iris, are common to all higher mammals, and indeed the cephalopods and fish. The squid eye is structurally like the human eye and may well date back to the ancient Orthoceras, which lived more than 450 million years ago. Today, the large carnivores contrast most dramatically with the corresponding herbivores. Cats' eyes are greatly advanced compared to those of a cow. When you examine other carnivores, you see the same situation. The eye of the squid has ten times the number of photoreceptors as the eye of a cow, and the eye of an owl or eagle eye has far more than the eye of a pheasant. Yet the contrast does not stop there. There is a huge difference between the total ability of an owl versus a pheasant, a leopard versus a goat.

This rigid separation of the species is not readily explained by chance, and such discrepancies were seen by Gordon Rattray Taylor as a cardinal failure of selection theory.[1] He criticised Neo-Darwinism with its "All sufficiency of Natural Selection". Indeed, he concluded, like Darwin, that there had to be another directive force in evolution; and both concluded it was the environment – Darwin's "Conditions of Existence" (see Chapters 2 and 3). Taylor was roundly criticised for this by Mark Ridley, a British Zoologist who studied at Cambridge with Richard Dawkins as an adviser.

Ridley pointed out that Taylor quotes from Darwin's *On The Origin of Species*: "*To suppose that the eye with all its inimitable contrivances ... could have been formed by Natural Selection seems, I freely confess absurd in the highest degree*". However, says Ridley, Taylor does not quote Darwin's next sentence: "*... the difficulty, of believing that a complexity could be formed by Natural Selection, though insuperable in our imagination, can hardly be considered real*". He concludes Taylor had no biological imagination.[2] The man had passed away by this time, so he was not in a position to reply.

As we discussed in Chapter 4, Gordon Rattray Taylor was not alone in siding with Darwin's "conditions of existence", as witnessed by Stephen Jay Gould and Niles Eldridge who brought "punctuated evolution" to our attention – long periods of nothing happening, and then sudden change.[3]

Watch television and your eyes will process 25 images a second. Look at the house across the road surrounded by trees and flowers. The image you see is in three dimensions and close to a 180 degree view. Good as it is, the latest 24 mega pixel Nikon is not a patch on this performance. If you are sitting in the passenger front seat of a motor car, the changing image you see is the consequence of billions of pixels or photons of light flooding your eyeballs at the speed of light. Yet even when the car is travelling fast, the moving image you see is being processed flawlessly. It is only when you board the TGV from Paris to Lyon running at 240k/hour that the image begins to blur, but even then the blur is only for near objects.

We take all that for granted, but it is truly awesome. And yet this is all done by photons, the tiniest of free-living particles known. Moreover, just one hits another tiny particle – an electron - in an outer orbit spinning around two carbon atoms in your photoreceptor, stunningly rich in DHA – to tell the brain you have seen something. These photons bombarding our eyes are so small that physicists cannot be sure if they are particles or waves. To get over this tricky problem of the very small, physicists have worked out that photons have a dual property, being both particle and wave.

## VISION – FROM THE POINT OF VIEW OF DARWIN'S 'CONDITIONS'

We have millions of photoreceptors in our eyes capturing these tiny weird photons to give us this wonderful thing we call vision, and moreover it is in colour. And if you think human visual capability is remarkable, consider the cat at night. As you step into the dark and crack your shin on the garden stool, the cat's eye has turned night into day and it is darting through the undergrowth in search of unsuspecting nourishment; in the meantime your own eyes are struggling to adapt to the dark.

At night the iris in the cat's eye opens wide to let every scrap of light impinge on its highly sensitive retina. Shine a torch at it and, at a speed almost faster than you can see, the iris clamps down to a narrow slit. It might be supposed that this rapid response is an immense advantage to the cat. Perhaps cats without this capability perished. On the other hand, it is highly unlikely that there were people, at night, shining electric torches at cats when they were evolving millions of years ago!

Although to our human mind such ability would seem to be an advantage, we must remember that darkness comes on gradually: sunlight is not switched on and off. Even a full solar eclipse takes its time! Hence it is difficult to see what advantage such a fast-response mechanism conferred. People discussing evolution see everything in terms of advantage or survival. Yet as we have described in this book, Darwin considered that *conditions* were the higher force. He was unable to frame those conditions in the light of modern physics and chemistry, but nonetheless his insight was mind-glowingly accurate.

It is difficult, for example, to see how the Nikon-like automatic-exposure setting of the cat's eye could have been created by selection bit by bit. Could it have been simply another example of Darwin's conditions of existence, or indeed conditions – i.e. nutrition – and selection acting together?

Vision requires vitamin A and DHA. Animals with poor night vision just happen to be the ones that do not eat foods containing either of these. Nor can they make them in any real quantity. Cats eat both. Owls eat both.

The animals with the most acute vision, such as cats and owls, have diets rich in DHA and vitamin A. It is possible that their diets provided them with the capacity for great eyesight, which so enabled them to exploit niches not available to other animals. The significance here is that it is once again the possibilities offered by *environment* that push evolution, rather than the more commonly accepted idea of a struggle for survival.

It is feasible to consider the development of a highly integrated mechanism, such as the cat's eye, in response to *a priori* encouragement of appropriate chemistry and physics responding to inputs: to Darwin's conditions of existence. Whatever the stimulus was, it does not seem that it was a chance putting together of a highly flexible iris under neurological control, a retina packed with photoreceptors and the capability of superb night vision together with an appropriate expansion of the visual cortex in the brain to cater for the input.

Had the process been a random accumulation of all these

separate things, we would expect to find highly flexible irises in near-blind species, but we don't; a plethora of photoreceptors and a rigid iris, but we don't; or light reflectors as in cats' eyes associated with a low number of photoreceptors, but we don't. We would find evidence that the visual processing region of the brain would be unaffected by deficiency of visual input, but we don't. We would find a retina highly populated with photoreceptors but with a tiny visual cortex, but we don't.

Colin Blakemore, a neuroscientist who became secretary of the British Medical Research Council, carried out experiments with newborn cats. He sutured one of the kittens' eyes so it remained closed. He then studied the animals' brains and found that the region corresponding to the sutured eye did not develop like the one corresponding to the eye that opened.[5] This experiment demonstrated that the input was important in development. Moreover, Blakemore considered visual input as essential to brain development.[6] If physical input is that important then chemical input must also be important. Physics and chemistry are inseparable twins.

The eye is one of the first protrusions associated with the developing brain. Once the ground-plan of the eye is established, it is not difficult to understand how consistent exposure to the necessary chemistry in the milieu intérieur of the mother could encourage that protrusion to develop epigenetically, whereas deficits would restrict it. Indeed, we know for a fact that deficits of the essential nutrients do indeed restrict neuro-development[7,8]. Consequently, provision must encourage development. We may not understand the full details of how cats developed night vision while cows are impoverished in this respect, but that does not alter the principle. Certainly Blakemore's studies demonstrate the effect of external stimulus. Putting stimulus and chemistry together, combined with epigenetics, provides us with an undeniable principle.

High efficiency brain control, as manifested in the articulated iris, developed in tandem with sophisticated development of the eye. The photoreceptor membrane is built with DHA, and DHA is essential for vision,[9] as well as for the brain and its development.[10] The evolution of multiple, super- sensitive photoreceptors, with nerves for a fast-response iris and a regional development of the brain to serve the lot and integrate its messages with motor and cognitive levels, all depends on chemistry, physics and input. It cannot be done without it. It does not look like a random process in the slightest. Blakemore showed that if you do not have the physical stimulation of a shower of photons you restrict development. The difference between the carnivores and herbivores shows the importance of the chemistry, as both types of animal are subject to the same shower of photons. The biochemical studies on adequacy and deficiency provide the confirmation. Brain development cannot reach its full potential without exposure to the required physical stimulus and chemical input. For example, the development of the part of the brain responsible for vision depends on the input of light (physics) and the presence of abundant DHA in the photoreceptor (chemistry/nutrition). Physical and chemical deficits restrict development of the eye and brain, just as they can restrict muscle or bone development.

Even human eyes are amazingly efficient at dealing with different degrees of light. If you look across a valley on  a clear night in the countryside, you can easily see a 60-watt light through an uncurtained window two miles away. Put your eye just two feet away from the same light and, though you would find it uncomfortable, you would be able to read the writing on the glass. It is a measure of the huge range to which our eyes can respond. The strength of light from the distant source is more than a billion times weaker than from the close one. Impressive; but the cat and the owl can do even better.

It is easy to imagine the advantage good night vision gives to a predator, and classical evolution theory has always supposed that this notion of advantage explains everything; and yet no one seems to ask why the animals preyed upon  by the cat family have not also developed good night vision. Surely it would have been a great advantage for an antelope to see a leopard in the evening shadows balancing on a tree branch waiting to pounce?

If evolution only proceeds through random mutations, why has this development not occurred randomly in a single herbivorous species? There must have been enough random events taking place. The bottom line is you cannot build a computer without chips, and, equally, you cannot build a photoreceptor without the molecules which make its biological 'chips'.

The importance of chemistry to the development of the eye and visual region of the brain can be illustrated by the owl and the pheasant. Both are bombarded with equal numbers of photons to stimulate eye and brain development, but no amount of photon stimulation will give the pheasant the eyesight of an owl, as it lacks the chemistry that gives the owl its extraordinary vision...

...Similarly, herbivores have never managed to evolve the acute vision of the carnivores that hunt them by night. This is simply due to a lack of vitamin A (retinal) and DHA in their diets. A buffalo converts only a part of the beta- carotene in its diet to the vitamin A essential for vision. The lion when it eats a buffalo liver (their first choice rather then the meat) gets the life time effort of its conversion to vitamin A at each meal!

This nutritional problem puts a limit on the potential of the buffalo's and other big herbivores.. If evolution proceeded merely through a struggle for existence, the prey would have evolved eyes to match the predator – but their development is restricted by nutrition.

## VITAMIN A - VISIONARY

A reminder of the importance of vitamin A to human vision came after the First World War, when Denmark exported all its butter in order to earn foreign exchange. For home consumption they made do with margarine. As a result there was a high incidence of night blindness, with even worse problems among Danish children. This t led to margarine being fortified with vitamin A, and that brought an end to the night blindness outbreak. At that time knowledge about vitamin A was fairly limited. We now know that this vitamin, is essential for the growth of nerves and photoreceptors in the eye. It is made by the conversion of beta-carotene (from plants such as in carrots and dark, green leafy vegetables like spinach, and some coloured fruits too) to the active retinal. Cats cannot do that. They have to get vitamin A by eating other animals which have already done the work of conversion.

Michael notes:

"One day, working on an African safari in south Karomoja in Uganda, I came across a recent lion kill – a cape buffalo. The stomach had been torn open and all the inside had gone – eaten. Lungs, heart, liver, spleen, intestines, stomach, kidneys – the lot eaten! Part of the rib cage had been eaten too, and a few chunks of the haunch had gone. But the bulk of the meat in the carcass remained untouched.

"The liver in these animals is large and is where the plant colour beta-carotene is converted  to vitamin A. Only a proportion is converted, as the process is inefficient. The liver is, an excellent source of vitamin A. It is also a good source of vitamin B12 and other B vitamins. The buffalo was of good size and still fresh – the absence of vultures or hyenas told us that. They were not long behind, though.

"It is interesting that the lions had  eaten the stomach contents, so they managed to get their helping of fruit and veg from that source as well. This was by no means the last lion kill seen where the bulk of the meat had largely been left for hyenas, dogs, jackals and the rest of the scroungers.

"The offal is the most nutrient-dense part  of the body, and in the olden days you would see it hanging from butchers' stalls in abundance. Now offal is confined to a few cheap items on the supermarket shelves. The nearest we get to eating offal is in haggis, which the Scots now seem intent on wrapping in plastic instead of the sheep's stomach lining. Some also seem keen on replacing their traditional fish and chips with deep fried Mars Bars, whose impact on health is another story for another time!"

## GENE DELEGATION

But here we encounter a curious paradox. Many animals can make their own vitamin A from beta-carotene in plants. Cats, which have such a strong need for the vitamin, cannot do that, which is just amazing. You would have thought they would be superheroes in the making of the vitamin so fundamental to their acute night vision! But no – they have to obtain it preformed and stored in the livers of their prey. What possible advantage can it be to cats that they are unable to produce a nutrient they need so badly?

Oddly enough there *is* an advantage, although strictly speaking it would be more proper to say an opportunity is created. Every function that an animal has to carry out demands an appropriate gene-driven mechanism and subsequent organisation within the animal. But there is a limit to the level of gene organisation that any particular animal can achieve, and also to what it can pass on through its genes. In a way this is like the limited disc space on a computer. If any function can be delegated to another organism to perform some new function or to perform an old one better, it frees up genetic disc space: the more complex the organism, the more DNA instructions it needs to carry all the information required for its construction and function. Mammals have 1400 times as much DNA in each of their cells as a simple bacterium, and despite the immense amount of information that can be encoded in it, there is still a limit to the use that can be made of it. For some reason, the total amount of DNA is the same for all cells in the same animal and, even more interestingly, from one mammal to another. There seems to be a fixed amount that is workable as a mammalian design.

Animals are limited by the capacity of their genes. Vast as the possibilities inherent in those genes may be, they still impose limitations, in the manner of disc space on a laptop. This explains why, for example, a cat does not use up "disc space" making its own vitamin A, "outsourcing" the requirement instead, and getting the vitamin second hand from its meaty diet. This is a common situation – humans, for example, can only get essential amino acids, vitamins and essential fats through diet. Our bodies can't manufacture them.

So it is with the cats, for if they had to synthesise their own vitamin A in large quantities from beta-carotene it would take up a significant amount of their 'disc space'. They may therefore be better off delegating the process to their prey: at one meal they can take in the whole supply of vitamin A that their victim has accumulated over many weeks or years, and do so at low cost to their own organisation.

But things may not be that cut and dry. For example, onions have vastly more DNA than humans, whose DNA is 40% similar to that of worms. To quote from The Harvard Gazette: "*Junk or not, scientists still don't know why some organisms get rid of it (DNA) faster than others. But at least we now know why having less DNA than an onion doesn't put us at a survival disadvantage.*"[11] (Note here the "survival" mind set – it is such a persuasive and convenient metaphor that it crops up all the time without due thought.)

Perhaps onions are simply better able to conserve junk DNA, which does indeed seem to be a large part of the story. Humans carry quite a lot of junk DNA too, for that matter. The bulk of the explanation, though, is epigenetics, steering the advance or retardation of specific attributes. Eventually the redundant DNA in cats associated with making vitamin A could be lost and replaced with more junk or something useful in the context of the animal's current lifestyle. Neither explanation is mutually exclusive.

Delegation of this kind is what seems to have allowed the whole hierarchy of animal life to be built up. Every species has certain compounds that it needs but cannot make for itself out of simpler compounds. Nutritional requirements were born the day tiny air-breathing organisms started eating phytoplankton. We now call these compounds vitamins or essential amino and fatty acids. We cannot, for instance, synthesise all the amino-acids that make up our protein; those that we cannot make – the *'ten essential amino-acids'* – we must acquire ready-made from the organisms we eat, as we must do with vitamins. It is the same with essential fats. You cannot reproduce without omega-6 and you cannot make a brain without omega-3.

The secret code for making these compounds is in the DNA of plants and bacteria. The more complex life systems evolved later than the simpler systems, and that basically is what evolution was about. The vegetable and bacterial systems had to be there, building up carbohydrates, amino-acids, lipids and vitamins, which included highly complex molecules like vitamin B12 that animals later came to use. The DNA of the new animal forms of life could be relieved of making stuff that was readily available in the food web, and could therefore deploy its powers of organisation in other ways. It is plausible that an availability of these interesting molecules in food made new developments in biology possible, not unlike the way in which oxygen made animal life possible and lipids made intracellular organisation and then specialisation possible.

Life has always made use of its nutritional environment.At the beginning of multicellular life on Earth, an organism which ingested essential nutrients did not have to evolve the genetic ability to make those nutrients itself. The "freed up" DNA could than organise itself in other directions, enabling evolution to progress hand in hand with the possibilities provided by environment.

The mechanism whereby the new came into being was almost certainly a mixture of mutation and epigenetics – more so than selection, which could not work anyway until there was a challenge. We side with Darwin and believe the epigenetic route was the dominant and most powerful force.

The reason for the pre-eminence of epigenetics is simply that it can operate on a whole population, not just individuals, and it occurs with lightning geological speed compared to a viable mutation.

During the Cambrian Explosion, as the various animal species 'forgot' how to make vitamin B12 and other nutrients, so they explored various ways of using the freed-up disc space. Yes, you could imagine a degree of randomness in this process, and this may explain peculiarities such as the duck-billed platypus. However, it quite clearly was not all random by any means. Although the lipids were absolute determinants of cellular organisation that came in with air-breathing systems, there is no genetic code for them.[50] And yet, surprisingly, they are deeply involved as activators of nuclear receptors and in epigenetics.

Epigenetics and mutation, rather than the "survival of the fittest", were the main drivers of evolution. But the leading role would have fallen to epigenetics, whose trigger – environment – impacts an entire community of creatures with great speed, enabling or ruling out gene-based mechanisms, compared to the slow progress of random genetic mutation.

## A STORY ABOUT VITAMINS AND WHY WE NEED THEM

Regardless of conditions, a world ruled by randomness would have continued to throw up new things. But it didn't! It is no coincidence that you almost always find that the same vitamins and essential amino acids are required, whatever animal is being studied. One species may require more or less of these than another, but the basic ground rules are the same. Although a cow is a vegetarian it requires B12, as do humans. The cow just has a different way of getting it in the bacteria producing fermentation in its rumen. Right at the beginning of animal life, the seeds of what was to become 'nutritional science' were sown: they took 600 million years to germinate in our text books!

The science of nutrition basically concerns this elaborate system by which advanced forms of life delegate the production of some of their biochemicals to less advanced forms. It is useful to look at some of the things this branch of science has discovered and why. In 1887 the Dutch government established a research laboratory in Java to study beriberi, a very serious disease common throughout the East, which brings on muscular weakness, nervous disorders and finally death. In the wake of the revolutionary discovery of bacteria by Pasteur it is not surprising that the disease was originally thought to be due to infection. However, a young army doctor named Christian Eijkman was placed in temporary charge of the research. When a new hospital manager decided that feeding the chickens on hospital scraps amounted to pilfering, Eijkman had to buy rice from the market for them. He then noticed that they developed a similar condition to beriberi. It was soon found that the chickens responded to different diets and that feeding them polished rice produced the disease, while feeding either unpolished rice or the polishings – i.e. the husk, bran and germ removed by the polishing process – affected a rapid cure. Later in 1905 Professor Pekelharing, who had originally been in charge of the Java laboratory, followed Eijkman's lead, gave up the search for a bacterial origin and published the results of conclusive experiments demonstrating that beriberi was related to a factor in the food: vitamin Bl.

At that time, it was believed that food consisted only of protein, fats and carbohydrates, and of these, protein was considered to be of the first importance (a premise encapsulated in the word, derived from the Greek *prows*, meaning first). It had been discovered that carnivores could live on a diet of protein without fat or carbohydrate, and there was a growing appreciation of the need for protein for growth. But in 1906, the year after Pekelharing published his results, an English biochemist named F. Gowland Hopkins (later Sir Frederick) also came to the conclusion that there was more to food than protein, fats and carbohydrates. He wrote:

"Scurvy and rickets are conditions so severe that they force themselves on our attention; but many other nutritive errors affect the health of individuals to a degree most important to themselves and some of them depend on unsuspected dietetic factors. I can do no more than hint at these matters, but I can assert that later developments of the science of dietetics will deal with factors highly complex and at present unknown."[12]

In 1912 Hopkins rose to fame by publishing the results of experiments showing that when rats failed to grow on a carefully purified diet, he could supplement their diet with a factor isolated from food, which restored growth. This led Hopkins immediately to the idea that specific constituents other than protein were needed for life. This was the beginning of an exciting period in the biological sciences, when chemistry gave birth to biochemistry and when the basic knowledge was provided for the present understanding of nutrition.

In the years since then, not only beriberi but scurvy, rickets, pernicious anaemia, vitamin A blindness and congenital iodine deficiency syndrome (formerly known as cretinism) have been largely eradicated except among some poor peoples. Interestingly however, vitamin D and iodine deficiency are now returning to the UK.

It is easy to forget how recent much of our present knowledge is, but within living memory the diseases listed above were widespread. In their 1969 book *The Englishman's Food*, Drummond and Wilbraham relate how an elderly American surgeon became convinced of the vital role of nutrition. As an eager medical student on the ward rounds  he had recognised the symptoms of pernicious anaemia in  the patient lying in bed in front of the class and, thinking to impress his teachers, he blurted this out. Far from being impressed, his tutor, with a dark expression on his face, took a firm grip on his arm and guided him out through the swing- doors. There he spoke in stern, deliberate terms: "You do not mention pernicious anaemia in front of a patient because the name is as good as a death warrant".

Only two years later, in 1926, G. R. Minot and W. P.Murphy, following a lead from experiments on dogs, discovered that feeding them raw liver effected a dramatic cure. The dread of pernicious anaemia vanished almost overnight by feeding liver to the suferers. It was not until 1948 that the active principle in the liver, vitamin B12, was isolated and crystallised. [13]

It is really astonishing to see how much was discovered and confirmed without the modern randomised clinical trial (RCT) alleged to be the pinnacle of proof. Often animal studies are claimed to be irrelevant and without an RCT you can forget it. This adulation of the RCT at the expense of animal evidence is unacceptable when so many lives have been saved and diseases relegated to the past simply on the basis of basic science and animal studies.

Man is not the only animal that has to obtain B12 from its food. Indeed, the need seems to be common to all mammals, and what were once thought to be exceptions have turned out to be further examples of higher animals delegating the task of production to lower organisms. The richest source of vitamin B12 is liver. It used to be believed that vegetarian animals did not need vitamin B12, but then it was observed that rabbits kept in a cage with a wide wire mesh for a floor, developed symptoms of B12 deficiency. The reason, it turned out, was that rabbits normally eat their own soft droppings sometimes known as night faeces (as opposed to the hard, darker variety). In the wild they leave these droppings at the mouth of the burrow and when they return after foraging they chew them. While the rabbits were away, bacteria have been busy producing B12 in the droppings.

Grazing animals also use bacteria to produce B vitamins for them. Cows keep a bacterial flora in their stomachs, where they produce B12 and many other nutrients. The fermentation that makes yoghurt and a number of other foods generates a significant amount of B vitamins. Because the need for B12 is common to all advanced animals, and because their successors have all inherited it, we can safely assume that mammals evolved with this need, or that B12 played an important role in stimulating advanced animal design. It is unlikely that the different species would have developed the need independently, just as it is unlikely that many different families of animals would have independently developed a need for the same essential amino-acids to build their proteins. The amino-acids essential for one species are also essential for all other mammalian species. It is all too much to be mere coincidence. So, in investigating the requirements for certain nutrients that we and other species have in common, the science of nutrition is also exploring fundamentals in the process of evolution. In human B12 deficiency, according to Wikipedia, "...nerve cell damage can result. If this happens, vitamin B12 deficiency may result in tingling or numbness to the fingers and toes, difficulty walking, mood changes, depression, memory loss, disorientation and, in severe cases, dementia. .... B12 deficiency can also cause symptoms of mania and psychosis, fatigue, memory impairment, irritability, depression, ataxia, and personality changes. In infants' symptoms include irritability, failure to thrive, apathy, anorexia, and developmental regression." In a word –irreparable brain damage.

One conclusion here is that during evolution and the increase in human brain size, we could never have been vegetarians or vegans. Lack of B12 would have put an end to the story. The vegan movement was founded by Donald Watson in the UK in 1944. Initially B12 deficiency was a serious problem for true vegans but this was sorted by supplements. During our evolution we would not have had access to supplements – unless we too had evolved the trick of eating our own bacterially-fortified faeces.

## AND SO WE COME TO THE BRAIN

At the Institute of Brain Chemistry and Human Nutrition, located at that time at the Zoology Society of London, we asked a very simple question. "Did different species that eat different foods use different essential fatty acids (EFAs) to build their tissues?" A study of 42 species of mammals from zebras to hyaenas, leopards and water buck in Africa to tiny viscachas from South America and dolphins showed that although different fatty acids were used for muscles and livers, all species used the identical profile of fatty acids in their brains. This held true despite wide differences in the fatty acids in food (dolphins versus cows, for example) or in other parts of their bodies.

The variable in the brain was not its fatty acids profile but its size. Indeed, the availability of the special long-chain fatty acids used in the brain was a determinant to the extent to which the brain was developed.

Were all species able to make the neural fatty acids from the nutritional starting point in plants? This is a question often asked today. Can we just eat vegetable-derived omega-3 and convert it to the long-chain stuff our brains need? In all small mammals like mice, rats and tree shrews, we found ample evidence of this conversion. However, in the large herbivores like cows, buffaloes and giraffes, which eat leaves and seeds, we could find plenty of the original linoleic and alpha-linolenic acids from plants in their tissues, but the conversion process to the neural fatty acids was not completed: it seemed to peter out. However, brain composition was the same.

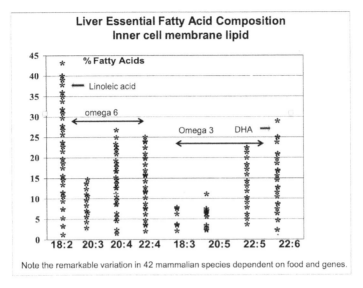

Note the remarkable variation in 42 mammalian species dependent on food and genes.

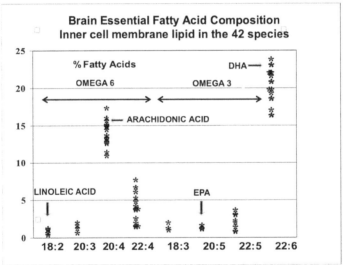

All mammal brains require the same long chain derivatives of the two 18 carbon EFAs. The defining factor is the environmental availability of those specific fatty acids the fatty acid composition of the brain does not differ from animal to animal – it is the size of the brain that differs. Without them, the upward possibilities of brain growth are limited. The large human brain must have evolved in an environment of abundant EFAs, while the small rhino brain (for example) reflects an EFA-poor environment. This illustrates a profound fact – the fatty acid composition of the brain does not differ from animal to animal – it is the size of the brain that differs The production of the most polyunsaturated fatty acid, docosahexaenoic acid (DHA, known by the shorthand 22:6 n-3 or even C22:6ω3 in physiological literature) was most affected. The tissues of the large herbivores accumulated only small amounts of these neural acids, whereas the animals which ate them had more.

This was interesting because carnivores have more sophisticated nervous systems and presumably a higher demand for neural fatty acids. In the cat, for example, the nervous system and control of function reaches to the extremities of the animal's articulated claws. This contrasts greatly with the hoofs of the corresponding herbivores. Other obvious attributes of a more advanced nervous system include high visual acuity, night vision, hearing, and acute sense of smell, in animals such as cats, dogs, hyenas, vultures, owls and eagles. The slow rate of making DHA from its parent essential fatty acids in green leaves, is largely overcome when the carnivores get a life times effort of the herbivore at one sitting! Although the carnivores have a more advanced brain, vision and peripheral nervous system compared to the herbivores, they do not compere with the huge brains of the marine mammals who get a rich supply of DHA from their marine food web.

## ESSENTIAL FATTY ACIDS DO NOT VARY IN THE BRAIN: SIZE VARIES!

Were carnivores perhaps better at making these neural fatty acids? Surprisingly, we found the opposite to be the case – just like the cats being unable to make vitamin A from the carotene plant precursor, as we discussed earlier. In 1975 John Rivers and Andrew Sinclair reported another peculiarity of cats: they did not convert plant EFAs into neural fatty acids.[15] Others have found that this same principle operates in carnivorous fish. The cat relies on eating the lifetime's accumulated efforts of its prey to get the necessary dosage.

Here is a mechanism to explain both the higher development of the nervous system in the carnivores compared with the herbivores, and the rigidity of the evolutionary lines.

The ready availability of preformed neural acids and vitamin A in the flesh the carnivores eat offers nutrients needed specifically to support more sophisticated brains, nervous and optical systems. They can afford the luxuries of widely adjustable irises in their eyes, along with the nerves and central control systems this demands. The herbivores cannot. Furthermore, the retinas themselves are directly affected. The retina appears very early during embryonic life as an extension of the developing brain. The photoreceptors, in rods and cones that receive and respond to the photons of light entering the eye, are, like the brain itself, built of structural lipids and proteins. A very high proportion of the structural lipid in the photoreceptor is DHA. Gene Anderson in Houston was he first to demonstrate a loss of electrical activity from a DHA deficiency in the retina. Dr W. E. Connor of Oregon found that monkey infants deprived of these omega-3 fatty acids lost visual acuity, which provides experimental evidence in favour of this mechanism. Evidence in Rhesus monkeys and preterm infant has described the same loss of visual acuity if the formula did not contain arachidonic and DHA. The evidence has really been in from the 1970s that DHA is an essential component for vision and the brain[16].

Let us now put the story another way. As with the increasing availability of oxygen leading to more efficient use of food resources, are we here seeing evidence of a greater availability and complexity of the building materials leading to a more advanced building? Are we seeing evidence of nutrients or substances in the form of vitamin A and DHA stimulating the development of the visual and nervous systems in the cats and owls but lack of them, restricting it in cows and rhinos? Is this evidence of substrate-driven evolution?

We suggest that what gives carnivores better eyes also gives them better brains, and it is consistently true over the whole range of species that carnivores are smarter than their prey. The spider has a more complex pattern of behaviour than the fly. The old male lion, standing upwind of a herd of gazelle and roaring and urinating at the same time, is showing a far more complex pattern of behaviour than the gazelles who break off grazing to run petrified in the opposite direction, straight into the claws of the lionesses waiting behind the bushes.

Think, too, of the vast difference between the buzzard and the pheasant. The cock pheasant looks very pretty, but all he can do is fly in such a straight line that he has evolved into a very successful target for a two-legged animal with a double-barrelled shotgun. The buzzard can control its flight so precisely that it can stand still in the air by sensing the forces of wind and gravity and fluttering its wings in response. Its visual acuity is such that it can see a mouse moving in the grass 50 or 100 feet below, and its judgement so rapid and precise that it can fold its wings, drop like a stone, calculate the exact moment to open its wings while falling at nearly 60 miles an hour, set the angle of the wings to the air to break the speed, extend its legs, open its claws, snatch the mouse and leap back upwards into the air without even touching the ground.

An owl has a night vision sensitivity ten to 100 times better than ours, and our night vision is not that bad. Moreover, the great grey owl can use its stereoscopic hearing to pinpoint a mouse under the snow without even seeing it. The barn owl does much the same. They detect the subtle high frequency sounds made by a nibbling rodent, sounds too high-pitched for any human ear but enough for the owl's sophisticated sensor and computer system to guide it blind through the air to the location in the snow or under leaves with deadly accuracy.

The palaeontological evidence tells us that throughout evolution the brains of the carnivores have been consistently in advance of the corresponding herbivores. For anyone who doubts that carnivores are more intelligent than herbivores, the argument can simply be based on anatomical differences. Comparing the anatomy of the leopard and the Uganda Kob immediately brings the contrast into stark relief. While the kob's hands and feet are in the shape of hoofs, the leopard has articulated claws. The business of using a soft foot for sensing and for controlling the claws demands a greater investment on the part of the brain and the nervous system than does the use of a hoof.

Random mutation and natural selection offer no clear and convincing explanation for a process that in terms of nutrition appears inevitable and identical in many species. Random selection does not explain why the carnivores and herbivores split into two streams; why these species, living in the same habitat, divide into two functionally and morphologically distinct groups; why herbivores have poor night vision and consistently less developed nervous systems. Most significantly, random selection does not explain why herbivores and carnivores are stuck in their grooves. Nutrition or substrate-driven change does.

This nutritional evidence answers a problem posed by Gordon Rattray Taylor (who we mentioned earlier), of the departure from randomness created by the rigidity of the evolutionary lines. *It can be explained simply as dependence on developments from the food chain. The carnivores and herbivores are held in the grooves by nutritional differences.*

## THE MORE THAN FISH OILS

Although the omega-3 DHA dominates the composition of the cell membranes in the retina, neurons and synapses it has been tested positively, for its effect on brain development, it is not alone. It needs to be remembered that fish and seafood also contain iodine, selenium, zinc, copper and manganese and some powerful antioxidants. Iodine is essential for the brain, something we have known for more than a century. Zinc is involved in the enzymes involved in the utilisation of EFAs and indeed is at the heart of DNA function. Zinc, copper, manganese and selenium all participate in nature's defence against peroxidative damage, to which DHA is especially susceptible and is concentrated in the most highly active and oxygen using regions of the brain, These do all the signalling work which enables us to see hear, touch, feel, think, act and dream. You get all of this when you eat a fish or sea food meal. A supplement of fish oils or even pure DHA is not the same. You may get some results with such supplements, and they can be important as the contemporary diet has become impoverished of the DHA that would have powered the evolution of our brain.. It helps if the rest of the contemporary diet has good amounts of B vitamins and trace elements.

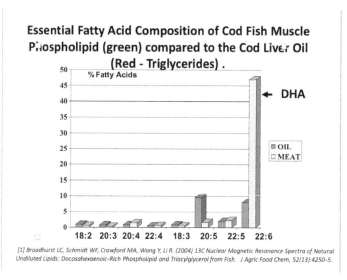

Essential Fatty Acid Composition of Cod Fish Muscle Phospholipid (green) compared to the Cod Liver Oil (Red - Triglycerides) .

[1] Broadhurst LC, Schmidt WF, Crawford MA, Wang Y, Li R. (2004) 13C Nuclear Magnetic Resonance Spectra of Natural Undiluted Lipids: Docosahexaenoic-Rich Phospholipid and Triacylglycerol from Fish. J Agric Food Chem, 52(13):4250-5.

Nutrients act in the body together, not in isolation. Any Randomly Controlled Trial (RCT) that isolates a vitamin, mineral or fatty acid to test its effects singly, is missing that fundamental point, and this can often render the results of such a trial not just useless, but a batch of misinformation. For example, we don't eat oil, we eat the fish that contains it, and in the process we also take in other essentials such as iodine, selenium and zinc and the meat contains the phospholipids. This is why RCTs on a single ingredient are not very useful for investigating nutritional issues.

Moreover, the oil is body fat whereas the tissues of the body and the brain exclusively use phosphoglycerides not the triglycerides of the oil, to build and maintain their cellular structures. So while supplements have an important use, eating fish and sea foods does two things. First it provides the phospholipids, anti oxidants and trace elements in a wholistic package. Secondly, they replace junk foods which can interfere with the supplements. ,

## A FAILURE TO ACCEPT EVIDENCE FROM BASIC SCIENCE.

In 1976, a joint International Expert Consultation of the Food and Agriculture Organization of the United Nations (FAO) and the World Health Organization (WHO) were called to review the literature on 'the role of dietary fats and oils in human nutrition'. It set out knowledge available at the time on the requirements for EFAs and in particular the long- chain omega-6 and omega-3 for cell membrane growth and function, together with their implications for pregnancy, foetal and early postnatal development of the infant, the brain and cardiovascular system.

To provide an image of what nature and evolution determined, the committee reviewed studies on the composition of human milk from five countries and five centres in the UK. A hundred studies since then bear out the major features of those early studies: that arachidonic acid (ArA) and docosahexaenoic acid (DHA) are prominent components of human breast milk. The section dealing with infant development concluded by laying down the sensible biological marker stating '...the ideal recommendation for milk substitutes (infant formula) would be to match the essential fatty acids of human milk from well-nourished mothers with respect to both parent and long-chain essential fatty acids' (FAO, 1978: 30).

The report further commented on the importance of dietary EFAs during foetal and infant growth, when there is a high 'demand for the synthesis of cell structural lipid'. This included the acceptance of the evidence that Michael Crawford and Andrew Sinclair published in 1972, namely that both long-chain omega-6 and DHA were essential to brain development, evolution and function.[17] That these were in abundance consistently in similar proportions in the milks of women from several different countries was consistent with that evidence and set the composition of human milk as the "gold standard" for anyone wishing to manufacture substitutes.

In addition, the report referred to the robust evidence that "... studies indicate that each type of dietary fatty acid influences the utilisation of the others" (FAO, 1978: 22 iv). At that time the significance of ARA and DHA was already established. This was especially true of the significance of DHA for the brain and visual structural lipid with deficiency experiments showing adverse outcomes of electrical function of the visual systems and learning and behavioural deficits due to impacts on vision and the central nervous system

Graham Rose (1972) reviewed "What We Eat Today" by Michael and Sheilagh in the Sunday Times, 05/11/1972, wrote that unless attention was paid to the relevance of the brain in the food system then we would become "a race of morons" – colourful language but nonetheless visible evidence that the message from science had penetrated the public domain.

Then in 1982 came the Nobel Prize for Sune Bergstrom, Bengt Samuelsson and John Vane for the discovery of the oxidative derivatives of ARA which controlled blood flow, reproduction and immune function, vascular relaxation, the prevention of platelet adhesion and indeed the opposite of responding to injury by sealing a wound, precipitating inflammation for the recruitment of white cells. Yet another derivative reported by Samuelsson acted as an agent resolving the damage, now a hot topic at the hands of Charlie Sherhan and others. 18

The discovery of these hormone-like substances completed a circle. Protein was considered essential for building cells, especially muscle. The amino acids of protein individually are used to make hormones to control functions  throughout the body. WOULD BE BETTER TO USE INSULIN = Better known than Melatonin, (examples being serotonin, thyroxine and insulin). Strings of amino acids are used to make others like insulin, growth hormone and several more, some involved in reproduction.

Fatty acids are used to build cell membranes which are at the heart of intracellular specialisation, as we discussed previously. The fatty acids are especially important in building the brain and nervous system. With the 1982 Nobel Prize we now had complimentary knowledge to protein chemistry and its hormones. Bergstrom, Samuelsson and Vane had described hormone-like substances derived from fatty acids, principally from arachidonic acid – called the eicosanoids.

There is however a fundamental difference from the protein hormones. These are made in a specific location – insulin being made in the pancreas, for example. However, their impact is at a distance – body-wide – virtually everywhere.

The eicosanoids are not like that. They are made at a site, and act at that site with surgical precision. Cut yourself and one eicosanoid clots the blood to stop you bleeding to death. Another causes inflammation which recruits white cells and an immune reaction to kill any foreign invaders through the wound and digest damaged and dead cells. This is then followed by the resolvins which tell the immune cells to clear up the mess. Their activity is very short-lived, which means they act at the site of injury but not elsewhere. This surgical precision is critical, because otherwise all your blood would seize up after even a small cut or bruise. The biological circle is closed.

It is a truly wonderful piece of organisation. So far, so good.

## THE COMPOSITION OF WHAT IS NEEDED TO MAKE A BRAIN AND ITS PROVISION BY HUMAN BREAST MILK IS IGNORED BY THE EFSA: UNBELEIVABLE BUT TRUE

But now we jump ahead to 2014, when the European Food Safety Authority (EFSA) published a report making recommendations for the composition of artificial milks for infant feeding. They concluded that arachidonic acid was not required for human milk substitutes. That is, the EFSA is saying that new-born infants do not need arachidonic acid, thus discarding human milk as the FAO/WHO gold standard. To make matters worse they conceded that DHA was still needed. The studies in the 1970s, remember, had made it clear that both ARA and DHA were building materials for the brain and essential for its function and were both universally present in human milk across the planet.

Astonishingly, the EFSA report declared that the authors only reviewed the literature from 2000 onwards. Hence, they ignored the Nobel Prize and its significance to arachidonic acid! They also ignored the original FAO/WHO 1978 recommendations and indeed the 1994 follow up which put numbers on the amounts recommended for infant formula (IF). Even more remarkably they ignored the 2008-2010 FAO/ WHO Expert Consultancy on Fats and Fatty Acids, which comes to a quite different conclusion to the EFSA, saying: "There can be little doubt about the essentiality of DHA and ARA (arachidonic acid) for the brain". The FAO/WHO reports went through a rigorous prior review of background papers, face to face presentation and discussion with the final conclusions being further reviewed before publication. In the last report there were 24 authors and 38 external peer reviewers.

We understand that for the EFSA report, just *one person* was charged to write the review! This is scientifically unacceptable.

**Human milk: a consistent source of arachidonic and docosahexaenoic acids**

It is accepted that the composition of human milk is the gold standard for healthy infants. Since the 1978 FAO/WHO report there have been various reviews covering several thousand milk samples from across the planet (e.g. Brenna et al., 2007; Drury and Crawford, 1990; Koletzko et al., 1992). There is a robust finding of a consistency of ARA and that includes its 20 and 22 carbon chain length family members. DHA is more variable but nonetheless constantly present so that the balance of long- chain omega-6 to long-chain omega-3 (which in the latter case is largely DHA) is in the region of 1 to 1 and 2 to 1. Dual labelled isotope studies by Andrew Sinclair in the 1970s, demonstrated that the biosynthetic capability for provision of long-chain polyunsaturated fatty acid (LCPUFA) for brain growth is low with the preformed LCPUFA being preferentially incorporated into the brain with an order of magnitude of greater efficacy than from synthesis. This was in rat pups and rats are far better convertors than humans.

Although it is not possible to do the same type of experiment on human brains there is convincing evidence that the same principle applies to both preformed ARA and DHA in human milk (Del Prado et al., 2001). Some maintain (without good cause) that before birth the foetus has the capability of synthesising sufficient ARA and DHA. It has been shown conclusively in preterm infants that the method of feeding resulted in a threefold rise in blood plasma of phospholipid linoleic acid (the plant precursor for ARA) and a threefold drop if not more of ARA itself in the plasma of the infants fed only linoleic acid. If the precursor climbs and the product falls, any biosynthetic capability is largely academic in relation to meeting demand. However, all of this was first published in the 1970s and in the FAO/WHO joint consultations was ignored by the 2014 EFSA reviewer.

## Arachidonic and docosahexaenoic acids have discreetly different functions

As readers of this book will know by now, DHA dominates signalling membranes in the photoreceptor, brain and nervous system. By contrast arachidonic acid is the principle unsaturated fatty acid in the inner cell membrane lipid of heart muscle, vascular endothelium (the cells lining the inner surface of blood vessels), T-lymphocytes (in the immune system), adrenal glands, kidneys, liver, placenta, and almost all other organs with the exception of the brain, testes and adipose fats. The cell membrane is the basis of organisation of the cell and its internal specialist structures,

The fatty acid and lipid composition of these membranes is species-, organ- and sub-cellular- specific, and even intimately specific in protein contact domains to meet the physico-chemical and thermodynamic requirements for optimum protein function. Change membrane composition in these regions and you alter function. In the brain, much of the ARA is in the glial cells which serve quite a different role to that of DHA. This specificity of lipid composition and the known biochemistry completely falsifies the EFSA analysis.

The lipid (i.e. fatty acid) content of cell membranes differs, depending on the organ and species in question. But the difference is not fixed, and is affected by environment – namely food, temperature and pressure. Changes in diet alter the lipid composition, which in turn alters protein function.

Here comes the rub. The EFSA claim is based on our old friend the Randomised Controlled Trials. These were done on IF containing both arachidonic and docosahexaenoic acids. The tests used for outcomes were based on the effects of DHA on, say, vision or learning, but no tests for the known functions of ARA were carried out. It may sound great to the press to hear that there were no effects observed for arachidonic acid from the RCTs; however, the press use what they are told and they were not told that none of the RCTs carried tests relevant specifically to ARA. This performance by the EFSA is simply unbelievable bearing in mind that in other matters they have functioned well.

This is the EFSA comment:

*... even though studies have shown that feeding an IF containing DHA alone (without addition of ARA) leads to lower concentrations of ARA in erythrocytes compared with the consumption of control formula without DHA, no direct functional consequences have been observed in relation to growth and neurodevelopment and this lower concentration of ARA in erythrocytes seems not to be associated with a decrease in concentrations of ARA in the brain. The adverse effects on growth which had been reported in one RCT in preterm infants have not been replicated in several more recent trials. Therefore, the Panel considers that there is no necessity to add ARA to IF even in the presence of DHA.*

Of course, no direct functional consequences of arachidonic acid were observed *because the designs did not test arachidonic function.* They were principally concerned with DHA function in the retina and brain. Studies consistently report up to 40% reductions in blood ARA levels in response to formulae providing DHA without ARA.[19] They concluded there was no decrease in concentrations in the brain when, quite clearly, they did not take biopsies of infant brains to find out the truth. It would have taken a Hannibal Lector to do a study like that! Funnily enough, Forester Cockburn, a paediatric professor in Glasgow *did* study the brains of cot death infants. He and his colleagues published a paper in the Lancet in 1992 showing there was a difference in the brains of infants fed with breast milk compared to those fed on IF, which at that time did not contain any DHA or ARA. Unsurprisingly the breast-fed babies had higher levels of DHA.[20]

Eileen Birch and co-workers from the Retina Foundation in Dallas, USA, have reported visual[21] and cognitive[22] outcomes of infants supplemented with DHA alone or in combination with ARA for 12 months at 4 years of age. While visual outcomes were found to be similar between groups at this age, the group with DHA but no ARA had significantly poorer verbal IQ scores compared with breast-fed infants. However, the infants supplemented with both ARA and DHA were statistically the same as the breast-fed infants.[23] This data suggests that depressed arachidonic acid in response to supplementation with DHA without ARA may well have had a functional consequence, even in brain function.

## Predictable infant health risk from the EFSA recommendation

The principle problem in the EFSA's analysis comes from a fundamental ignorance of the subject: specifically of the difference between DHA and ARA. By not reviewing the literature before 2000, *they omitted reference to the 1982 Nobel Prize* (see above) and of course all the earlier evidence referred to in the FAO/WHO 1978 and 1994 report.

When a child is born, the area of vascular endothelium which lines the blood vessels might be likened to the area of a football pitch. That area will grow rapidly as the child advances into young adulthood when it has an area of six football pitches. That is, there is a prodigious velocity of endothelial development to line the blood vessels in the newborn. For 99.9% of the time, arachidonic acid will be converted to a hormone-like substance – an eicosanoid called prostacyclin. (It was for the discovery of prostacyclin and its action of suppressing blood clotting activity and ensuring good blood flow that John Vane was included in the 1982 Nobel Prize.) Its activity prevents rogue cell-adhesion to the endothelium with blood clotting, ensures vascular relaxation and good blood flow vital for organ development and health.

If you suppress arachidonic acid and prostacyclin, vascular problems follow which can kill.

## A sobering story of drugs

The 1985 Congress on Essential Fatty Acids and Eicosanoids was held at the Zoological Society of London, where this book's joint author Professor Michael Crawford was working at the Nuffield Institute of Comparative Medicine. He, Ralph Holman from Minnesota, and Jim Willis from Hoffman la Roche organised the conference to celebrate the 1982 Nobel Prize. The proceedings were published in *Progress in Lipid Research* volume 25, 1986.

A dinner was held by the chief representatives of the pharmaceutical industry hosted by John Pike of Upjohn. During the dinner, the discussion turned to the novel idea of developing a drug to stop the conversion of arachidonic acid to its eicosanoids to treat inflammation, especially for rheumatoid arthritis, and to prevent thrombosis. Hugh Sinclair, Jim Willis and Michael Crawford all said *do not do this. You will stop the synthesis of prostacyclin. Prostacyclin stops the blood from clotting, and that could lead to death.* That cry was based on the existing animal experimental data. Well, the pharmaceutical people said they would of course conduct an RCT before selling.

The RCTs were done and great excitement followed as pain in rheumatoid arthritis was dampened dramatically. Sales of the COX2 inhibitors (e.g. celecoxib or rofecoxib, made by Merck) boomed. But after a while it became apparent that cardiovascular and stroke events were higher in those using this drug. An article in the *New Scientist* reviewed the situation and claimed that up to 140,000 people may have had increased cardiovascular and stroke events as a result of using a COX2 inhibitor. The US Food and Drug Administration (FDA) stepped in and Merck voluntarily withdrew its drug. Pfizer withdrew Bextra from the US market on recommendation by the FDA. According to Wikipedia in 2010, the national US case against Vioxx and Merck was resolved with a $4.85 billion settlement. There were quibbles about the legal fees, but this experience underlines the importance of listening to the animal studies and the basic science derived from them.

We are not recounting this story to knock pharma companies. They make life-saving drugs and are an important element of health care. The point to be made here is that the RCT is not all it is pumped up to be. For the drug industry it is of course an essential tool; but when it comes to nutrition and health it is of marginal value, at best.

Systematic reviews are often carried out by people with statistical competence but little knowledge of nutritional science or biology. For example, breast milk contains good amounts of DHA and arachidonic acid for the growing brain. A systematic review of the impact on feeding infant formula with and without DHA concluded there was no effect on IQ. The trial outcomes were heavily influenced by one very large trial carried out by an American infant formula company. In it they quoted that the DHA range varied in human milk from 0.1% to 0.9% (it actually goes higher). They chose a dose of 0.13%, just nudging the absolute lowest level (which came from disadvantaged, low socio-economic status mothers). Any sensible person would have chosen the middle of the range, i.e. 0.45%. But no, they chose the lowest possible – wonder why?

Trials done at the higher level of 0.35% produced measurable increases in visual acuity and mental test scores. The systematic review did not consider a dose response, nor indeed the form of DHA added to the formula. The net result was that the FDA did nothing, and the media duly reported that DHA or omega-3 did nothing too! We now have a serious problem. A 2015 commentary by L. Lauritzen et al on dietary arachidonic acid in perinatal nutrition concluded that "the question on whether preformed ARA in infant formulae is of any importance (good or bad) is still unanswered..."[24] The authors of this paper were members of the Working Group on Dietetic Products that contributed to the EFSA Scientific Opinion. It is difficult to reconcile the key message in the Lauritzen commentary that it is not possible to give an evidenced-based opinion on the need for preformed ARA in infant formulae, with the apparent equivocal EFSA opinion that there is no necessity to set a minimum requirement for ARA in IF. The precautionary principle at the least should insist on the inclusion of ARA. However, we simply submit that the science base, the universal presence of arachidonic and DHA in human milk across the planet, their presence in dominant amounts in the structures of the brain and essential for brain growth (which was not discussed by either Lauritzen or the EFSA), is too strong to consider the question unanswered.

The EFSA admits that providing DHA in the absence of ARA will diminish the circulating arachidonic acid. *DHA is in effect like a COX2 inhibitor.* Infant formula without ARA but with DHA could plausibly lead to infant cardiovascular events, stroke or even death. The EFSA, by rejecting the need for ARA and accepting DHA, goes against what human evolution designed and what the three FAO–WHO Expert Consultations took for granted – namely, that the composition of breast milk from well-nourished mothers was the gold standard.

Human physiology, and indeed evolution, has firmly pronounced its choice of a significant presence of ARA and its partners at similar molecular concentrations to DHA. There is now abundant science to explain the reason. And yet the EFSA opinion became enshrined in European legislation. Their departure from the decisions taken by human physiology could come at the cost of lifelong disability, if not lives, and its recommendation on arachidonic acid should be rejected. This is an example of the wilfully selective use of science. The mother feeds the foetal brain selectively in a special way.

We can take this line of argument a step further by looking at the way all mammals first come into the world, carnivores and herbivores alike, and so gain a greater insight into our own species. In reproduction, the brain is the first organ to develop after the heart, which provides the flow of blood for its growth. Seventy per cent of the total maximum number of brain cells that any individual has was built inside the mother during foetal life. Inside the womb the foetus 'eats' the food that the mother supplies; this food has previously been processed by the mother's own digestive system, including her liver. Just as a carnivore eats the end-products of another animal's efforts, so a foetus is nourished entirely by the end-products of its mother's work.

There is more to it: between mother and offspring there is a placenta. In our research we studied the concentration of nutrients on the maternal and foetal sides of the human placenta and discovered that it was selecting specific fatty acids used in the brain from the mother's blood: arachidonic and DHA, and passing them on at higher concentration to the foetus. We can see a foetus – even of a vegetarian animal – as a kind of super-carnivore. The process of bio-magnification applies to other nutrients as well, but in the case of the essential fatty acids, it specifically selects arachidonic and DHA, the neural, and not the parent plant varieties.

From this evidence one would predict that, as most of the brain's development takes place in the womb, long gestations should favour brain development.

The placental mechanism for concentrating the nutrients used specifically in the developing brain offers an explanation as to why egg-laying species have tiny brains. Instead of a steady flow of blood from the placenta continuing over the weeks or months of pregnancy, the growing creature inside the egg is presented with a once-for-all package. Then, once it is clear of the egg, it must take its food from the surrounding environment without having it first concentrated inside its mother's body, concentrated a second time by the placenta and then again through its mother's milk. One of the keys to the relatively large brains of placental mammals lies in the fact that the foetus receives constant nutrition from its mother over a long period, rather than via nutrients deposited in an egg yolk. For brain growth, the placenta selects specific fatty acids from the mother's blood, and concentrates them through a process of biomagnification. This concentrated good stuff remains available after birth through the mother's milk.

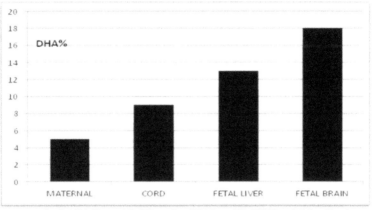

**Biomagnification of DHA**

Mid-term elective abortion data

Crawford, M.A., Hassam, A.G., Williams, G. and Whitehouse, W.L. (1976) Essential fatty acids and fetal brain growth. LANCET (i): 452-453.

Note that by contrast all DHA precursors including EPA are returned to the mother[19].

We would maintain that it is this inferior system of nourishing their developing progeny that condemns the egg-laying species to perpetual inferiority of brain power. No fish, bird, snake or other reptile has ever evolved a large brain. However big a bird's egg (and they are, of course, enormous compared to those of fish), none has ever cracked open to reveal a big-brained chick. The ostrich can weigh as much as a fully grown human: its brain is the size of an infant's fist.

Marsupials occupy a place between the egg-laying species and the placental mammals. The kangaroo has a very short gestation period of just two weeks or so before the baby moves into the pouch. They end up with bigger brains than

19    Crawford MA et al 2023, doi: 10.1016/j.plipres.2023.101222. Epub ahead of print. PMID: 36746351.

egg-laying species, but smaller than placental mammals with longer periods inside the mother. When the mammals reached South America, they ousted the marsupials (with the exception of the possum), so that Australia became the last haven of the pouched mammals.

The gestational period of the cow is the same length as that of the human. A newborn calf, however, weighs as much as a teenager. At two years old a calf can weigh 200kg, but with only 350g of brain; a human infant at the same age weighs about 15kg, with a 1 to 1.2kg brain – three times the size of the calf's, and, in proportion to total body size, around 60 times as big. The body growth of the fetal and new born calf is too rapid and outstrips brain growth.

## Maternal malnutrition restricts brain development permanently

The comparative data would be weak without some experimental evidence demonstrating nutritional effects on brain size and function. Experiment does more: it shows just how critical the period of brain growth is. Professor John Dobbing and Dr Elsie Widdowson reallocated newborn rat pups so that some mothers had 14 and others only four to feed with their own milk. The result was that the pups in the larger litters became microcephalic (they had small brains), whereas those in the small litters had much larger brains[25]. No matter what they did afterwards, the difference in the brains *remained fixed*, showing that the rat's brain develops mainly during the period the pups are suckled.

Dobbing concluded that there is a 'vulnerable' or 'critical' period of brain development during its early growth. Any deficits or distortions that occur during this period cannot be corrected once it is over, a principle demonstrated in humans who are born blind or educationally subnormal due to some distortion in development: the defect cannot be put right later.

The developmental period is critical. It is during this period that brain growth can either be stimulated or stunted, and the effect is permanent in the lifetime of the individual.

Nature can only grow a brain once. If that first attempt meets with problems, the owner of the brain will suffer. This window of opportunity for optimal brain development occurs during gestation and throughout weaning, with the pre- conception health of the parents having an important impact too.

Several laboratories have now shown in experimental animals that specific alterations of dietary essential fatty acid intakes can influence brain development, synaptic function and, as we have seen, visual acuity. In 1973 Dr Andrew Sinclair, working at the Institute of Zoology, tried feeding female rats on a diet with a low concentration of EFAs. Without any they failed to reproduce at all, so he gave them enough to allow reproduction but not enough for safety. The experiment was continued over three generations and resulted in low brain cell counts in the third-generation pups.

In Milan Dr Claudio Galli similarly showed that if lactating rats were fed on a diet deficient in essential fatty acids, their pups got deficient milk and suffered permanent learning defects which could not be reversed by giving them a correct diet after weaning [26]. Like Dobbing's experiments, the EFA under- nutrition during brain development led to permanent deficits.

Fats have another special characteristic: they are stored in the body. They are passed from mother to infant, and specific effects of changes in dietary fatty acids are delayed by the buffering capacity of the store, but later can be multi-generational in their effect.

Dr Galli's work also underlines the importance of another source of nutrition for the developing young: milk. Although no milk contains the high concentrations of EFAs found in blood leaving the placenta (especially neural fatty acids), it still contains an important amount and keeps the 'carnivorous' feed style going after birth. (As a proportion of the calories in human milk, the EFAs are present in a much larger quantity than the essential amino-acids.) Work at the Institute of Zoology has shown that species such as nesting rodents, which leave a large part of their brain cell division to be completed after birth, have higher proportions of the neural acids in their milks than those born more fully developed and ready to go, like guinea pigs.

There is a similar contrast between cow's milk and human milk. The young cow does a lot of growing but will end up with a small brain. Its mother's milk has three or four times the amount of protein found in human milk, and five to seven times the mineral content: protein for fast body growth and minerals for bones. Human milk, on the other hand, has the least amount of protein compared to other large mammals but, by contrast, has six to ten times the amount of EFAs essential for postnatal development of the nervous and vascular systems. Gorilla milk has more linoleic and alpha- linolenic acids and fewer long-chain neural acids than human milk. In practice, the milk of each different species is uniquely tailored to its postnatal requirements. Biology and food have long worked together to shape the different designs.

## Evolution of the horse: from toe to hoof

This story of milk also contains the solution to the second conundrum about the herbivores. The first was their failure to develop good night vision; the second concerns hoofs. If hoofs were developed to give them speed, how is it that the fastest four-legged animal is a soft-footed carnivore? The cheetah can hold a speed of 100kph for 60 seconds. Of course, one can see the advantage of paws and claws to a lion: you cannot easily bring down a running buffalo by dragging at it with a set of hoofs. In that form the argument is convincing. Natural selection would have provided these species with claws. It is when you turn it around that it fails. If hoofs bestow speed, why can't the gazelle, zebra, giraffe or buffalo run as fast as the cheetah, when the extra speed would give them an inestimable advantage for survival in neo-Darwinian terms? It would be hard to convince a cheetah racing across the ground that it would do better if it let you fasten a set of hoofs over its paws.

Biochemistry and nutrition offer a different origin story for the hoof: not speed, but economy. Hands or articulated claws need a vascular system to nourish them and to supply chemical energy to the muscles that move them. They need nerves and synaptic junctions to send and receive messages, and they need corresponding parts in the brain to deal with those messages. In short, hands and claws need a big chunk of brain volume to serve the articulated control and a large vascular area to ensure a supply of oxygen and nutrients. These two systems depend on long-chain, EFAs: arachidonic and DHA. Unlike the herbivores, the carnivores get these premade in their food.

The horse provides a good illustration of all this, as its earliest form the Eohippus, which lived about 50 million years ago, had toes – four on its front feet and three on its back feet. As it evolved into later species these toes were reduced first to two and then to one. In his delightfully titled book *Hens' Teeth and Horses' Toes* Stephen J Gould expresses his dissatisfaction with the traditional explanation of evolution as the summation of small changes that adapt populations ever more finely to their local environments.[27] Yet here, in the evolution of the horse's hoof, is surely a convincing demonstration of a theory which, at least in its negative form, can hardly be denied. The argument is simply this: *whatever the mechanism that brings about evolutionary change, no new life-form can come into existence if it needs a type or quantity of food that it cannot get.* If there is anything strange about that very obvious thought it is only that its significance appears to have been missed by so many evolutionists, past and present.

The absence of individual toes in hoofed animals is not about evolution selecting in favour of speed and efficiency. After all, a cheetah, with toes, can outrun any hoofed animal. It is, rather, a matter of economy based on the principle of "you can't have everything". The body design will always reflect the nutrients available during its evolution. The nutritional resources required for the development of sophisticated digits and paws, and the maintenance of the vascular and nervous systems, muscles, and brain power to use them, involve quantities of long-chain essential fatty acids that hoofed animals simply had no access too.

Some understanding of what happened to the horse can be gleaned from a disease that afflicts human beings. Peripheral vascular disease, sometimes associated with heart disease or diabetes, can cause the capillary circulation to degenerate. An important sign is a 'clubbing' of the fingers, which appear to shrink and thicken. Tiny blood vessels at the ends of the fingers, which have a large surface area relative to their diameter, can no longer be properly maintained. They collapse, thrombose, or in some other way are put out of action. The tissues they should support are affected, cells that have reached the end of their life spans cannot be replaced, and the diseased part becomes shorter and thicker as inactive material accumulates in it. In diabetes, the nerve supply to the feet can atrophy. It has happened that people with diabetes have sat in front of the fire in winter to keep their feet warm and tragically the first they know of the disaster is the smell of burning feet!

It is not difficult to see the relevance of this to the horse. We have discussed before how the embryonic development of the brain, the heart and blood vessels takes place at the earliest moment. Similarly, the evolution of the brain and the vascular system go together and, biochemically, they use similar fats. The fast growth and food pattern of the horse do not favour an extensive vascular or nervous system; this would have become ever truer as the evolving horse grew larger. By comparison with animals of a similar size it is biochemically the worst off. In theory, the horse and other large vegetarian mammals can make arachidonic and docosahexaenoic acids. A squirrel, mouse, rat and rabbit can do so easily. They have a fast metabolic rate and limited growth. The problem is that to make DHA from the green leaves and arachidonic from the seeds is a slow process. The greater the velocity of growth and protein manufacture, the more that outstrips the synthetic process. DHA has 22 carbons and six double bonds, arachidonic has 20 carbons and four double bonds. Consequently, it is more difficult to make the former.

The liver is the place where incoming substances are metabolised. When we studied the membrane chemistry for the livers of the horse and other herbivores, we found that they had plenty of the green leaf and seed precursors but relatively small amounts of arachidonic and DHA. The latter was particularly affected. The giveaway evidence for the rate limitation was that its immediate precursor, with only five double bonds instead of 6, was present in quite significant amounts, as though it got that far before the business of growth demanded it was assembled with the rapidly acquired proteins to form new membranes or maintain the old. It got as far as 5 double bonds but not much further. The brain and nervous system can only use the six double-bonded full DHA.[28] The likely reason, we propose, is that its unique electron configuration of six methylene interrupted double bonds can act like a semi- conductor, as in our phones and computers.[29]

Hence not just the peripheral nervous system but also the brain is under the stress of too few building materials. As it can only be made with the correct materials it has to shrink in relation to the rapid expansion of body size. The horse in consequence has what is often called a walnut sized brain. That the DHA content of food makes the difference is amply illustrated by the dolphin, which has 1.7kg of brain, although roughly of the same bodyweight as the horse.

### Liver inner cell membrane (ethanolamine) phosphoglyceride from Syncerus caffer (Cape buffalo) and Tursiops truncatus (Dolphin)

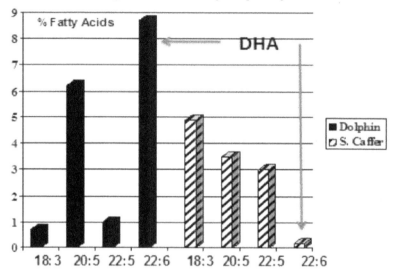

*Williams, G. and Crawford, M.A. (1987) Comparison of the fatty acid component in structural lipids from dolphins, zebra and giraffe: possible evolutionary implications. J. Zool. Lond. 213: 673 - 684.

At its first recognisable appearance the horse was no bigger than a Labrador dog, and in that form it had toes. It can be suggested that the larger it grew, the more demands were made on its lipid food supply and the less there was to spare to build vascular and nervous systems in proportion to its new bulk. Hands and feet demand a huge investment in nervous 'hardware' and software. In the human species, the hands are developed to the point where they can perform the most delicate micro- surgery, intricate needle work or carvings, or execute a Liszt rhapsody on the piano. The volume in the brain occupied with controlling the hand is out of all proportion to its apparent size. It is huge. The same is true of the vascular network. Since the horse had to economise somewhere, the toes and fingers were a sensible sacrifice, bringing about a disproportionately large saving in return for a seemingly unimportant loss.

The importance of this saving is clear if we look at the horse's brain. It takes up a mere 0.05 per cent of the animal's total weight (compared with the 2 per cent taken up by the human brain), and from the fossil record it appears that, using this relative size as the measure, the horse's brain has shrunk as its body grew larger. As N. W. Pirie [30] has pointed out, small mammals like squirrels have roughly the same relative brain size as man, and it is significant too that none of them have hoofs: all have little toes and fingers.

The horse is as pure a vegetarian as they come, whereas the cow unexpectedly turns out to be partly carnivorous. The technique adopted by the straight herbivores, like the horse and the zebra, is simply to process vast quantities of vegetable foods. They are selective feeders, using green leaves to provide the protein and minerals they need, and the vegetable fibre to push it all through and make excellent manure. By contrast, the ruminants such as cows, sheep and goats hold the vegetation they eat in their stomach, where a beautiful symbiotic relationship exists between resident bacteria and protozoa and the beast itself. These micro-organisms, fauna and flora, can digest the cellulose of plants - an impossible task for other species as they do not possess the digestive enzyme, cellulase, which the micro-organisms do. Hence the bacteria break down plant fibres; protozoa eat the bacteria; these are filtered in an additional stomach and then passed on to a 'true stomach' and digestive system. Here, the microbes and protozoa provide the cow with a high protein diet: as protozoa are tiny animals, the cow and other ruminants are in this sense carnivores! Why then do they not have sophisticated nervous systems?

The answer lies in the fact that the micro-organisms – the bacteria and protozoa – are reproducing without access to oxygen. There is little or no free oxygen in the cow's stomach, so how do they burn the carbohydrates to make energy for growth? Instead of combining hydrogen and oxygen, which is the way aerobic systems produce energy, they rely on the energy derived only from breaking down quantities of cellulose and carbohydrates in the plants. The large amounts of hydrogen produced in the process are then 'dumped' in any willing molecule.

At this point, the understanding of the nature of polyunsaturated fats becomes rewarding. The EFAs are polyunsaturated, which means they have double bonds from which the hydrogen is missing. Because they have lost hydrogen, these unsaturated bonds make excellent hydrogen acceptors in place of oxygen. In this way the micro-organisms get rid of their hydrogen, produce masses of proteins but in so doing, destroy much of the double bonds and hence the essential polyunsaturated fatty acids of their food turning them into saturated fats and trans isomers. Seeds, especially from bushes and trees, may escape this process. Being oil-rich, they tend to float through. The protected seeds and incomplete hydrogenation means that some EFA molecules escape. Those that do are precious and used for cell membranes; there is certainly not enough to spare for the body fats, though, which is why beef fat is full of non-essential, saturated fats. The carnivorous cows gain the advantage of a rich supply of protein, but the cost is the irrevocable and simultaneous destruction of the EFAs needed for brains, nervous systems and hands, big and small toes. Hence a huge body and little brain and again, like the horse, no hands.

## Bodies and brains: the race is on

Of the mammals, the large herbivores are the worst affected by this phenomenon of body growth outstripping brain growth. However, the secondates (such as cows and lions) are worse off than the primates (monkeys). The primates have much larger brains relative to their body size than the secondates. They have gone down a different pathway, that of slow growth, long gestation and lactation; and they do not destroy their

EFAs in their stomachs as the cows and other ruminants do. The biochemistry shows that the primates are much more richly endowed with the long-chain EFA derivatives than the secondates, and their milks have much less protein and fewer minerals. So the group differences in relative brain size of the egg-laying birds and reptiles, the marsupials and then the mammals, and the differences between the herbivores and carnivores, whether they are birds or mammals, can be explained by the flow of nutrients in the food chain.

Needless to say this example is of great relevance to the emergence of the human brain, which weighed 1.45 kg by 160,000 y.a. compared to the vegetarian chimpanzee, which has only a 340g brain. Note that our genome differs by only 1.5% from that of the chimpanzee! We shall be looking at the significance of this fact to Homo sapiens later.

This evidence, that a paucity of DHA in food is a limiting factor for brain growth and development, learning and vision, has been well confirmed in different guises repeatedly. The concept was first claimed in the 1972 paper by Crawford and Sinclair; it was confirmed at the joint FAO–WHO International Expert Consultation on Dietary Fats and Oils in Human Nutrition.[31] Later reports in 1994 and 2008-2010 added further confirmation, if needed. There is abundant evidence described in these reports, first from experimental animal studies and then studies on pre-term infants, with quantitative assessments of requirements. For example, the 2008-2010 report recommends 200mg/day of DHA or 250mg/day of EPA plus DHA for pregnancy. That really has to mean beforehand, probably back to puberty when physiology is getting its reproductive act together. There will also be a continued need after birth to maintain levels in the mother's milk. A whole book would be needed to review all the evidence, but there are two bits that are notable in the context of DHA and neurodevelopment.

Effect of DHA deficiency on brain cell migration cannot change colour

**Maternal DHA deficiency in the brain of the developing fetus restricts migration of cortical neurons in rat fetal brain. Staining specifically reveals migrating cells.**

Diet 59                                    Diet 61 (D)

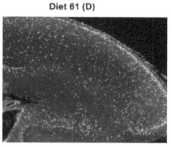

Data from Ephraim Yavin, et al. Neuroscience. 2009 Sep 15;162(4):1011-22. doi: 10.1016/j.neuroscience.2009.05.012. x4 Epub 2009 May 14. PMID: 19447164.

cortex. The image on the left shows the dense migration in the foetal brain of a rat from a mother fed omega-3. The image on the right is of a control foetal brain from a mother without the omega-3.32

Hee-Yong Kim and Arthur Spector, working at the National Institute on Alcohol Abuse and Alcoholism, NIH, Bethesda, USA, demonstrated conclusively the function of DHA in stimulating the outgrowth of nerve fibres and synaptic connections.[33] Professor Ephraim Yavin, working in neurobiology at the Weismann Institute for Science, Rehovot, Israel, showed how if a pregnant rat was fed a diet deficient in omega-3 then neurogenesis (the growth and development of nerve tissue) in the developing brain of her pup was delayed.[34]

During early brain development – around week 12 in humans – the newly arrived brain cells migrate from their focal region and move outwards to form the cortex and other regions of the brain. In Professor Yavin's histological image of the foetal rat pup's brain you can see how the yellow dots of the cells have moved out to the cortical region in abundance. Viewing the image of the developing pup's brain from a mother fed a deficient diet, it is clear that the concentration of neurons is sparse: neurogenesis has been adversely delayed.

Yavin later confirmed by lipid analysis that there was a deficit of DHA in the brains of the deficient pups.[35]

The results from the work of Kim and Yavin together with the Hungarian data on DHA stimulating gene expression[36] in the brain provide a robust mechanism both for a DHA requirement for neurodevelopment and for the way in which nutrients from a marine food web, eaten generation after generation, would have enhanced brain development. It also points out that a deficiency would reduce brain development generation after generation, as we have seen in the shrinking brains of the savannah animals.

What we have been looking at in this chapter is a contrast in strategies that animals of different sorts adopt to get nourishment. The strategy could result in substrates driving change in different directions and could explain, in simple terms, the puzzle of how rigid 'lines' were developed and maintained. One strategy led perhaps to a more specialised development, whereas another led to regression. In the long run there is a lot to be said for not becoming committed to an overly specialised lifestyle. The fact that *Homo sapiens* uses what is perhaps the most diverse food selection pattern and is, in its own eyes, by far the most successful of the primates, may be a good advertisement for compromise and diversity. However, within that diversity there can be no doubt that during the evolution of the big brain our ancestors had to have access to a rich food source of DHA with accompanying iodine, selenium and zinc. With mental ill-health now going through the roof, we need to worry about that!

## Conclusion

In conclusion, epigenetics was a more powerful shaper of evolution than has been previously thought. Indeed, it is consistent with Darwin's "Conditions of Existence" as the more powerful force, more powerful than selection and the struggle for survival. The latter is a seductive concept, but it is an end game. It does not tell you about the beginning; and, like everything else, evolution had a beginning.

We know people will be reluctant to hear this conclusion, but that is what the evidence and common sense tells us. Natural selection works on a mutation. Survivable mutations are claimed to take place rarely. By contrast, epigenetics can act simultaneously on a whole population, as was witnessed by the impact of the WWII Dutch hunger,[37] and the increase in average height that started in 1900 in England and is continuing. Moreover, epigenetic changes will occur every time there is an environmental and/or nutritional change.

You have to think about beginnings – the beginning of placental mammals, for example. That had to start with a pretty small beast. When the arachidonic acid precursor became abundant its adhesion molecules did their job in making the fertilised ovum stick to the uterine wall; blood vessels proliferated, stimulated by the same; and the rest is history. This, then, is an example of Stephen J. Gould's punctuated evolution. It may well challenge your belief system, as it challenged Gould's own beliefs when he first put forward the idea. But there is evidence all around us, witnessed by the different disease patterns seen in cultures with contrasting dietary systems, along with differences in height, shape and size. Then think of the earliest of mammals foraging under the feet of the dinosaurs. When the crunch came, whether by asteroid or starvation, it led to a radical change in the vegetation, and the epigenetic response to this change in conditions would have quickly changed the mammals. Eventually some would settle on meat for their sustenance, and others grass. Perhaps some found themselves with a lot of dead or ailing dinosaurs in a place ravaged by the great impact, and so developed a taste for meat. Who knows?

There are many ways one can speculate on changed conditions having an epigenetic impact on the early mammals, leading to the major differences seen in the many classes of animals found today. And although it remains speculation, it is founded nonetheless on evidence-based knowledge of the behaviour of various molecules. After all, whichever narrative you want to believe in, they are all speculative. We have no time machine to transport us back to the Cambrian Explosion and test our ideas. We cannot go back and watch a group of apes separating from the horde and finding the new ecological niche that set them on the path to becoming H sapiens. It is all science-based speculation, unprovable perhaps, but nonetheless interesting.

If epigenetics really was at the base of evolution the question that remains is this: does the epigenetic influence remain a reversible system, or does it become at some point irreversible? The dolphin foetus has vestigial legs and has the bones of a hand in its flipper. It must therefore have the genes for legs and hands, but they are suppressed. Could they be released? With time new genes may have developed to take the place of those that have become redundant. Although the genes for legs must be there, a great many other instructions are needed to restore a working leg with feet and five toes together with their sensory systems: a tall order. Perhaps if humans became extinct, the shorelines would restore their phenomenal wealth of food. Perhaps some dolphins would then investigate and enjoy the shoreline harvest. Then the opportunity to sleep on land would release the full power of the 1,7 Kg of brain. Then the planet could, at last be occupied by a super-intelligent species.

## More concluding comments

The evolution of the carnivores with their articulated claws and the herbivores with their hoofs was separately co-ordinated and discontinuous. Gould offers a mechanism for the major leaps in a few words and probably better than anyone else:

*"Genetic systems are arranged hierarchically, controllers and master switches often activate large blocks of genes. Small changes in the timing of action for these controllers often translate into major and discontinuous alterations of external form." (Gould, 1983).*

The thrust of his comment is similar to ours. There can be no doubt about the role of genetics, but there can equally be no doubt that genetics alone cannot direct evolution without the materials. Add the possibility of the genetic switches being set by nutrition in one way of expression or another and we have a potential explanation for co-ordinated evolution in response to the environment: that is, to Darwin's *'higher' law of conditions"*. As we have commented before, no matter how good the architect's plan, the building cannot be constructed without the materials: planning and availability of materials and their quality, go together.

We now have a mechanism whereby nutrients could alter gene behaviour and ultimately release genetic space to modify the genetic scene. Moreover there is evidence that both arachidonic and docosahexaenoic acids manipulate gene function.

Mutations are necessary but not sufficient. Useful ones probably appear over and over again in inopportune circumstances and do not get selected. Most are lethal. Everything has to wait for a potentially opportune mutation to occur at a time, in a place and in circumstances congenial to it. Epigenetics by contrast will act across a whole population simultaneously with speed far faster than any mutation. Darwin would surely have agreed with this model. It took 3.5 or so billion years for the anything serious other than the single cell anaerobic life to exist. When oxygen came on the scene in sufficient quantity, the change was fast when all the phyla of airbreathing animal life we know today, appears in the fossil record: the Cambrian Explosion.

There is, however, a fundamental deviation from the classical view as it is commonly understood today. *Alteration in nutrition changes shape, form and function before mutation occurs*: the horse, the cat, the elephant, dolphins and whales and our own dramatic recent increase in height and disease pattern, shape and size, in less than a century, acts as incontrovertible evidence for this effect.

The conclusion is that substrates could have driven change either forwards in progressive development, or backwards, in retrogression or degeneration. The "self-sufficiency of natural selection" for advantage in the Wisemannian - neo-Darwinism interpretation just does not stack up. Why would whole swathes of animals degenerate brain size? That feat has exposed them to annihilation. What advantage is there in turning useful hands into a single toe? We hear you say to run faster and escape predators. Give us a break – the cheetah runs the fastest and it has soft feet. This is not to say natural section is redundant, far from it but its an end game and not the beginning. Moreover the beginning would be in the midst of plenty in a new rich diversity resulting from the extinction of the old. Too much credence has been given to it at the expense of understanding the forces such as nutrition and epigenetics which can work far faster than any process governed by random mutation and selection.

More importantly, the random process *ipso facto* has no predictive value. The driving force of conditions and nutrition offer a precise, predictive ability which is testable with time and even with experiment. For example, the brain evolved in the sea 500-600 mya. It only had marine nutrients for its purpose. We can test if marine nutrients encourage brain development. Indeed, this has been done and validated by the study of over 14,000 pregnancies. Note that the bulk of brain cell division takes place before birth. The researchers, led by Dr Joe Hibbeln the at the National Institutes of Health in the

USA, Dr Jean Golding from the Centre for Child and Adolescent Health, University of Bristol where the study was done, found that the proportion of fish and sea foods eaten by the mothers during the pregnancy enhanced markers of cognition, motor function and behaviour. The more fish and sea food eaten the better the outcomes in the children at 8 years of age.[38]

Hypothesis, prediction, and testing is the hallmark of science. Exactly the same principle holds true as we come to explore the origins of what must be for us the most interesting of all animal species: ourselves.

# CHAPTER 7

# Reptiles versus mammals: a tale of nutrition

## DINOSAURS – DEAD ON IMPACT?

There may well be an interesting similarity between the present crisis of elephant survival in Africa and the problems that beset the dinosaurs. Sixty-five million years ago they, and many species associated with them, went out of existence so rapidly that theories of global catastrophe have been put forward to explain the suddenness of their extinction at the end of the Cretaceous period.

One of the more controversial of these theories made headlines when Luis Alvarez and his colleagues at the University of California suggested that the Earth had been hit by a huge asteroid. This would have produced a vast cloud of dust which, blasting off from the point of impact, would have drifted through the atmosphere across the globe, blotting out the sun and cutting off its life-giving energy. The effect would have been like the 'nuclear winter' that is supposed to freeze the world after all-out nuclear war. The impact of the asteroid could also have tilted the Earth's axis, which again would have meant dramatic changes of climate in different parts of the planet. It would have caused havoc in the oceans, sending shock waves up to the North Pole and wrecking coastal regions. The evidence for this collision is the existence of an anomalously rich and narrow band of elements of the platinum group, such as iridium and osmium, in the rock strata at a depth that corresponds to the time at which the dinosaurs became extinct. The surface of the

Earth contains little iridium, but interstellar material is rich in it. The narrowness of the band of rocks containing it suggests an instantaneous event.

However, Alvarez's fellow countrymen Charles Officer and Charles Drake of Dartmouth College, New Hampshire, have put forward an alternative hypothesis that the iridium band is volcanic in origin, brought up from the interior of the Earth, which is much richer in iridium than the surface. Alvarez did not consider a volcano to be a possibility because it would have meant an eruption some thousand times greater than the biggest known to us, the Krakatoa eruption of 1883. However, violent volcanic activity was characteristic of the earlier days of the planet's history.

More recent studies suggest that the iridium band is not as continuous or as sharp as would have been expected, and was in fact deposited over a period of 100,000 years. While volcanic activity diminished as the planet cooled, there is evidence of late activity in the Deccan Traps of India, one of the largest piles of lava on Earth. They cover an area of more than half a million square kilometres and the volume of lava has been estimated at about a million cubic kilometres. The activity occurred between 60 and 65 million years ago, which is about the right time for the final extinction of the dinosaurs; but the lava is low in iridium. As Peter Smith said in *The Guardian*, "Until the crucial piece of evidence is found (if it ever is), the debate will continue..." [1]

The evidence for an asteroid impact has since then strengthened. The Chicxulub Impact Crater in the Yucatan fits the bill nicely. Its centre lies out to sea in the Gulf of Mexico but with much of the 180-240 Km diameter crater inland. Estimates of the size of the impactor vary widely, but even the smallest estimates are huge – some 10-15 km in diameter.[2]

There are still critics, some claiming that the impact actually predates the K-T boundary of mass extinction by 300,000 years.[3] The opposite view is held by Schulte and others, who write *"The temporal match between the ejecta layer and the onset of the extinctions and the agreement of ecological patterns in the fossil record with modelled environmental perturbations (for example, darkness and cooling) lead us to conclude that the Chicxulub impact triggered the mass extinction."* [4]

The frogs and cockroaches and Gingkoes were amongst the survivors, with recovery apparently relatively fast. However, as we shall see later, the recovery was associated with a changing panorama of life.

## THE CHANGE IN LIFE AFTER THE GREAT EXTINCTION

As with the punctuated evolution theory of Gould and Eldridge (chapter 2), the reason for great periods of stability would be the fact that conditions of existence remained stable. That would be the case until a population reached its logarithmic phase of growth and outstripped the slower plant production of essential nutrients required for the animals' sustenance. A Malthusian catastrophe would then put paid to the affected species. Malthus asserted that the growth in animal populations can become exponential, but plant growth remains linear. In such circumstances demand outstrips resources. Although catastrophic for the affected animal species initially, the Malthusian pattern actually returns populations to a sustainable level in the long term. The term derives from the surname of the Reverend Thomas Robert Malthus (1766- 1834), a political and economic theorist whose fame rests on his 1798 publication *An Essay on the Principle of Population.*

Catastrophe theorists also have suggestions for extinctions. There have been five major extinctions and several smaller ones in the history of Earth. Each time, new life appeared. The trilobites have gone, the eurypterids have gone, but that was a long, long time ago. This extinction of the dinosaurs was more recent and so provides us with a better chance of obtaining evidence on which to speculate. Following their demise there were worldwide changes. The fossil record charts the emergence of flowering plants with protected seeds, the bees, and the mammals – a beautiful, symbiotic example of planetary renewal after the extinction of the giant reptiles and their food resource: giant trees. [5]

That example was clearly a response to the changed Darwinian conditions of existence. Although, an asteroid impact could have finished off the giant reptiles, they were on the way out anyway. The massive vegetation they relied on was suffering from predation. Just think of the number of calories to keep one of those giants going! Despite the efforts of the carnivorous raptors, tyrannosaurs, ornithomimids, large and small theropods, they clearly grew bigger and bigger and reached the giant proportions familiar to us from Hollywood films – hence demanding more and more primary plant food. A *Mamenchisaurus*, for example, ate about 100,000 calories per day of leaves and other vegetation! How could the plants keep up with that degree of predation?

Notably the gingkoes, giant ferns, cycads and the like are still with us. They did not suffer the disaster that sorted out the dinosaurs.

But, (and it is a big but) these plants are now much smaller: shadows of their former selves. There can be no doubt that conditions changed for plant life. Whatever random mutation was taking place it was going nowhere. When the environment changed, not all changed as with our Gingkoes. The question arises – could there have been a physicochemical mechanism for the shift from reptiles to mammals? Perhaps we shouldn't, but nonetheless we will, quote from *Skeptical Science*: [6]

- The first great mass extinction event took place at the end of the Ordovician (about 438 mya) when according to the fossil record, 60% of all genera of life, which would mostly be marine life, was exterminated.
- 360 million years ago in the Late Devonian period, the

environment that had clearly nurtured reefs for at least 13 million years turned hostile and the world plunged into the second mass extinction event.

- The fossil record of the end Permian mass extinction reveals a staggering loss of life: perhaps 80–95% of all marine species went extinct. Reefs didn't reappear for about 10 million years, the greatest hiatus in reef building in all of Earth history.

- The end Triassic mass extinction is estimated to have claimed about half of all marine invertebrates. Around 80% of all land quadrupeds also went extinct.

- The end of the Cretaceous mass extinction 65 million years ago is famously associated with the demise of the dinosaurs. Virtually no large land animals survived. Plants were also greatly affected while tropical marine life was decimated. Global temperature was 6 to 14°C warmer than present with sea levels over 300 metres higher than current levels. At this time, the oceans flooded up to 40% of the continents as we know them.

What caused these mass extinctions? To find the major driver of coral extinction, in 2008 J.E.N. Veron[7] looked at the possible options and eliminated many as the primary cause. A meteorite strike can create huge dust clouds that lead to devastating darkness and cold. However, if this were the cause of coral reef extinction, 99% of the world's coral species would be wiped out in weeks or months. The fossil record shows coral extinction occurred over much longer periods.

Warmer temperatures cause mass bleaching of corals. Even in a warmer world, deep ocean temperatures would remain well below surface temperatures and there would be safe havens where cooler water up-wells from the deep ocean. That's not to say meteorites or global warming played no part in coral extinction - both have been contributing factors at various times. But they cannot fully explain the nature of coral extinctions as observed in the fossil record.

What Veron found was each mass extinction event corresponded to periods of quickly changing atmospheric $CO_2$:

*When $CO_2$ changes slowly, the gradual increase allows mixing and buffering of surface layers by deep ocean sinks. Marine organisms also have time to adapt to the new environmental conditions. However, when $CO_2$ increases abruptly, the acidification effects are intensified in shallow waters owing to a lack of mixing. It also gives marine life little time to adapt.*

Needless to say, this narrative is too John Veron and his colleagues. How long was 'dramatic'? What do you mean by decimated? What about the evidence on volcanism in the Siberian Traps, and volcanism close for comfort to the present-day $CO_2$ increase and oceanic acidification. Just as today, there were some violent opponents. What about asteroid impacts?

The asteroid that caused the Chicxulub impact crater in Yucatan is widely claimed as being responsible for the extinction of the giant reptiles. Recent findings as we discussed earlier, suggest the Chicxulub bolide impact is implicated in the Cretaceous-Paleogene (K-Pg) extinction approximately 66 million years ago. Researchers from Department of Geosciences, Princeton University, Princeton, NJ, USA estimated Deccan eruption rates with uranium-lead (U-Pb) zircon geochronology and resolved four high-volume eruptive periods. According to this model, maximum eruption rates occurred before and after the K-Pg extinction, with one such pulse initiating tens of thousands of years prior to both the bolide impact and extinction. These findings "support extinction models that incorporate both catastrophic events as drivers of environmental deterioration associated with the K-Pg extinction and its aftermath". [8]

The problem that catastrophe theories set out to solve is why 75 per cent of other species were wiped out along with the dinosaurs. Certainly, this does sound calamitous; but in fact, although a large asteroid has doubtless hit the Earth in the past, the extinctions are explicable *without* the need or apocalyptic asteroids and volcanoes. We need only think about what is happening today to understand with painful clarity how easy it is for one species to displace and eliminate many others. Perhaps so, and perhaps demise for an already weakened fauna could be precipitated by such a catastrophic event.

In the last few centuries 5,000 species have become extinct. The Red List of Threatened Animals, published by the Union for the Conservation of Nature, contains a long, sad roll-call of species either recently extinct or endangered. The tiger, snow leopard and African elephant hang on precariously. The whales have been offered a dubious last-minute reprieve from being eaten into extinction. Less well known, the aye-aye in Madagascar, the sole surviving representative of a whole primate family, has been reduced to the point where it is feared that fewer than 50 still survive. The gorilla has been driven back into a few forest habitats.

In the meantime, the human primate population has exploded to 8 billion in an instant of biological or geological time. This population explosion has brought the world to a state where only a few hundred of those magnificent primate cousins of ours can still find room to live. Species after species has been extinguished, hunted for food, trinkets, skins and aphrodisiacs. More are simply forced out of the world by the sheer pressure on space, specialist resources and habitat destruction, exerted by the expanding population of the dominant animal, *Homo sapiens*.

As recently as the Roman period, hippos and lions were living where London now stands. Their remains were found, with a happy touch of serendipity, when a corner of lion-flanked Trafalgar Square was being excavated in 1962 to build the Ugandan High Commission.

We can imagine extra-terrestrials colonising our deserted planet in the future and delving into its geological history and fossil records. They will record the current path to extinction of 90% of the planet's land-based fauna as happening in a blink of geological time. It will appear to them to have happened so rapidly as to suggest a massive and sudden catastrophe. That's how swiftly we are, in reality, destroying the animal world around us. So it is that we, of all the generations in history, should find it easy to see how the dinosaurs could have devoured some of their fellow animals, destroyed the vegetation so eliminated the habitats of others and driven so many species to extinction before bringing the final ruin down on themselves in one very thin seam of geological time.

Catastrophe theories involving huge asteroids and volcanic eruptions have been invoked to explain the extinction of the dinosaurs and other species 65 million years ago. And yet the current mass extinction of species taking place on Earth today, the result of human-induced environmental crisis, shows that catastrophic extinctions can take place in the geological blink of an eye. A collapse in environmental systems brought about by giant herbivores outstripping their food resources could have finished off the large dinosaurs without the need for extra-terrestrial projectiles or super-volcanoes. Indeed, both forces could have done the trick.

## DID THE DINOSAURS EAT THEMSELVES OUT OF EXISTENCE?

This may be the simple explanation: that the dinosaurs may have been responsible for their own extinction, just as we are responsible for the present mass extinction of our fellow inhabitants of this planet – and, indeed, threatening our own survival. Apart from their voracious appetites, the weight of the giant herbivorous reptiles must have been destructive. First, they would have needed considerable quantities of food – a 40-ton dinosaur could have eaten 46,000,000 kg of plant life each year. The trampling of their huge feet would have destroyed much of what they did not eat and inhibited its re-growth. As their numbers grew the time would come when even the giant-sized plants of that time could no longer keep pace with the demand of those voracious appetites. Plants grow much slower than animals. This period was one of the hottest and it may be that the dinosaurs created their own hothouse effect. The Malthusian end of story had come.

The leaching of minerals from the soil into the swamps, rivers and seas, would have added another dimension not generally considered. Even today something like 39,000,000 tons of minerals and salts are washed annually by rain into the oceans. We can even see the effects of this in our towns and cities – one litre of rain water saturated with carbon dioxide will dissolve one gram of lime from the cement and stone of our historic buildings.

It needs to be remembered that at the beginning, the planet's surface was rich in chemicals created in the original super nova. That cocktail provided a fertile soil for massive plant growth in the primordial oceans and on any land that poked above the ocean surface. The fact that plant life was characterised by giant ginkgoes, cycads, ferns and their allies, testifies to this fertility. It was an age of giants, and the animals that lived on those huge plants became, in time, gigantic themselves. However, the young and fecund planet was already showing signs of environmental deterioration when the dinosaurs reached their peak.

There are many examples of depleted ecosystems at play today. One example is the Nile Delta. The river carried a rich load of minerals and elements, washed by rains from Ethiopia and Central Africa. This transfer of richness to the Nile Delta created the Granary of Rome and, until recently, nourished the Mediterranean sardine grounds. In recent years the Aswan Dam, by retaining a high proportion of the silt, has restricted the constant fertilisation of the Mediterranean upon which the sardine fisheries depended. The collapse of the sardine population caused by the Aswan Dam, holding back the riches of the soil, testifies to the significance of this washing process.

We can see here the rich marine community with its reliance on the nourishment flowing from the Nile being severed, and in doing so we can also appreciate the sheer amount of nutrients, everywhere being lost from the land.

This process was operating during the reign of the dinosaurs. The dinosaurs themselves would have contributed by eating the plants and defecating and urinating: in this form the minerals and trace elements would have been more easily washed away, especially where swamp lands connected to the sea. A dinosaur's faecal output would have been quite prodigious. It would only need the population growth to reach its exponential phase, combined with a continuous undermining of soil fertility as nutrients washed into the sea, for the time bomb to tick down to zero.

This is not to refute other lines of argument regarding the extinction of the dinosaurs. There is little doubt about the realty of the meteorite impact, and little doubt that it would have had a catastrophic effect on climate and life, both animal and vegetable. But with soil and plant nutrient depletion combining with population growth, the giant reptiles could already have been in a precarious position from environmental deterioration when the meteorite hit. This could have tipped them to the point where environmental destruction was over-riding any chance of natural selection and survival of the fittest finding a way out of the mess. Once the critical point was passed, the acceleration of the destructive process would have been rapid.

It is most significant that there are still ginkgo survivors: indeed, the Viale Baptista in Modena, Italy, and the road that circuits the Emperor of Japan's estate in Tokyo are lined with them, and there is a specimen outside the offices of the Zoological Society of London. However, these are tiny compared to what they once were: Bonsai ginkgoes!

During the reign of the dinosaurs the planet was clothed in ferns and allied species. Today there are 15,000 of them, compared to 250,000 flowering plant species. Some giant ferns can still be found, usually in new habitats created from recent volcanic activity. Indeed, many of the volcanic hillsides in New Zealand (a land of recent origin, geologically speaking) are cloaked in ferns which, if not gigantic by dinosaur standards, are certainly huge compared to the average species found in European woodlands and hillsides. The upper slopes of the Ruwenzori (Mountains of the Moon) in Uganda are clothed with giant heathers. In these rare spots, the giant-nurturing mineral bounty of the land has not yet been washed into the sea.

The epigenetics fostered by the soil at the time before and during the rise of the reptiles led to their great sizes. That nutrient wealth, creating the land-based giants, was relocated into the seas by rain and river. piss and shit. It may be no coincidence that the only comparable giants living today are in the sea: the great whales and the whale shark.

Our idea that the great appetites of the giant dinosaurs would have contributed to their extinction has been supported by a new study which "support an environmentally driven decline of non-avian dinosaurs well before the asteroid impact". [9]

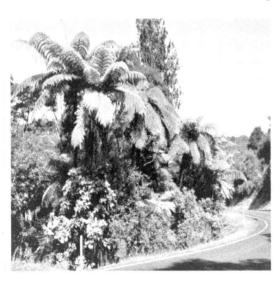

GIANT FERNS AT THE ROAD SIDE, COROMANDEL, NEW ZEALAND Volcanism can bring a rich set of trace elements providing good conditions for plant life.

# ELEPHANTS AT MURCHISON FALLS NATIONAL PARK – THE ROAD TO EXTINCTION

Just how rapidly a large animal can destroy its own habitat when the amount of space available to it falls below the critical point can be seen in the plight of the East African elephant. In the days of the Protectorate of Uganda, National Wildlife Parks were established to encourage tourism and conservation. One of the localities chosen was around Murchison Falls where the whole weight of the Nile squeezes itself violently through a 2.74 metre (19-foot) cleft in the rocks. Legend has it that if a man jumps the gap, he can possess the woman of his choice. It is claimed that some have taken the challenge and succeeded, suggesting an Olympian level of fitness.[20]

The Murchison region had been cattle country until, at the turn of 1900, a rinderpest epidemic from imported cattle swept through Africa and destroyed most of the livestock. The area round Murchison Falls was left as a mixture of forest, scrub and open grassland, and this, together with the presence of the Nile and the Falls, recommended it as a site of scenic interest with open country where the local wildlife could be readily seen. The new National Park was home to buffalo, hippo, crocodile, hartebeest, kob, waterbuck, giraffe, bush-pig, wart-hog, lion, hyena, leopard and of course elephant. Many of the animals moved freely in and out of the area, unlike humans, who were moved out and told not to return.

By any standards the park was a good size, with 2,000 square miles on the south bank of the Nile. Soon settlements became

20    The current Olympic record for a long jump is held by Mike Powell of the USA, who chalked up 8.95 m (29 ft 4¼ inches) at Tokyo in 1991 – easily enough to jump the Nile at Murchison. The women's record is up to the challenge too, with Galina Chistyakova of Leningrad, USSR, achieving 7.52 m (24 ft 8 inches) in 1988. Interesting from the point of view of the Murchison leap, the long jump is perhaps the longest known competitive activity in sport, having originated in Greece during its heyday and before the great Olympic festivals. Perhaps they were practicing for the Murchison leap!

established around the park boundary. No doubt people were attracted by the thought of having a source of meat wandering nearby – a valuable commodity. A combination of growing populations and influxes of refugees from various disputes in other regions resulted in a cordon of people, very happy to make use of the chance of any food, leather or ivory that might pass nearby.

Hunting was illegal without a licence and the penalty was a term in what was called Kingi Georgi Hoteli – the local prison. The consequence of this peripheral enclosure was the disruption of the elephants' traditional migration route (from the Nile basin to the forests on Mount Elgon in the east of Uganda).

Once the elephants were penned inside the park boundaries the pressure on its woodlands and forest began in earnest. At first there was a swift increase in the number of elephants, but soon it became clear that the park's woodlands could not support such a growing population on their own. The elephants were quickly turning the forests into grassland, eating the trees, pushing some over for exercise and stripping the bark from others, which results in the death of the tree through a process called ring barking: the loss of even a small amount of bark can spell death for a tree. Eventually it was noticed that the park woodland was giving way to more grassland, and although there was plenty of grass, some of it six feet high, the elephants' health was noticeably deteriorating.

Studies of the elephants showed that there was a lowered fertility, longer calving interval, increased neonatal mortality, reduced growth rate and delayed sexual maturity. Frequent mouth infections produced large bony abscesses on the jaws with pus draining to the outside.

Dr Sylvia Sykes, who was working with Michael Crawford, at the Nuffield Institute of Comparative Medicine (a research wing of the Zoology Society of London (ZSL) at the time) studied the pathology of these elephants. She reported that the elephants living on the grasslands suffered to an extraordinary extent from hardening of the main artery, the aorta, while those on the scrubland suffered far less and those in the eastern forests not at all. The elephants, initially confined to the park by the actions of men, were now destroying their own food supply and bringing about a fatal change in their environment.

The story was being repeated in Kenya as well as Uganda, and so the last populations of the largest of our land mammals was showing just how a species could become extinct – and how quickly.

In a paper presented to the ZSL in 1966, the ecologist, Dr Richard Laws (who was later to become Director of the British Antarctic Survey and Secretary of the ZSL) and Ian Parker wrote, "*The evidence presented suggests that the extinction of many elephant populations over the next fifty years is a strong possibility in the absence of population and habitat management.*"

The graph below is taken from Laws' paper at a symposium of the ZSL in 1966. The data from 1953-1965 illustrate the collapsing elephant population in Murchison Park. A total collapse is predicted.

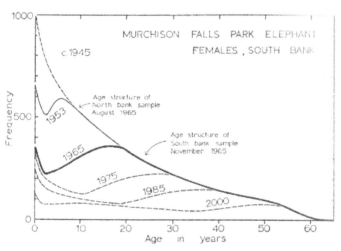

FIG. 9. Population age structure from samples (———) and hypothetical age structure (- -) for previous and future populations (see text for explanation).

Laws' solution was cropping the elephants, but this was met with powerful resistance from conservationists who ignorantly, lobbied for their protection. Some also felt the parks would lose their key attraction (which, ironically, was a problem that the proposal to cull the herd sought to address). However, the health of the elephant populations declined so rapidly that even the tourists began to recognise their poor health, and a cropping programme began. In parts of Kenya it was too late to save thousands of elephants from dying in front of the colour supplement cameras from sickness and malnutrition.

The natural habitat for the elephant is woodland, where they can reach into the trees with their trunks and eat the leaves, nuts, fruits and fresh wood growth. The possibility that the elephants might adapt to meet the new conditions of smaller plants was never suggested by Laws and Parker. From the evidence before their eyes it was clear enough that they would not. It was painfully obvious to them that the elephants were heading for extinction due to population explosion and the resultant habitat destruction, deforestation and the animals having to rely on grass rather then the browse to which they were adapted.

This recent lesson in extinction has relevance to the fate of the dinosaurs. There was no Sylvia Sykes around to cull the poor beasts with her double-barrelled 600 and 375 Winchester backup. Similarly, no amount of rapid adaptation or struggle for survival or waiting for a random mutation could have seen the dinosaurs through the crisis. Once their numbers reached the critical point, the evolutionary cycle followed its inexorable course. The pressure of numbers led to irreversible environmental change, the destruction of the ecology and food supply, and final extinction.

The dinosaurs' end may have been aided by a meteorite impact or massive volcanism; but the death of the elephants and their race towards extinction was happening visibly without any extra-terrestrial or volcanic intervention.

Confirmation that there was a difference between the nutrients provided by trees and grass was supplied by a group of researchers at the Nuffield Institute of Comparative Medicine with the Uganda Game Department. They found that the tissues of woodland elephants were richer in vascular essential fatty acids than were the tissues of grassland elephants. They found the same when comparing woodland and grassland buffalo. [10] It is not hard to see how the population explosion of the dinosaurs, some of them far larger than elephants, could have borne at least as heavily on their land food chain, to their own cost.

## GIANTS WITH TINY BRAINS

There is another twist to this tale. The demise of the dinosaurs and the shrinkage of the giant plants were followed by the development of a new wave of vegetation: the flowering plants with their protected seeds. The seeds of flowering plants in the main contain linoleic acid. Linoleic acid is an essential fatty acid and is the parent of the omega-6 family. The mammals which evolved rapidly after the demise of the dinosaurs are, as science tells us today, dependent on linoleic acid and its omega-6 family for their reproduction. Before the flowering plants took over, the dinosaurs and all before them had to rely largely on an omega-3 food web based on the photosynthetic part of the plants.

Flowering plants and their seeds provided an abundance of important omega-6 linoleic acid building blocks, central to the reproductive system of mammals.

Also, arachidonic acid (ARA), the long-chain derivative of linoleic acid, is one of the principal fatty acids used in the brain. Before the K-T extinction, it had not been particularly abundant. But the brain is consistently built with the same fatty acids in the same amounts, with the balance of omega-6 to omega-3 in all species so far studied between 2 and 1 to 1. [11] We discussed previously how the study of 42 mammal species revealed that the difference in the chemistry of the brain between species is not its composition but the extent to which it has evolved or degenerated. It is always built with the same materials in the same proportions.

The parent omega-3 essential fatty acid, alpha-linolenic acid, comes mainly from green leaves. The dinosaurs would have enjoyed a great abundance of this, but little linoleic acid, as the flowering plants with their protected seeds would have been tiny and in minimal supply. The oceans are much the same. There are no flowering plants in the oceans, the biology of which is initiated by photo-synthesis; hence the fact that seafoods are rich in omega-3 with relatively little omega 6.

As we have underlined many times in this book, the king of the omega-3 family is docosahexaenoic acid (DHA). It is the universal and irreplaceable and only omega-3 fatty acid used in brain structures. [12] It is essential for nerve signalling, neurogenesis and maintenance. Most interestingly it is highly susceptible to peroxidation, and people have gone as far as to say that it can actually damage the brain because of this. That is not true – Nature pumps it into the foetus during human brain development, and it would hardly do that if DHA was harmful. Nicholas Bazan, who heads the Neuroscience Center in the University of New Orleans, has discovered that Nature has a trick up her sleeve to counteract DHA peroxidation. The brain makes a highly potent antioxidant from DHA, neuroprotectin D1, and in this manner it protects itself. [13]

DHA derived from the green leaf fatty acid is made in a tortuous and slow manner. Nonetheless, the dinosaurs would have had great quantities of its precursor, leafy fatty alpha-linolenic acid, in their diet. We do not know how good they were at converting the green fatty acid into DHA for their brains, though it is unlikely that they were very efficient, if the fast growing animals of today are anything to go by. Animals' capacity for DHA synthesis diminishes with velocity of growth and ultimate body size. Maybe the early, smaller dinosaur species were more efficient in this respect, just as the mice, rats, squirrels and rabbits of today are able to make good amounts of DHA and indeed, have high brain sizes as a proportion of their little bodies. However, as the velocity of protein acquisition and body growth escalated, the capability would have more and more outstripped by the acceleration in deposition of body mass protein. [14]

Even so, before the mass extinction of the K-T boundary, there was an abundance of omega-3 and a paucity of omega-6. The study of the brains of 42 different species at the Institute of Brain Chemistry and Human Nutrition (IBCHN) in its early days at the Nuffield Institute of Comparative Medicine tells us that the right balance of between 2 and 1 to 1 of omega-6 ARA and omega-3 DHA is critical. Without much linoleic and arachidonic acid, the dinosaurs would only have been able to build tiny brains. ARA has a role in glial cells, while DHA is more concerned with neurons and synapses. [15]

## THE RISE OF THE PLACENTAL MAMMALS

After the collapse of the giant gingkoes, ferns and their allies, the flowering plants were liberated and emerged in great profusion. With them came pollinating insects such as bees.

That is, the land food web became enriched with omega-6 fatty acids and, yes, that would have filled the gap of previous systems in the needs for brain growth. Could the availability of the omega-6 fatty acids, in a concentrated form in the protected seeds, have led ultimately to a proper omega-6/3 balance, and a mechanism whereby a larger brain could have evolved, as it undoubtedly did?

For that to happen, there would also have been a need to enhance vascular and immune function. In both, ARA is a major component of the inner cell membrane phosphoglycerides and essential for their function. We remind you again, also, of the 1982 Nobel Prize given to Samuelsson, Bergstrom and Vane was for the discovery of the physiological role of arachidonic acid derivatives and their function in the blood flow and immune function.

We have seen how the placental system is a key to foetal growth in mammals. It may again be no coincidence that the placenta is a highly developed blood system. Linoleic acid, its long-chain derivatives, and prostaglandins are crucially important for the health of the blood system and proper blood flow, muscle development, immune function and cell adhesion. In particular ARA is also dominant in the placenta. [16]

Now we have a brand-new interpretation of the dinosaur collapse and the emergence of mammals. Omega-6 is not essential for reptiles and fish, but is essential for mammalian reproduction. Think about an egg, whether bird or reptile. Everything that is needed is packed into a shell. The fertilised ovum sits in a yolk of food. There is only one squirt of food for the ovum, the embryo and the developing new life. Think now about a mammal. The fertilised ovum develops into an embryo and soon a heart appears, to pump blood around so that organs can develop. The embryo sends out blood vessels to seek food from the mother who in turn sends another set towards the foetus. The result is an entanglement of the blood vessels to form a new organ, the placenta. The placenta then miraculously sets itself up as a gateway determining which components of the mother's blood should be allowed access to the foetus. Once formed the placenta grows swiftly, reaching its peak velocity of growth around the beginning of the third trimester. This is the time when the foetal brain growth spurt begins and, in humans, it will use up 70% of all the energy the mother sends to the foetus! The placenta by now is a rapidly growing network of blood vessels processing vast lakes of blood from the mother and foetus. [17]

## The emergence of the heart and blood vessels in the embryo

One of the most interesting aspects of embryo development is that you can see a formed heart at 24 days after conception. Hence the heart and its connecting blood vessels start work before the foetus is formed.

This early appearance makes great sense, as organogenesis cannot occur without a flow of blood. Put another way, in mammalian development the heart and the blood vessels are critical to everything else that happens. Then again, the placenta takes over as the supplier of energy and nutrients for foetal brain and body growth. All are ArA rich systems.[21]

As we've said before, the visual system and the brain has a high requirement for DHA. The human foetus benefits not just from a supply of mother's DHA, but from the placenta actively selecting DHA from any other omega-3 fatty acids and amplifying its concentration for the foetus. For example, the mother's choline phosphoglycerides are the principle DHA- rich fraction in the plasma, containing about 4-7% DHA, but when this reaches the foetus the level has reached 8-12%. Examining the foetal liver shows the level to have been enhanced again to 10-15%. Finally, on reaching the foetal brain we see the higher content of 18-22%. When it reaches the synapses and photoreceptors, we see the highest levels of all, which in the latter reach some 50%-plus!

At the same time the placenta massively favours ARA over its precursor. The plasma choline phosphoglyceride ARA content may be about 7-9% of the total fatty acids. In the foetal serum it is doubled to 18-20%. However, its precursor linoleic acid

---

21    See proof on line at the time of writing: Crawford MA, Sinclair AJ, Hall B, Ogundipe E, Wang Y, Bitsanis D, Djahanbakhch OB, Harbige L, Golfetto I, Moodley T, Hassam A, Sassine A, Johnson M. The imperative of arachidonic acid in human reproduction. Prog Lipid Res. 2023 Feb 4:101222. doi: 10.1016/j.plipres.2023.101222. Epub ahead of print. PMID: 36746351.

has its proportion slashed by more than half. This process illustrates the selectivity of the placenta to prioritise ARA which will support vascular and immune cell development and growth, and DHA, again to support brain neuron development.

It is a beautiful system for a key ingredient needed for the business of the brain's communication in sensation, seeing, hearing, mood, thought and action. The blood vessels and immune cells are different. Unlike the brain, these are dominated by omega-6 arachidonic acid (ArA). People seldom realise just how significant these specialised cells are. The major fatty acid constituent of the inner aspect of the vascular and immune cell is ARA, not DHA, which is present in relatively small proportions. The blood vessels are lined with endothelial cells which are long and flat. In total the cells weigh 1kg and have a surface area of 4,000 to 7,000 square metres. [18] Lined up they would stretch for 96 kilometres (60 miles).

What is fascinating regarding bio-magnification is that, unlike the mechanism for DHA, the step from mother to foetus for ARA is huge. In the mother you can find about 18% or more linoleic acid in the plasma choline phosphoglycerides and only 7-9% of its product arachidonic acid. Across the placenta the situation is reversed. The product ARA reaches 18-20% in the foetal plasma choline. By contrast, DHA is amplified by the placenta by a small amount. However, by the time it reaches the brain it has been biomagnified sixfold and close to tenfold when it reaches the photoreceptor that will enable the child to see. This selectivity was described in 1976, when it was first called bio-magnification. [19]

This narrative fits with the notion that the heart must develop first, followed by the blood vessels, to initiate and nourish the various organs including the brain. In the last trimester brain growth is so rapid that it consumes 70% of the energy fed to the foetus by the mother. That prodigious feat demands a good heart and set of blood vessels. That means arachidonic acid.

In the early days of foetal development, the heart and blood vessels form. Without them, there can be no growth elsewhere in the foetus. The blood vessels are lined with millions of cells, and the major fatty acid inside these is omega-6 arachidonic acid, which is provided in huge amounts via the placenta. Later in the development of the foetus the emphasis switches to the rapid development of the brain, and the placenta then switches its fatty acid provision predominantly to omega-3 DHA.

The biomagnification of DHA from food to the photo-receptor. At each interface the phosphoglycerides are broken down and re-synthesised with a preferential re-incorporation of DHA.

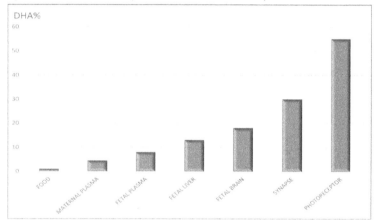

LINOLEIC ACID & DHA PRECURSORS:
Disallowed by the placenta.

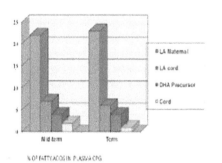

BIOMAGNIFICATION ACROSS THE PLACENTA
Placenta is an AA super pump for vascular development.
(Nb: gradient achieved by selection not conversion).

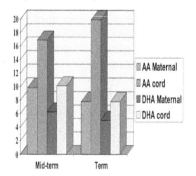

The mammalian reproductive system is, with its continuous flow of energy and nutrients, vastly different to the egg-laying systems of the fish or giant reptiles with their one- squirt-does-all system. Note that there was little restriction on body size with the dinosaurs, but brain size was so small they needed booster systems along their spinal cord to ensure messages to and fro reaching its rear end.

The secret of mammalian evolution, then, was to abandon the strategy of laying eggs and keeping the egg inside the mother until it was ready for life outside the womb. Did the advent of the seed-bearing plants and their components have anything to do with that shift of strategy? Did their nutrients provide the change which made possible the evolution of the optimum balance between ARA and DHA to facilitate the evolution of mammals' larger brains? DHA had been there before, but not ARA. Could the latter have been relevant to the very origin of the mammals, and eventually the big human brain?

## Plant seeds are rich in omega-6, and mammalian evolution requires omega-6 – a coincidence?

### The missing bit of Nature's puzzle to build a big brain
Linoleic acid is essential for mammalian reproduction; and the importance of omega-6 fatty acids in this respect is well embedded in the scientific literature. It was even a topic of the United Nations joint consultation of the FAO and WHO in 1976.[20]

It seems that just as oxygen coincided with the evolution of animals which became dependent on essential amino acids and vitamins, or just as cell organisation and specialisation became dependent on membrane lipids, the arrival of linoleic acid in plant seeds at the K-T boundary, saw the introduction of a new chemical building block – one that coincided with the arrival of a new wave of species dependent on its components for reproduction.

Once we begin to ask what the connection was between nutrient and user, and whether the presence of this nutrient, linoleic acid, could in some way have influenced the arrival of the mammals, we get into very difficult ground. The standard neo-Darwinian answer would be that the series of mutations that produced the mammals was purely random. Similar mutations might well have occurred many times in earlier ages, but since the resulting animals would have been unfit to survive in an environment that did not contain their essential needs they would have immediately died out. There is nothing to quarrel with in that account, as far as it goes. But does it go far enough? Is it plausible? Up to a point, over geological time, maybe. Nevertheless, with the advent of the placental mammals we have an evolutionary explosion which, like the Cambrian Explosion, heralds a new way of life, a new way of reproducing. Was there a more positive influence at work, an active driving force and environment that would explain the sudden all-change? It was not just the new wave of mammals that appeared. There were other newcomers, such as the pollinating insects. The pollinating insects were a vital cog in the system, ensuring that the flowering plants were fertilised and developed those omega-6 linoleic acid-rich seeds.

In due course new forms of life settled into these new conditions. Of these newcomers, the most relevant to us was that revolutionary new family to which we ourselves belong, the placental mammals. Of all the things that distinguished these mammals from any other animals of the same or earlier times, the most significant were their reproductive systems and their brains.

Was the inherent potential for the mammals already there, simply waiting to be unleashed? It is certainly the case that conditions had been changed and were now appropriate to organisms that could take advantage of the products of a new range of plants: a new chemical environment. It would be a far-fetched coincidence if, at the same time, there arrived on the scene animals who depended specifically on a new nutrient found in rich supply in plant seeds. And yet this is exactly what happened.

That nutrient, linoleic acid, is essential for the reproduction of mammals but not, interestingly, for the first vertebrates, the fish. Marine phytoplankton and algae largely produce alpha-linolenic acid and/ or its higher long-chain omega-3 derivatives. This family of essential fatty acids is synthesised in the photosynthetic system, hence its appearance in phytoplankton, algae and green leaves. The first animals to evolve did so in the sea and emerged into a food chain in which these omega-3 fatty acids dominated the nutritional scene for lipids. The balance was not right for a big brain, which also requires omega-6. Up to this point, there were no large brains on sea or land. It is worth noting that the first large land animals had access to huge amounts of protein, giving rise to massive size (i.e. the dinosaurs) but the tiniest of brains – a brawn-over-brain system that still manifests today in animals such as the rhinoceros.

Fish, and probably all the vertebrates that preceded the demise of the giant reptiles, depended on this omega-3 family for reproduction and growth. The mammals depended on omega-6. The proliferation of flowering plants became the key to the evolution of the placenta, the mammals, larger brains and ultimately, *Homo sapiens*.

## DIFFERENCE BETWEEN REPTILES AND MAMMALS

The fundamental difference between reptiles and mammals is that reptiles reproduce by laying eggs. Mammals keep the egg inside. Given a male sperm and a female ovum making contact, the fertilised egg either gets extruded as in the fish, reptiles and birds. Or it sticks to the wall of the mother's uterus and joins with blood flow.

What could make it stick instead of being encased in an envelope of calcium carbonate and extruded? *The simple answer is arachidonic acid.* The omega-6 ARA with its adhesion derivative, which won Bengt Samuelsson his Nobel Prize in 1982, could well have been the trigger that made the egg adhere to the wall of the uterus and so initiate the evolution of the placental mammals. That biochemistry explains the emergence of the mammals coincident with the appearance of an abundance of the omega-6 rich protected seeds of the flowering plants.

In 1930 gynaecologist Raphael Kurzrok and pharmacologist Charles Leib identified prostaglandin derivatives in semen with many powerful functions. Sperm are fascinating because they have a tail that drives them to their destination. The sperm tail is particularly rich in DHA and without the tail it is dead in the water – not going anywhere. We have proposed that a function of DHA in the photoreceptor and synapses of the brain was electrical. It is plausible that its role in sperm tails is similar, with electricity involved in the lashing of the tail which provides the thrust for the sperm to swim to its destination. The presence of prostaglandins in the ejaculate almost certainly provides for muscle contraction which aids the movement of the sperm in the right direction. Hence, we not only see ARA accompanying DHA in the brain, but also in fertilisation.

Bergstrom and his colleagues at the Karolinska in Stockholm in the early 1960s followed up this work and described the prostaglandins that induced uterine contractions. These were first used for therapeutic abortion in May 1969, and they are still used for that purpose today.[28] In the 1960s it was already known that omega-6 essential fatty acids were vital for mammalian reproduction and here was a clear mechanism for one of their actions. It was also found they were involved in cervical ripening. Bergstrom described a leukotriene made from ARA which is produced in the pituitary gland of the female brain and stimulates ovulation: again, a key in reproduction, but notably the work was done in mammals.

Bengt Samuelsson, egged on by the older Bergstrom, described and characterised several such prostaglandins as derivatives of ARA with widely different functions. Thromboxane, for example, caused platelets to stick together and adhere to the blood vessel walls. The signal for its synthesis was collagen or other intracellular material released in response to injury. Hence this action stops us bleeding to death. Moreover, Samuelsson described another group of ARA derivatives called leukotrienes.[29,30] These again had varied functions, with one – LTB4 – causing cell adhesion and movement of white cells from the blood into a site of injury or bacterial infection within cells and tissue, so as to destroy the invaders and allow for repair.

Prostaglandins are lipid compounds derived from fatty acids, ArA in partriular. They have diverse, hormone-like effects, and a huge structural variety that accounts for their different biological activities. A given prostaglandin may have different and even opposite effects in different tissues, determined by the type of receptor to which the prostaglandin binds. Importantly, the presence of prostaglandins in the first place is dependent on a diet containing omega-6 linoleic acid and its conversion to arachidonic acid.

The best-known activity of the other arachidonic acid derivatives is involved in the response to injury by restriction of blood vessels, thrombus formation, white cell infiltration to protect against and kill foreigners, and lipoxins to clear up the mess. They were the first resolvins to be discovered. Bengt's work has been extended by Charlie Serhan of the Center for Experimental Therapeutics and Reperfusion Injury at Harvard, who has described resolvins, also derived from DHA.[31]

Not to be outdone by this stunning and wondrous array of substances for responding to injury, John Vane, and Salvador Moncada discovered yet another derivative of ARA – prostacyclin, for which John shared the 1982 Nobel Prize with Bergstrom and Samuelsson.[32,33] Prostacyclin is made from the ARA in the endothelial cells that line your arteries, stimulated by the beating of the heart and the pressure waves that lead to expansion and contraction (which you can feel in your pulse). The platelets in the blood are being pushed around at speed and high pressure. As they bump into the arterial walls, and especially at the places where their vessels divide, they tend to feel aggravated and start the process of responding to perceived injury. Prostacyclin prevents them from doing this, or from sticking to the cell walls, thus keeping the blood flowing. With another trick it also keeps the blood vessels wide, preventing constriction and a rise in blood pressure.

The endothelium that lines the blood vessels covers an area which, as we said before, in an adult human is equivalent to six football pitches. Moreover, when we analyse the inner cell membrane of this immense network, we find that the dominant fatty acid is ARA. Another feature of this story is the body's defence against anything noxious or living getting into the blood system. The immune cells play a dominant part here. When a baby is born, the membrane lipids are also soaking in ARA ready to participate in any challenge from the new world outside the comfort zone of the intra-uterine sea. There is very little DHA.[34] Put it to the test and you have an army of defenders, killer cells and resolvins at your disposal as soon as you emerge from the womb.

Moreover, as we have commented previously the placenta is a very fast growing network of blood vessels rich in ARA. So much so, it occurred to researchers that perhaps during its growth the placenta accumulated ARA until it reached a critical point at which prostaglandins were excreted and initiated parturition.

Dimitrios Bitsanis, working at the IBCHN, wondered if he could test this idea. By studying the earliest stages of the placenta, from elective abortions at 12-14 weeks, he could compare this with full-term placentas. If, as in the diagram below, the placenta built up its concentration of ARA to term, we would see very low levels in the earliest ones.

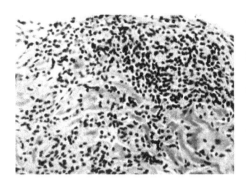
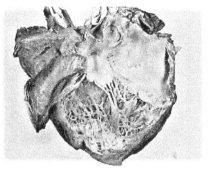

*Arachidonic acid-rich immune cells (the black dots) infiltrating a diseased section of heart muscle from a study of experimental Endomyocardial Fibrosis (EMF) in guineapigs [35]. On the right is a postmortem picture of EMF. The white fibrosis which led to heart failure can be seen at the apex base of the heart. EMF was the most common cause of death from heart disease in Kampala, in contrast to the coronary heart disease (CHD) of the UK. This contrast in nutrition based non-communicable disease included a lack of CHD, breast, and colon cancer in Uganda. This is an example of the thesis of this book on the power and influence of the nutritional environment affecting whole populations*

The placenta is a fast growing vascular network: does arachidonic accumulation result in PG production and parturition.

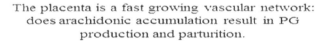

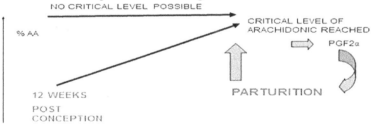

## II. Placenta/embryo Inner Cell Membrane (Ethanolamine) lipids

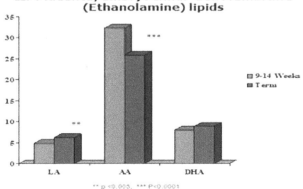

227

The results showed that was *not* the case. Indeed, early placentas were even richer then the term ones. Possibly the supply of ArA was being stretched.[36] You can't have organs developing without a flow of blood, which has to come first.

The relevance of this to the difference between reptiles and mammals should be clear. The reptile extrudes its egg, which develops inside a shell. In a mammal the egg adheres to the uterine wall and blood vessels start to invade the mother and she reciprocates. Thus forms a blood processing system to continuously feed the product of conception. Not just one squirt of nutrients into an egg yolk, but a continuous perfusion for 9 months, in the case of our own species.

When the time comes and the foetus is ready to be delivered, contractions are aided by an ARA derivative PGF2alpha.[37] This prostaglandin has been used for abortions or bringing on labour if the baby is reluctant to make its exit. PGF2alpha and others act by causing the muscles to contract. Once the contractions start, the squeezing of the placenta sets up a fail-proof delivery system through waves of prostaglandins from the ARA-rich placenta with its blood vessels.

The mammals had been evolving long before the collapse of the dinosaurs, although very much on the side-lines. That does not change the argument regarding their proliferation when the flowering plants took over, creating for the first time an abundance of linoleic acid, which could be made into ARA and prostaglandins with adhesive properties, so the egg stuck to the uterine wall initiating the evolution of the mammals. With arachidonic acid as a major component of the vascular cell membranes, it again does not stretch the imagination to envisage the proliferation of blood vessels at the interface of the developing egg and uterus leading to the development of a blood supply in the form of the placenta.

It stretches credibility too far to suggest that these two events – the new abundance of omega-6 fatty acids with their known role in reproduction and blood flow, and the emergence of the placental mammals in great quantity. A food chemical appears in abundance in the food web where it had previously only been present in minimal amounts. At the same time we have the appearance of a group of animals which need that specific chemical for reproduction. This seems to us as again an example of Darwin's conditions of existence. We see here the driving force of chemistry – or, if you prefer, nutrition: nutrition-driven gene expression and epigenetics at work: substrate-driven evolution.

## In summary

The biochemistry explains why and how omega-6 influenced – and was indeed essential to – the evolution of the mammals. Omega 6 is essential for mammalian reproduction – not so for fish and possibly the early amphibians and egg laying reptiles. There is no science fiction here: it is rock solid stuff which won the Nobel Prize in 1982.

Anyway, the point of this discussion is that after the collapse of the dinosaurs, the giant gingkoes, ferns and their allies were replaced by an abundance of flowering plants. Although the gingkoes and ferns are now dwarfs compared to their dinosaur era, they are still with us. Perhaps the bonsai like state of our present gingkoes and ferns is due to the loss of mineral wealth of the soils, by the piss and shit of giant reptiles washed out to sea. Their replacement by the gentler flowering plants with protected seeds, rich in the then novel omega-6 linoleic acid, provided the ArA and its derivative to make the egg stick and so laid the ground work for the evolution of the mammals. The new appearance of the ArA to accompany DHA in neurogenesis, and long gestations, set the stage for the enlargement of the brain. The rest is history.

# CHAPTER 8
# The Origin Of The Big Brain

## Homo vs Heidelberg

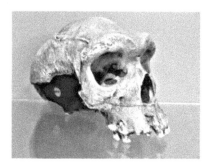 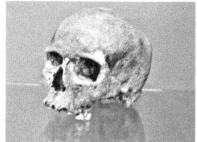

Homo Heidelgergensis. Cat no Broken Hill 1 125,000-300,000 y.a Cranial capacity 1,100cc - ate no fish On the right, early homo sapiens (Cro Magnon) 32,000 y.a. Cranial capacity 1,550 cc ate fish and wore necklaces of sea shells. The Dolní Věstonice 14 at 29,000ya was assessed to be 1,663 cc. Today, the average is about 1,336 cc[22]. We have lost an amount equivalent to the size of the chimpanzee brain with which we started 5-7 mya!

22  Neubauer S, Hublin JJ, Gunz P. The evolution of modern human brain shape. Sci Adv. 2018 Jan 24;4(1):eaao5961. doi: 10.1126/sciadv.aao5961. PMID: 29376123; PMCID: PMC5783678.

# WHEN AND WHERE DID THE BRAIN EVOLVE?

## Every one knows if they think about it.

Everyone knows if they think about it! Life evolved in the sea. The brain had to evolve in the sea. Perhaps most would not be able to put a date on it and anyway what we know is a guess, but it would have had to have been about 500-600 million years ago or more. That is when air breathing life of the sort we are first evolved on our planet. As far as nutrition and the evolving brain is concerned, the only stuff available at the time was stuff from the sea – sea foods.

Another fact that people would know is that those who decide on nutrition and food production policies base their principles on providing us with protein: good for body growth and body builders. Sadly, policy has not caught up with common sense, with its strong support by science. Namely that our biological priority is brain growth, not body growth. The dinosaurs were very good at body growth.

Common sense tells us that it is the brain which makes us different from other animals. We also know there are and were some very big animals as in Jurassic Park, which had very little brain. Body builders buy protein, and protein rich supplements to nourish and build their bodies. So we know protein is good for body growth. Then, if it is the brain not the brawn which characterises us humans, then surely it would be common sense to have nourishment of the brain as top priority rather than protein. So what is good for the brain? Science tells us the brain is mostly made with very special fats. But fats are bad news and a television advert has a couple of young beautiful people tasting a food and shouting with joy "and no fats."

Whoppee!.

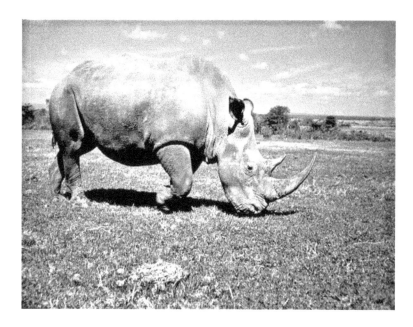

Above is a picture of an animal - a white rhinoceros – taken in Kenya. It reached a 1-ton body weight in four years after birth. It gets all the protein it needs to support that prodigious velocity of body growth from the simplest foods namely, grass. And yes... as the body builders and most of us know, protein is very good for body growth.

But hang about a minute, what about its brain? It is largely made with fats. DHA is a vital component of the eye and the brain's signaling systems. So that means the neurons and synapses where information is processed. The brain evolved in the sea and the marine food web is rich in DHA but the land food web is not. It does have the parent essential fatty acid called alpha- linolenic acid which we cannot make so it has to be obtained in the food. It occurs in the photosynthetic parts of the plants: that means in our green veg. It can be converted into DHA, but it is a slow process. So the faster an animal grows eating green stuff the less DHA it can make. DHA is essential for the brain and hence brain growth. Hence the brains of all the land-based mammals shrank with increasing body size, without exception.

Well, a PhD student of Michael's, Dr. Laurence Harbige, seized an opportunity when a rhino died in London Zoo. "Lets see if our boss is right!!" He says special fats are good for the brain not protein. He persuaded the Chief Veterinary Officer that here was an opportunity not to be missed. With this phenomenal and rapid acquisition of protein rich tissues, would the rhino also have a big brain, inside its huge head? After all it has a huge head. So, they took a bandsaw through the head of the rhino and see for yourself the clear evidence. You must search to find the tiny brain inside this massive head.

Biochemistry then showed the Rhino did not accumulate the special fats including of course DHA, needed to build a large brain. It did not get them from its vegetarian diet. Nor indeed has it evolved an advanced peripheral nervous system such as we have to control our hands or make much DHA!

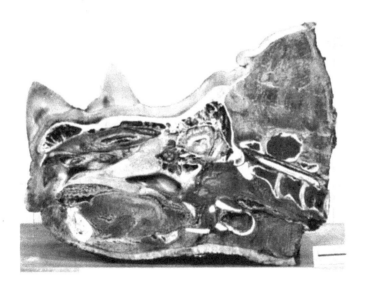

## The Cod in English history

## So what are these fats?

To cut a long story short, remember the brain evolved in the sea so you need to eat foods from the sea of all sorts to grow your brain and keep it in good health. Britain as an island Nation was once a major sea faring nation, which came about from the fishing boats. At the time of Queen Elizabeth, the First, some 50% of the English income came from the fishing, mostly cod from the rich cod banks near New Foundland. Cod muscle (the flesh we eat) has fat in it even if it is small in amount: it contains 47% DHA[1] which we need for our brains,

The cod banks were discovered by Admiral John Cabot (1450-1500) on one of his expeditions. Recovering from a lengthy and severe storm in the North Atlantic he commanded his sailors to wash the decks. They were in a very disgruntled state after a long voyage with no land and being battered and soaked by this lengthy storm. The sailors were deeply unhappy as the decks had already been washed by tumultuous rain and thrashed by massive waves.

The Admiral wanted to assert his authority to prevent any ideas of mutiny. So, they threw their buckets over the side to collect sea water. Then Cabot standing on the bridge, could not understand why all of a sudden there were shouts of joy and roars of laughter. The reason he soon discovered was that the buckets pulled from the sea were full of cod. They had discovered the cod banks. They had been discovered before by Basque fishermen, but they had kept it a close secret. Sadly, that wealth has been eroded and lost to today, although the Icelanders have been busy trying to repair the damage.[23]

## Fats for the brain

Now that we have established that there are different nutritional principles of protein for the body and fats for the brain, what are these special fats? Scientists call them lipids. Just as essential amino acids are needed to make protein, there are essential fatty acids are needed to make the lipids. We have already

---

23    *Cod: A Biography of the Fish That Changed the World by Mark Kurlansky* | *28 Feb 2011*

encountered these essential fatty acids in the discussion of the transition from egg laying to mammals. Like the essential amino acids you cannot make the essential fatty acid (called EFAs for short even if it also means European Fighter Aircraft, they were first!) and have to acquire them in the food you eat.

The snag is there are two families of the EFAs. One starts with linoleic acid which we met in previous chapters in the discussion on the evolution of the giraffe and the appearance of flowering plants and mammals. We saw that the richest source of linoleic acid is in seeds of the flowering plants. Then we met arachidonic acid (ArA) which we make from linoleic acid and is very important for building arteries, keeping blood flowing, in the response to injury, helping to stop the people bleeding to death and then help repair the damage as the precursor of "resolvins"[2,3].

Then the brain needs a lot of energy which is supplied by the blood so arachidonic is important in that respect and funnily enough it is important in the structure of the brain and is importantly concerned with the glial cells which keep the myelin and much of the rest of the brain in order. It occurs in warm water sea foods and in the meat and offal of land-based mammals, birds and birds' eggs.

Then there is the very special marine fat, DHA, which was a key to the origin of vision. It is found in dinoflagellates which have an eye spot. They, or some single-celled, oxygen using thing like them, used it to capture sunlight and turn it's energy into electricity at the beginning of air breathing evolution.

As you know if you ever had an electric shock, electricity makes things jump, When facing towards the sun, that would make our little flagellate jump or at least its tail and hairs twitch and so it would move towards the surface and that is where the food was. That is most likely how the evolution of the nervous system started. The creation of electricity from sunlight is a well-known affair, hence solar panels.

Today, in the photoreceptor of the eyes, the neurons

and synapses you will find the same extraordinary, high concentrations of DHA used to build the cells that now enable you to see, feel, hear, sing, play a musical instrument, think, catch a ball, dance, remember things, work out problems and dream.

It is always the same chemistry, in the nervous systems and brain in all the studies done on the many different animal species. And moreover, workers at the Laboratory of Functional Genomics, Biological Research Center, Hungarian Academy of Sciences, Szeged,, Hungary and the School of Exercise and Nutrition Sciences, Deakin University, Victoria, Australia, have reported that DHA actually instructs the DNA, the genome, to turn on energy use and the synthesis of many constituents needed for brain growth and function[4].

If that is not amazing, there is another amazing fact. Nicholas Bazan and his co-workers, at the Neuroscience Center of Excellence, Louisiana State University Health New Orleans, were concerned that DHA was highly susceptible to oxidation yet was situated in the cell membranes of components that had the highest oxygen use in vision and the brain. The newborn brain uses 60% of the energy from its mother's milk. During the fetal brain growth spurt in the last trimester the brain uses as much as 70% of the energy available to it. So it is a heavy oxygen user which runs the risk of peroxidative damage. Nicholas and his co-workers astounded science by reporting the discovery that DHA makes its own protective molecule. They called it neuroprotection D1[5] and have recently described its importance in recovery from stroke.[6] So this wonderful molecule has its own protective agent.

There is not much DHA in the land food web, and there is really none in the products of intensively produced land foods. So again, we really need to eat our sea foods and as we shall see shortly it would have needed sea and freshwater foods to power the evolution of our brain. from the 340 gram of the chimpanzee to the 1.45 Kg of the Herto people who lived 160,000 years ago before humans became fixated on land based agriculture in the fertile crescent,10,000 years ago.

Incidentally, it is worth noting that the shortage of land-based foods and increasing populations, encouraged the development of agriculture and animal husbandry at the beginning. There was no need to do anything about the fish as the rivers and Mediterranean were seething with them. Their abundance could well have been why Jesus of Nazareth decided to feed the many who gather to hear him speak with loaves and fish..

## Iodine and trace elements are also critical

In addition to essential lipids including DHA, the brain also depends on trace elements such as iodine, copper, manganese, selenium and zinc. These metals form part of the enzymes which protect the brain from peroxidative damage. They are especially rich in oysters and mussels which would have been present in abundance and easily harvested as the many pre- historic, shell middens across the planet testify. Indeed, Google will tell you that " When Henry Hudson arrived in 1609, there were some 350 square miles of oyster reefs in the waters around what is today the New York metro area…..European settlers wasted no time in turning this natural resource into a powerful industry."

And "One million: That's roughly the number of oysters New Yorkers ate, every day, in the mollusks' 19th-century heyday." Again, the richest source of this trace element cluster is in the marine food web. Mussels, oysters and scallops are particularly good sources. These filter feeders are especially rich in iodine, the deficiency of which causes congenital iodine deficiency syndrome and mental retardation. Maternal iodine deficiency during pregnancy can lead to cretinism which can be so severe that the shape of the face and eyes of the new-born are distorted. The reason for the distortion is that the brain which gives shape to the skull, has not grown as it should in utero. Deficiency causes the thyroid gland to swell which is seen by a swelling on the neck. The thyroid hormone uses iodine and is important in energy production, hence critical for the brain[7]. Have a look at the picture taken by a PhD student of Michael's, now Dr Izzeldin Hussein, who was working on iodine deficiency in the Sudan.

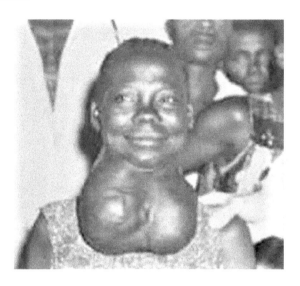

*The above photo taken by Dr Hussein in 2008. After being awarded a PhD for his work Dr Hussein went on to initiate programmes for iodine supplementation in the Sudan and became a member of the international effort to eradicate iodine deficiency[8].*

It gives pause for thought to learn that some 2 billion people are at risk of iodine deficiency. They are almost certainly at risk to DHA deficiency as well. Maybe also deficient in zinc another trace elements. Both DHA, iodine and other trace elements occur together at their richest in the marine food web. The effect must be to cripple brain capital.

The importance of iodine is common knowledge. It was common in the Alps of Switzerland and Northern Italy, but a century ago, and well known to cause mental retardation. Yet, how many people know that the brain cannot be built without DHA? The number of scientific papers which refer to DHA on PUBMED – the data-base for such matters – was 18,474 on the [22] July 2023. Iodine, knowledge of which goes back much further, clocked up 145,282 references, Not all of these papers would have dealt with the brain, but the point is that in science and medicine a lot of attention is given to both DHA and iodine. The number of researchers involved is even greater than just the number of published papers, as most of the scientific papers will have several authors. Moreover, their papers will be read or seen by many more people.

Hence it is both surprising and puzzling to realise that no food policy embraces this knowledge of what is needed for brain health, to make it, enable it to function, and maintain it into old age. It was discussed by and FAO - WHO joint expert consultation in 1976,[9] but few pay any attention even though attention was drawn to brain health in follow-ups, detailing the requirement in pregnancy and for the composition of infant formula in 1994 and 2008-10.

## APE'S 340 cc BRAIN TO EARLY HOMO AT 1,500 cc or more.

So we come back again to this central fact: the brain evolved in the sea 500 – 600 mya when obviously only marine nutrients were available for Nature to work its magic. We know it still requires these nutrients, especially DHA and the trace elements. You just cannot build a brain without DHA and if your mother does do not get enough iodine before you were born, you will be mentally retarded and facially disfigured through congenital iodine deficiency syndrome.

The time has come to return to a subject we touched on in Chapter one: the origin of *H. sapiens.* When it comes to postulating about how an ape with a small 340 cc brain became a human with a large cranial capacity of 1,500 to 1,700 cc around 30,000 y.a. the dominant argument over the last 100 years is based on the Killer Ape theory or Savannah hypothesis.

Since the 1950s adherents of this theory maintain that our ancestors left the forests and hunted game on the savannahs of

Africa. In this environment it is claimed:

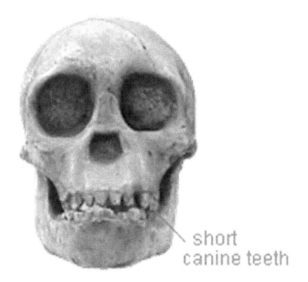

short canine teeth

"*Fierce competition with the top carnivores led to the expansion of the intellect*", to quote Raymond Dart . He discovered and presented the fossil skull of the Taung Child in the 1920s as evidence of the origin of H. sapiens in Africa: He proclaimed "*For the production of man a different apprenticeship [from forests] was needed to sharpen the wits and quicken the higher manifestations of intellect – a more open veldt country where competition was keener between swiftness and stealth, and where adroitness of thinking played a preponderating role in the preservation of the species.*"[10]

One of the arguments to support the Savannah hypothesis was that we assumed our upright stance through the need to stand up and see over the tall grasses to throw spears or shoot arrows at game for food. If that was the case, we must have to be smart already, if we were able to make spears, bows and arrows. So that is a naïve argument and does not work. Moreover, Darwin comments in his book "The Voyage of the Beagle" which is his account of a voyage around the world that ended on 2nd October 1836 when HMS Beagle anchored at Falmouth. He recounts that when the Australian Aboriginals went hunting for game, they crawled forward making themselves almost invisible even on bare ground. Not unlike the way the cats stalk their prey.

Interestingly, those supporting the savannah view of human evolution do not consider nutritional input in any qualitative way that is relevant to the brain. The idea that competition and the need to hunt resulted in adroitness, etc, is baseless. There is no biological mechanism, no science here! Like building anything, the brain needs nutrients to build it in the same way as a house needs bricks. Make no mistake – it is the brain that makes us different from other animals. So, to become *H. sapiens* our ape ancestors had to eat food which contained the building blocks for the brain: it is basic and elementary. The brain evolved in the sea and its building blocks came from the sea. So *ipso facto*, we had to be eating aquatic foods. But anyway, by the time you were able to hunt animals with arrows and spears, you were already quite smart.

Despite the sheer logic and simplicity of stating that we must have evolved beside water which means lakes, rivers, estuaries and coastlines, the Savannah hypothesis supporters have simply ridiculed the idea of any aquatic connection. Some are quite senior in their professions; hence the ridicule is difficult to understand, particularly because it is bereft of any science. Evidence of the controlled use of fire in cooking fish has been carbon date to 780,000 years ago at Gesher Benot Ya'aqov, Israel.

At a meeting, in the Nobel Forum, held at the Karolinska Institutet, Stockholm, Sweden on 4th-6th September 2019., Michael had been invited to give a talk on the brain. An individual, who shall remain nameless to save embarrassment, gave a talk on human evolution. We were told how our ancestors left the forests and evolved a big brain by eating meat on the savannahs. Michael put his hand up to speak; but Birgitta Strandwick got there first. Birgitta works at the Karolinska and has done notable research on cystic fibrosis and bone metabolism. She asked "have you not heard about fatty acids and the need for docosahexaenoic acid for the brain? There is little or none of it in meat. You get it from the marine foods so we had evolve at the coastlines and not the savannahs". To give credit, his response was one of interest, so not all is lost.

And there you have the reality in a nutshell. Large brains require huge amounts of DHA. The sea environment was the only one that could have provided that abundance. Hominids who strayed from the coastal path survived, but the relatively small brains of specimens in the fossil record show how they unwittingly never gained or lost the brain power that defines our their species.

At the same time' we also needed food from the land A crucial part of being a mammal is that you stay inside your mother for several months and it is the placenta that feeds you as a foetus. The fish, reptiles and birds reproduced by laying eggs. The secret to mammalian evolution was that the fertilised egg stayed inside the mother. We have discussed in the last chapter, about the emergence of the mammals coincided with and explosion of the flowering plants with protected seeds. This protected bundle of nutrients contained vegetable oil rich in linoleic acid. Now to repeat, surprise, surprise, we now know mammals require the linoleic acid family of fatty acids for reproduction. These are omega 6 fatty acids. Before that the fish require omega 3 for reproduction and the same would likely have been true for the reptiles.

As we discussed, we now know that arachidonic acid which is made from linoleic acid, produces molecules in the eicosanoid family, which make cells stick. That is of course the first step to becoming a mammal you need the fertilised egg to stick to the mother's uterus. We also saw how the first organ to appear in the subsequent embryo is a heart, essential to push blood around in the blood vessels to enable the embryonic organs to develop. The heart and blood vessels are rich in arachidonic acid.

Then we need to feed the fetus. This is done by the placenta which is and network of blood vessels and is again rich in arachidonic acid. Come to think of it, the birth of the child is traumatic. Not only is it transferred from a greatly protected environment into a world full of potential infective threats, but the artery also that fed it has to be cut. Before we had doctors, midwives and anti-biotics, especially during our evolution, the new life was on its own. So, we find the immune system at birth is particularly rich in arachidonic acid whose eicosanoids are again involved in the regulation of immune function. Then yet again we find arachidonic acid at similar proportions[55] to DHA in the brain[11]. Both DHA and arachidonic acid are needed to build brain structures. Hence the flowering plants, linoleic and arachidonic acid provided the missing piece in Nature's puzzle of how to build a big brain. The brains of the mammals were a major step forward after the small size of the fish, reptile and bird brains which lived before. The absolute essentiality of DHA for vision and the brain has been well researched and has been non-negotiable since the beginning of air breathing life on this planet. Whatever, random mutations or whatever DNA was wanting to do it could not change this chemistry. *It is as though DHA was the master of DNA!* But arachidonic acid was also essential to build brains.

Hence the coincident emergence of a new abundance of flowering plants and the mammals was not a coincidence but a strongly intertwined, event in biological chemistry. The message here of course is that the species which became H, sapiens, would have had to benefit from foods both from the land and the sea. We had the best of both worlds.

There is a mountain of evidence now from experiments, epidemiology, and studies on preterm and term infants supporting the essential role of DHA in vision, memory and cognition, eg the joint expert consultation by FAO and WHO on the Role of Fats and Fatty Acids in Human Nutrition (Report no 91 FAO Rome, 2010, ISBN 978-92-5-106733-8).

The evidence since 2010 has only added to the wealth of information. Preterm birth, is the strongest predictor of brain disorders. The prevalence in the UK and likely the USA is the same if not higher than 1950. That is despite the great advances in science and medicine. With it comes the escalation of mental ill-health. This is a scandal. None of our leaders in the government of the planet seem to care about food policy, nutrition and brain health. There is perhaps some kind of stigma attached to the brain and mental ill-health. A bizarre reluctance to seek information, the science and understand the principles behind the very biological development that made us and make us different from other animals.

Despite the incontrovertible nature of the evidence on a dependence on a marine food web as part of the stimulus which propelled us from a 340 gram chimpanzee brain to the large brain we have today, there have been slings and arrows shot at those who supported the thesis of a need for a connection with the aquatic environments. Vituperation is unintelligent and has no place in science:

Grand Master Ray Keene OBE, wrote in one of his articles[12] that Aron Nimzowitschm, a Lavtvian-born writer and one of the best chess players of the 1920s. (7 November 1886 – 16 March 1935), once wrote: "Ridicule can do much, for instance, embitter the existence of young talents; but one thing is not given to it, to put a stop permanently to the incursion of new and powerful ideas"

## THE SCARS OF EVOLUTION

Elaine Morgan was a Welsh writer of books and scripts for television. Algis Kuliukas wrote a fine book as a tribute to her life and work[13]. She read an article by Sir Alistair Hardy in the New Scientist. Hardy was a marine biologist and he gave a talk at the British Sub-Aqua Club which was published in New Scientist, 17 March 1960, as a short article called "Was

Man More Aquatic in the Past?" Elaine was impressed and considered it made real sense. Aware that the sense had not reached the public mind as it should have done, she wrote a book. "The Aquatic Ape Hypothesis: The Most Credible Theory of Human Evolution". Her defence and extension of Sir Alistair Hardy's notion of a semi-aquatic phase in human evolution was environmental and physiological. It was based on hairlessness unlike the savannah species and more like aquatic mammals, a diving reflex, presence of eccrine glands to control body temperature unlike many savannah species which do not waste water in this way, and that bipedal movement instead of knuckle walking might have been developed from wading and diving for food. It was simply and hotly ridiculed by leading paleoanthropologists.

Had the ridicule contained any scientific merit it might have been challengeable. The feeling was that Elaine "is not one of us" (her background was in the arts rather than the sciences), and moreover a feminist to boot. Her books elicited the same androcentric attitude that denied Rosalind Franklin her rightful co-authorship in the report on DNA as the harbour of genetic inheritance, not to mention the deliberate omission of any posthumous recognition at the Nobel ceremony in 1962 by neither Watson or Crick despite the fact that is was her x-ray crystal photo 51 (which they stole from her lab) and was the key to solving the structure of DNA. .

The problem facing Elaine was that the criticisms and defamation were more to do with hysteria and bigotry than science. There was nothing but hot air and prejudice. Indeed, Elaine at a meeting in Sun City, South Africa in 1998, organised by the late Professor Philip Tobias, pleaded for a simple, evidence-based debate or straightforward, scientific counter to her arguments. Philip was activist for the eradication of apartheid and one of South Africa's most renowned scientists. He held the chair of Palaeoanthropology originally occupied by Raymond Dart, at the University of Witwatersrand. Johannesburg.

In April 2005 Sir David Attenborough hosted a two-part programme "*The Scars of Evolution*." on BBC Radio 4 to explore the controversy and the attacks on Elaine Morgan. Sir David, introduced the programme as follows saying that they looked "*...at the history and current status of the 'aquatic ape hypothesis' (AAH), first proposed 45 years ago by Sir Alistair Hardy, then elaborated and developed by Elaine Morgan and others.*

*The hypothesis proposes that the physical characteristics that distinguish us from our nearest cousin apes - standing and moving bipedally, being naked and sweaty, our swimming and diving abilities, fat babies, big brains and language - all of these and others are best explained as adaptations to a prolonged period of our evolutionary history being spent in and around the seashore and lake margins, not on the hot dry savannah or in the forest with the other apes. The programmes explore the varieties of response to the theory, from when it was first proposed to the present day. Why it is seen by many as a very provoking idea, and at the accumulating evidence of recent years that seems to be tipping the mainstream towards assimilating many of the AAH proposals. Programme two ends with dramatic new biological evidence suggesting that water-birthing was a very early human evolutionary adaptation".*

The first *Scars of Evolution* programme featured Morgan and her many antagonists, and it is fair to say her argument stood up well to the scathing comments levelled at her, largely because her tormentors used mockery rather than science. (The programme can still be heard online).

Elaine was dismissed as just an ignorant, silly woman. Being a non-scientist, everything she said had to be non- scientific mumbo-jumbo. Moreover, she was a feminist. In Attenborough's Scars of Evolution you can hear ridicule in the voice of Leslie Aiello, then editor of the Journal of Human Evolution as she says "...what do they mean? Putting a toe in the water?"

Attenborough started the second part reminding the listener of the controversy surrounding the theory. He commented on

Elaine's presentation and the antagonism against any idea of an aquatic link during our evolution. He then said the foundations of antagonism were shaken by new evidence – "...on the brain". The programme then brought in Professor Michael Crawford, pointing out that the brain requires DHA for its growth construction and, function. That is, it would have been impossible to develop a large brain on the savannahs where there was little DHA to speak of in the food web. Consistent with this fact is the progressively smaller brains of the savannah and woodland mammals as they evolved larger and larger body sizes. On the other hand, DHA is present in abundance in marine foods. The marine mammals were the only large mammals which approached *H. sapiens* in relative brain size.

The logic is so simple and elementary it is amazing how it was dispelled. Unsurprisingly, the brain still requires the same marine nutrients today and makes it clear that we also needed brain specific nutrients from the land – as we say "the best of both worlds"

The brain requires the same nutrients today as it did when it was first evolving in the sea tens of millions of years ago. To imagine otherwise is the same as thinking bones can form without an adequate calcium supply, or that muscle can build to Arnold Schwarzenegger-like proportions without protein. The brain cannot escape what it is – it formed in a rich soup of fatty acids and nutrients, and it needs that same soup today.

## From being small to becoming big

When animals evolved on land, they obviously started out very small and ended up with huge body sizes but not much brain. Triceratops weighed in at 9.4 metric tons but had the tiniest of brains at 70g. Brachiosaurus was even better at 35 metric tons but a mere 154.5g of brain. Apparently, they needed to have power stations along the spine to boost the signals.

The principle of big bodies and small brains on land was

true for the giant reptiles, and it applies to modern land- based mammals too. The placental mammals achieved a greater brain size than the reptiles. Their evolution obviously started off very small and then split into various branches with increasing body size. As we have discussed, a small mammal with a high metabolic rate, had excellent efficiency of converting the DHA essential fatty acid parent in the vegetation, alpha-linolenic acid, into DHA itself and had high brain to body weight ratios.

As they evolved bigger bodies with faster growth rates so the velocity of protein accumulation outstripped their ability to make DHA for the cell membranes. The squirrel for example has a brain to bodyweight ratio of 2.4, bigger than ours! But when we reach the size of the rhinoceros reaching a 1-ton body weight in 4 years, then as we saw at the beginning of this chapter, it really was unable to achieve much in the way of brain size.

The only large mammals that achieved anything approaching *H. sapiens,* were those which had DHA preformed in their food as for example, the Dolphin. To test the hypothesis that preformed DHA was better than having to make it, our colleague, Andrew Sinclair when working at the Nuffield Institute of Comparative Medicine in the 1970s, used different radio isotopes to trace the conversion of alpha-linolenic acid into DHA compared to feeding DHA itself. By analysing the isotope in brain DHA he was able to quantitate how much came from the alpha-linolenic parent or from the preformed DHA. The DHA, as used for the growing brain, performed with 10 times the efficiency of conversion[14].

Tom Brenna, who is head of the Department of Paediatrics', Dell Pediatric Research Institute, University of Texas at Austin, has described how the FADS enzymes responsible for the conversion of alpha-linolenic acid to DHA, operates with different efficiencies, in different peoples. None the less, whatever you are, there is the same preference for DHA preformed[15].

This biochemistry explains why none of the land-based mammals achieved anything remarkable in the way of brain size. DHA built the original signalling systems of the eye and brain right at the beginning and is still essential for the brain and its signalling system today[16,17]. It is predominantly found in the marine food web where it is associated with iodine, copper, iron, manganese and zinc which we discussed earlier are essential for the health of the brain.

So it is no surprise to see that the mammals with the largest relative brain size are found in the sea: that is apart from *H. sapiens*. Body size for body size, the marine mammals have fared far better than their land-based cousins. As we are at pains to point out, the lion, a land-based carnivore has a similar bodyweight to a dolphin, a marine carnivore. The lion has only 320g or so of brain.[18] The dolphin brain weighs 1.7kg. Admittedly the dolphin only uses half of its brain most of the time whilst the other half sleeps. If it let the whole brain sleep it would drown. None the less they are considered to be intelligent, have a good capacity for learning and can recognise themselves in a mirror, an apparently sure sign of high intelligence. Both the Russian and US Navies have trained dolphins for use in war. It is known they were trained to detect swimmers and mines but what else is secret? The Romans used them to coral fish. Indeed the Romans were keen of fish and sea foods as they are to this day. A Roman Senator used his slaves to peel oysters to feed the fish in his fishpond. Another cut a tunnel in a hill so he could pump fresh sea water for the fishpond in his summer residence.

## We are born with a waxy layer of vernix caseosa

In the concluding moments of *Scars of Evolution* Sir David muses on *vernix caseosa*, a waxy layer that covers the skin of a newborn baby. It appears on the foetus at around 18 weeks after conception. No primate other than humans, nor any other land mammal, he says, is born with vernix. When he first heard of this peculiarity, Attenborough wondered if marine mammals were born with vernix, which would seem sensible for an animal born in water. However, the professors he contacted on the subject could shed no light.

Just two weeks before *Scars of Evolution* was due to be aired, Sir David received a phone call from a professor in British Columbia. He had heard that Attenborough was interested in the subject of vernix and marine mammals. Yes, he said, the harbour seal is indeed born with vernix. He had handled newborn pups, and each time his hands became covered in a waxy substance. The programme ends there, hanging in the air assumedly Attenborough leaves you to draw your own conclusion. However, we can now add to the story.

A close friend of ours, Tom Brenna of Austin, Texas, who we mentioned earlier, is a world class, expert in mass- spectrometry which is used to identify single substances and groups of substances with robust identifications. Previously head of biochemistry at Cornel University, his expertise was such that he has been called in to analyse samples from athletes accused of doping.

One day we discussed this vernix question with Tom. So off his own bat he did just go and do the analyses of human vernix and that of some marine mammals. The data was presented at a meeting in Stockholm in June 2014 and has since been published in the peer-reviewed literature.[19] Vernix turns out to be a complex mixture of waxes and fats. Despite its considerable complexity human vernix has the same chemical composition as the three marine mammals Brenna studied. No more really need be said.

## Disbelief in homo aquaticus

The story of *vernix caseosa* seems to us to be a clincher. It can only be explained by a relationship with water at some distant, formative time in the past. How else could this have happened?

The children of the Austronesian tribe called the Moken are born to a semi-aquatic lifestyle. The Moken children wean themselves with food gained from diving to the seabed. They learn to walk on land at four years of age. The Moken have remarkable underwater visual abilities and can see stuff other people cannot see even with goggles.[20]

The point here is that while the Kalahari Bushmen or the Hadza hunters and gatherers are often quoted as evidence for the Savannah hypothesis, here is evidence of a different sort illustrating a connection between *H. sapiens* and the sea. Moreover, it is evidence which connects with the present day, in the prenatal preparation and birth of new members of our species. Moreover, newborn babies can swim. They have to learn to walk on two legs.

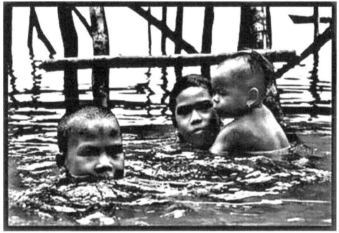

*Picture from Anna Gislen Department of Cell and Organism Biology, Zoology Building, Lund University, Helgonavägen 3, Sweden.with serious thanks*[21]

The photo below, is courtesy of British Gas, Originally, it was used in an advertisement. Michael saw it and asked for a photo which was gladly given. Newborn babies if submerged, can hold their breath underwater and paddle with apparent nonchalance. On reaching the surface, they put the head on one side and breath again. A healthy newborn carries a lot of fat which helps with being in water, especially sea water. This likely does not work with a low birthweight or brain damaged infant.

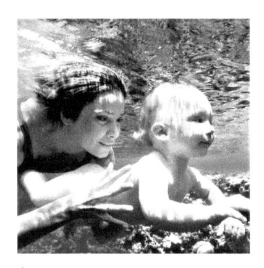

Tom Brenna might have found that the chemistry of human vernix was different to that of the marine mammals he studied. But he did not. To all intents and purposes, they were identical. It is difficult to beat that revelation. Mark you, there is probability that the vernix arose with the evolution of mammals as the fetus, after all has to grow in a water filled cave. It is likely that birth association with water would have emphasized the trait. It is possible that a hippopotamus is born with some vernix or even a dog if one looked carefully enough. No one thus far has looked. On the other hand, you do not have to look carefully to see the vernix in the newborn human or in marine mammals. It is a striking feature.

As we have already mentioned with reference to the "Scars of Evolution", The weight of the physiological evidence, was suggested by Sir Alistair Hardy in a talk at the British Sub- Aqua Club in 1960 (subsequently published in the New Scientist under the title "Was Man More Aquatic in the Past?"[22]). Now the evidence of vernix, makes one agree with Algis Kuliukas of the University of Western Australia who commented on the cynicism of the Savannah hypothesis adherents:

*It just shows me that the only argument they have against the AAH (aquatic ape hypothesis) is to amplify it to such an extreme point that it becomes absurd. If they take it as it was originally intended, it is simply irrefutable.*[23]

One reason for disapproval of the water-edge hypothesis is that it does not fit with Crick's Central Dogma. In a way, the Dogma was no different from Weismann's 'all sufficiency of natural selection' (which we discussed in Chapters 2 and 3). It was all part of the 'Modern Synthesis' which was at the root of the Savannah Hypothesis mind-set. It was a concept based on fierce competition on the African savannahs furnishing the laboratory which led to the emergence of *H sapiens* as the alpha species: shades of *"We are the greatest"*! It was an idea that suited the patriots of Victorian Britain; and a world map dominated by the red colour of the British Empire surely affirmed that they were indeed the greatest! Being genetically superior is a powerful and self-serving idea.

The enthusiasm that surrounded the Human Genome Project acted as a bastion of support for that lingering mind- set. With so much hope involved in the gene-centric story one can understand how. There is of course, nothing wrong intrinsically with gene studies and applications which have promise of much benefit to gene disorders and health.

## Sir David Attenborough is attached because he chaired a conference on the aquatic origin theory

In May 2013 an international conference was held in London, *"Human Evolution: Past, Present and Future: Anthropological, Medical & Nutritional Considerations"*. It was organised by the late Dr Peter Rhys Evans of the Royal Marsden Hospital in London, along with several colleagues. Sadly Philip Tobias, one of the greatest figures in palaeoanthropology and a supporter of the aquatic link, had just died. Elaine Morgan was unable to attend due to ill-health and she too died a short while later. In spite of these high-profile absences, the scientific evidence presented by many well recognised scientists was overwhelmingly in favour of the aquatic or waterside hypothesis.

The conference brought distinguished scientists from across the world to present evidence. Chaired by Sir David Attenborough the conference, despite the presence of doubters, basically vindicated Alistair Hardy-Elaine Morgan's position and extended it with further evidence.[24]

The conference ended on a sombre note with Attenborough summing up and commenting on the implications for the future. Note: the predictive value of the Savannah hypothesis is nil as it is based on random mutation, and randomness does not lead to prediction. By contrast the aquatic hypothesis is based on science with its predictive value. It predicts for example, that if fish and sea food consumption of a population, falls significantly, then intelligence would diminish, and disorders of the brain increase. This we will see later is just what has been happening recently.

At the conference, Sir David discussed the rise in global population as the most serious threat facing humanity. He has been consistent in his approach to population. In his foreword to the book "*The Earth in Danger – Pollution and Conservation*" by Ian Breach and Michael Crawford, he wrote:

*...the root cause of our ecological problems is overpopulation... Whereas at one time men could easily find space for their homes and had no difficulties in finding the raw materials... today we have overrun the Earth and carelessly devastated vast areas of its surface denuding it of valuable resources to meet our short term purposes... Now there are so many of us that the seas and the sky are not big enough to cope with the overwhelming quantities of waste and we are choking in our own filth. The yearly increase in population shows no signs in slackening, but it cannot continue*

*indefinitely without ending in disaster.*

He wrote this in 1976 before holes in the ozone layer and global warming became common parlance. The population was about 4 billion. Since then the global population has boomed, reaching 6 billion in 2000, 7 billion in 2011, and rapidly approaching 8 billion and counting. At the time of writing Sir David appears on the Wellcome Trust website saying much the same, but with added urgency, and with the crisis of climate change added to his warnings.

Meanwhile, Elaine Morgan's critics now had a new target. After the 2013 conference *The Times* ran the headline *"Attenborough under attack"*[25]. The article begins "Scientists rounded on Sir David Attenborough yesterday for lending credence to the theory that humans evolved in water".

This is a typical example of ridicule under false pretences. No one said humans evolved in water. The thesis is that we evolved at the water's edge. Most great forests have rivers flowing through them, so the apes would have had access to waterborne foods from the beginning. For example, water snails and other water creatures, water weeds, and algae such as spirulina were in huge supply for the populations living around Lake Chad, Congo.[24] The aquatic foods of the lakes and rivers of Africa still today provide brain foods including DHA.[26] Thus via a progression from rivers and lakes our ape ancestors would have made it to the coasts. The sheer abundance of the food resources in the estuaries and coastlines at that time would have been staggering. Moreover, the food would have been so easily accessible. Lessons would have been gained from the sea birds opening oysters and diving into the water to catch fish, enticing our ancestors to investigate more than the rocks. Off the coast just south of Mombasa, in Kenya, the shallows of the water, behind the reef were in Michael's days, teaming with fish

24    Being shallow, Lake Chad has seen great variation in size over the years; but at its largest, before 5000 BC, it is estimated to have covered approximately 1,000,000 km$^2$.so what it would have been like a million or more

and sea food. If you stood still for a moment only waist deep, the fish would come and nibble at your feet. Wading out deeper or swimming in the waters, kept calm by the reef at low tide, you could look down at rocks and spot the feelers of the cray fish twitch out from the holes. This was the 1960s, years ago. It simply boggled the mind with its beauty and abundance.

One could imagine the boss of the troop of apes that stumbled on an estuary or the reef protected coast, saying "Hey people, we don't have to climb trees any more".

The Times' article commenting on the conference said Sir David claimed *"that the theory made more sense than the conventional "savannah" narrative, and provided a further incentive to conserve the oceans and marine life today."* Quite right,

He is further quoted as saying that *"Gathering molluscs is far easier than chasing elephants and wildebeests across the savannahs."* Also absolutely correct! See also David Marsh on Water's Edge Evolution.[27,28]

Dr Todd Rae, a renowned expert on primate evolution at the University of Roehampton, UK, laments in the article in the Times Newspaper that the evidence *"...flew in the face of reason!"* He affirms that *"Adding in an aquatic phase in the evolution of people is like adding yo-yo strings to gravity to explain the movement of planets".*

Funnily enough "string theory" does incorporate gravity and becomes a candidate to provide a much sought- after theory of everything. Perhaps Dr Rae should have chosen a different analogy if the intention was to rubbish the aquatic thesis! Perhaps he should also have attended the conference and then challenged the evidence with other evidence, or perhaps even logic rather than vituperation.

Dr Joe Parker, an evolutionary biologist at Queen Mary University, London, was equally dismayed: the hypothesis was *"seriously flawed"*, he said. *"If our transition to an aquatic or semi-aquatic environment was so successful, why aren't we still there?"* That at least is a question, and it can be answered. We *are* still there.

Sixty percent of the global population lives beside rivers, lakes or the sea coasts. There are two billion people today at risk to iodine deficiency, the simplest way to make people mentally retarded. None of these are to be found in the fishing villages! The high spots of iodine deficiency are inland. The richest source of iodine is in the marine food web where it co-exists with DHA and other marine nutrients important for the brain. And where do many go on their holidays? Look at the window of any tourist office and you will see a galaxy seaside resorts on offer with glossy pictures of sand and sea. They go to swim, play on the water and enjoy fresh seafood? We are still there.

## Incontrovertible Evidence of the first humans using the marine foods

John Parkington[29,30] and Curtis Marean[31] have given us incontrovertible evidence that humans were exploiting the marine food web at their earliest emergence from South Africa. Stone hand axes have been found in oyster reefs on the coast of Eritrea, too.[32] Chris Stringer of the British Museum presented evidence in his paper, *Coasting out of Africa*, showing how humans populated the planet by migrating around the coastlines.[33]

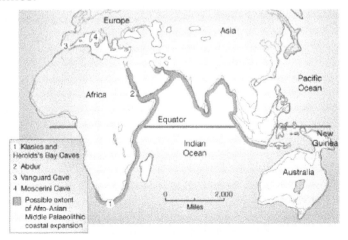

In Helsinki, Finland, the museum contains a fishing net. It was found preserved in a bog. It is 35 m long 1.5m deep, with Sinkers & Floaters: dated to 10,000 years ago. The museum describes the culture of extensive use of the marine food web which included conservation management of the seal populations following an excessive over kill. On the rocks beside the Alta river in northern Norway there is a collection of rock art depicting various ways of catching fish including the person with a fishing rod and a line drawn all the way down the cliff face to a whale or some other large marine mammal at the bottom. Then there is the fishing boat below with the mother holding aloft her lobster pot just like the man in the campanion picture taken on the beach of Dar-es Salam in 1963.

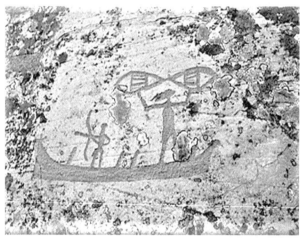

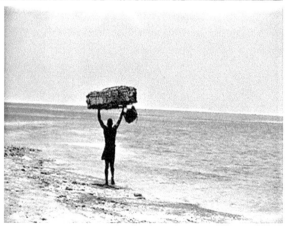

The fishing net dates to a time when people in the Fertile Crescent were abandoning hunting and gathering and busy domesticating plants and animals. They also had access to the great rivers, the Euphrates and the Nile which would have had an abundance of fish, a fact that was true until recent time.We also have evidence of the five original written languages being developed beside water.

Origin of the five written languages were beside water.
(Yangtse, Euphrates, Nile, Ganges & Tiber)

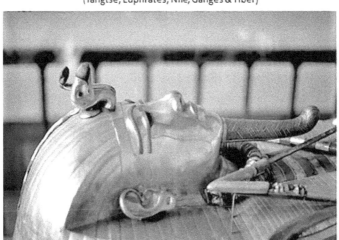

Photo taken by Michael, Cairo Museum 1965

Australia was almost entirely occupied around the coast (beginning more than 50,000 years ago). In more modern times people have excavated the sewers of Herculaneum, which tell of the rich seafood diet of the Romans. (Tragically, in stark contrast we have the modern sewers of London blocked by 'Fat Burgers', with the biggest of them all, in 2017, said to be as heavy as 11 double decker buses.[34])

In the Museum of London, you can see amphora which the Romans used to transport fish oil from Spain to London. In London at the beginning of the 1800s, Lord George Cavendish built a shopping arcade around one wall of his garden, as he was fed up with people throwing their empty oyster shells over his garden wall. In 1900, the barmen in the East End of London provided oysters from the Thames estuary free with the purchase of beer. Today you have the Moken tribe, who we mentioned earlier, as a relic of coastal occupation along the coasts of Thailand, the Philippines, Sabah, Malaysia, Brunei, Indonesia and parts of Sarawak. They still live virtually in the sea and subsist on its food, free from malnutrition and iodine deficiency which is returning in the UK school children.[35] You could write a whole book about this aspect of our story alone! The simple fact is that *H sapiens* could not have arisen without a rich source of DHA, iodine and the other trace elements so poor in the savannah food web and so rich in the marine foods. We would not be here without DHA and aquatic foods.

All of which makes the knee-jerk reaction of *The Times*, attacking Attenborough without attending or having heard the evidence, very disappointing. *The Daily Mail* took a saner approach, referring to the London conference as "*... the resurfacing of a theory after years of being drowned out by scornful academic laughter*". It included a picture of two human babies swimming under water, as they are able to do after birth. Indeed, it can be said that we are all born able to swim under water and only later learn to walk on land. *The Daily Mail* adds this quote:

*"Apes sink like rocks," says Ohio State University chimpanzee specialist Professor Sally Boysen. "They don't have much body fat to help flotation, and they have dense muscle and a heavy, robust skeletal system. If you were to drop an infant orang-utan in water, it would sink to the bottom. A human baby, however, will close its larynx and automatically paddle its arms and legs."* [36]

Much of what favours occupation of the ecological niche at the waterside is actual hardnosed science depending on experimental and human clinical studies. To specify:

the distinguished set of scientists at the London, evolution conference included Marc Verhaegen and Mario Vaneechoutte, presenting evidence from anatomy and physiology, including the bone cortex for aquatic adaptation. Dirk Miejers discussed the physiological reflexes in Homo attuned to diving and swimming, Pierre-Francois Peuch discussed fossil and modern dental evidence consistent with fish consumption. And Kathlyn Stewart described how much hominid fossil evidence is linked to water. The uniqueness of our fat storage, which is akin to marine mammals, was tackled by Stephen Cunnane, who described the vital role of fat biology in meeting the energy requirements to fuel a big brain and float a newborn child. Leigh Broadhurst of the USDA, Beltsville, MD, USA, gave the fossil evidence in relation to aquatic foods which leads to the highly specific molecular biology of nutrient requirements for brain development. Conference organiser Peter Rhys Evans talked of how *"Surfer's Ear Provides Hard Evidence of Man's Aquatic Past".*[37] The conference ended with a session on the global crisis in food security implications for the future of mankind. This line- up of evidence was dismissed by critics as flying in the face of reason and seriously flawed. Clearly the accusers should have attended the conference.

## CONCLUSION

### "We Were Profoundly and Unutterably Wrong"

A few simple words of wisdom can help crystallise acres of debate and knowledge. The late Philip Tobias, was one of the greatest paleoanthropologist alive. He organised 2,000-strong conference in Sun City, SA in 1998. It was at the 'Dual Conference' of paleoanthropologists and biologists. It included a session with Elaine Morgan, Marc Verhaegen, Leigh Broadhurst, Stephen Cunnane and Michael Crawford. It was here that Morgan challenged the deriders to come up with science rather than derision. Tobias sat in the audience and at the end, he summed it all up neatly saying: "Wherever humans were evolving they had to have water to drink." He then declared, as he had apparently declared on a previous occasion: "We throw the savannah hypothesis out of the window." The evidence presented strengthened Tobias' convictions. Back in 1995 at the Daryll Forde memorial Lecture at University College, London, he had declared "We were finally and utterly debunking." [38]

*Philip Tobias at the McCarrison Society's conference in 2000 at the lecture hall of the Zoological Society of London. "The revenge of the Taung Child" following its original dismissal in 1925 by Sir Arthur Keith, who was in favour of Piltdown Man –"We have evidence of human origins here in England!"*

It takes a great man, and in this case one who grew up under the mentorship of no less a figure than the great anthropologist Raymond Dart, and who inherited Dart's Chair at Wits (University of the Witwatersrand, Johannesburg) to make such an about turn in his later years. Lesser mortals might take note – there is still time! Moreover, it is important to understand the force which propelled encephalization as it tells us about what the brain needs for health and is relevant to the escalation of mental ill-health today.

The brain evolved in the sea starting with vision which turned the photons from the sun into electricity. We can analyse the structure which does that in single cell representatives of that time 600 million years ago, which are living today. They are rich not just in DHA but double DHA molecules as are in the photoreceptors of our eyeballs today.

This extreme conservation of DHA in photoreceptors has been found in the fish, the squids, amphibia, reptiles, birds, and all mammals so far studied. Similarly, DHA is found to be present and as a functional component of the brain in neurons and synapses in an identical composition across again all mammalian species so far studied. With experimental studies and epidemiological evidence telling of its importance not just to vision but also to learning and cognitive function. This is a supreme witness of the essentiality of DHA for the brain.

It is time for recognition of our bio-chemical heritage, which began in the sea 600 million years ago, handed down through time. Doubtless the expansion of our brains was supported by making use of the abundance in the warm coastal waters of Africa and the bounty of land, giving our ancestors the best of both worlds. The wild foods they ate helped shape our genetic heritage since we parted from the great apes.. The evidence on the role of the aquatic food web, presented in this chapter has a predictive value absent from the Savannah hypothesis. The latter involves inductive reasoning in contrast to the deductive logic of the aquatic thesis. We ignore the simple logic deduced from the chemistry of the brain and its origin in the sea at our peril.

## POST SCRIPT

On a happy note, on Elain Morgan, the miner's daughter, has been honoured by a bronze statue of her in her home town Mountain Ash, Rhondda Cynon Taf.. The statue was unveiled by her sons, Gareth and Morien Morgan in the 18th March 2022. It was designed and created by the sculptor Emma Rodgers. The BBC said that the bronze statue is not just a figure of Elaine Morgan, but includes elements that point to her life and career, where she excelled in both the arts and science. She wrote well-loved dramas including How Green Was My Valley and The Life and Times of David Lloyd George and several books including The Descent of Woman which was an international best seller. Elaine Morgan challenged the scientific establishment with a new theory of human evolution as we have described above. Elaine Morgan's son, Gareth Morgan, said "his mother's work had inspired women everywhere".

## CRO-MAGNON AND CONCLUSION

After 50,000 years before present, there was a rapid cognitive and cultural expansion of Homo sapiens into Europe. With the ice age, they faced the challenge of varying temperatures often below freezing with brief summer weather. They had a widely diverse and sophisticated blade technology. They hunted reindeer and small animals for food, skins and fur for clothes and boots. They fashioned tools which included spear throwers, bladelet technology for knives, chisels, spear points, harpoons tipped with bone points, and long needles for sewing garments for multi-layer clothing enabling them to be comfortable when out in severely cold weather. They are known to have occupied caves along side rivers, where animals came to drink and where they had access to the salmon runs which they caught in large numbers and dried for eating later, there would also have been a constant supply of other fish. They wore decorations made from seashells. Their caves are famously painted with artworks[25]. Cranial capacities reported were larger than today

---

25      Cro Magnon life is elegantly  described by Professor Brian Fagan of the Inverarity of Califormia, USA.
ttps://www.bing.com/videos/search?&q=cro+magnon.u-tube&docid=60350914
2102675070&mid=62C7B17D2E930901F57C62C7B17D2E930901F57C&view=d
etail&FORM=VDRVRV&ajaxhist=0

and the people are sometimes referred to as *Homo superior*.

How the cognitive capacity of these people compares to the earlier anatomically modern humans at Pinnacle Point or Herto or even with present day humans is difficult to assess.

The cranial capacity of skulls of that period have been assessed at as much as 1,700cc. Today, the average is about 1,336 cc. The brain has been and is shrinking.

e.g.

- **Geologic Age:** 32 Ka 30 Ka, **Discovery Date:** Mar 1868
- **Discovered By:** Louis Lartet & Henry Christy
- **Discovery Location:** Abri Cro-Magnon, Les Eyzies, France
- **Cranial Capacity:** <1,600 cc
- **Specimen Age:** Adult. **Sex:** Male

See also 1,660 cc at *www.prehistoric-britain.co.uk/brain-capacity*

We have lost a chunk of the brain nearly the chimpanzee size of about 340cc, with which we started with 5-7 m.y.a. It is argued our brains have become smaller but more condensed and more efficient. However, the escalation of mental ill health and decline in IQ since 1950 belies this excuse.

The physiological force which powered that increase in brain size could only have come from *wild foods.*

Wild food will have included foods both from the seas, rivers and lakes and from the land. That is, the omega 6 foods from the land essential for human reproduction, and the omega 3, especially DHA from the sea, which is required for making the signalling systems of the brain that enable us to think, reason, touch, dance, talk, and dream.

It can only be the failure of the modern food system to supply the ingredients required for brain growth, function and maintenance that can explain the shrinking brain and shrinking intelligence.

There is a precedence for the reversal of brain evolution

which we have already discussed. Small land mammals like the squirrel have a high brain to bodyweight ratio at 2,4%. As the land-based mammals evolved larger and larger bodies so brain size in relation to the body size, shrank, without exception. The small mammals were able to make DHA from the parent fatty acid alpha-linolenic acid that occurs on land in green foods and some beans. But the rate of synthesis is limited. Hence increasing velocities of body growth outstriped this ability leading to deficiency of DHA and shrinking brain size.

We site the rhinoceros which achieves a bodyweight of one ton in four years after birth. It gets all the protein it needs from the simplest of vegetable foods, namely grass. But its brain is no more than about 350cc which is less than 0.04% of its bodyweight. They do not have the marine, brain specific nutrients which have served the evolution of the brain in the sea for over 500 million years. Unlike the squirrel at 2,4% they cannot make enough DHA.

As no Government pays attention to the requirements for the growth and maintenance of the brain, this situation is hardly surprising but can be corrected.

### "The Global Crisis in Brain Health"

This book describes the role of the environment and nutrition in the evolution of the brain. This included the fact that the brain evolved in the sea 500 or so m.y.a.identifying the importance of sea foods. It was wild foods, including aquatic foods that powered the evolution of our primate brain from the 340cc to the 1,600 or so cc of 28,000 y.a. In recent time, with no attention to the requirements for the brain, it has been shrinking, mental ill-health escalating and IQ falling.

In the Spring of 2023, the European Brain Council's Brain Awareness Week, at last, recognized that "Brain health conditions have become a global health emergency". A key theme of the meeting "was the need to grasp the extent of the problem,"

Recognition of the crisis in brain health was recognized over 13 years ago. Five audits of the burden of ill-health have *brain disorders as the highest cost,* EU 2005, 2010, UK DoH 2007, 2010. The Welcome Trust 2013.

At a meeting of the US military in Washington DC, 2013, to discuss the crisis in brain health and the implication of DHA, fish, and seafood, to brain health, the chairman, Vice Admiral Richard Carmona who had served as the seventeenth Surgeon General of the United States, said *"We do not have time"*[26]. Ten years later with no action, that message is even more important and we will refer to it again.

May we remind the reader that in 1972 Graham Rose on the 5th of November wrote in his review of What We Eat Today[27] in the Sunday Times, that unless action was taken to care for the nutrition of the brain *"We will become a race of morons!".* He understood the message of the book. 51 years later and no action, that prediction is being proved true.

This reversal in the evolution of our brain is a more serious threat to the sustainability of humanity than global warming important as that is. Action is needed now. We shall present some solutions next.

### Footnote

*We are grateful to Dr. Kathlyn Stewart of the Canadian Museum of Nature, P O Box 3443, Stn. D., Ottawa K1P 6P4, She brought the casts of the skulls for the exhibition organized by Stephen Cunnane at the 2010 celebration of DHA at the Royal Society of Medicine where we photographed them.*

---

26   *Mil Med (2014) volume 179(11S): PMID: 25373088*

27   *pages 147-148 in "What We Eat Today" By Michael and Sheilagh Crawford, Neville Spearman, London. UK 1972, SBN 85435 360 7.*

# CHAPTER 9
# The Three Crises

**Humanity faces three crises:**

1. Exponential population growth, with limits to food and fresh water
2. Pollution and irreversible climate change
3. The global rise in mental ill-health and the decline in IQ

These issues are existential threats to the survival of humanity, but they are brushed under the carpet as we all go about our daily lives and politicians make hollow reassurances or denials. In spite of grassroots environmental movements and sobering mental health statistics, there is still no real sense of urgency except amongst the few. Never before has the phrase 'action not words' been so pertinent. Never before has the need for action and fundamental change been so strong; but what would it actually take to muster the required focus, cooperation and willpower to act? The pandemic of Covid-19 and its inequality of mortality is a wake-up call. But it has been use as a scape goat for the inequalities of health that abound.

In 1985, during the Cold War, US President Ronald Regan asked Soviet Union Premier Mikhail Gorbachev if the Soviets would set aside differences and assist the US if it was attacked by aliens from outer space. "No doubt about it", Gorbachev replied, and Regan concurred that the US would do the same for the USSR.[1]

In a Jimmy Kimmel Live TV interview in 2014, former US President Bill Clinton commented on the possibility of an extra-terrestrial species invading Earth. "It may be the only way to unite this increasingly divided world of ours", he suggested. It is divided and fractured even more so today.

In the context of the Presidents' musings, the prospect of extra-terrestrials carries an implied threat of annihilation. Individually, the three crises we are currently facing threaten us with annihilation. Combined, the implications are terrifying. Set this challenge beside the fact that the single greatest investment being made today globally is in making things that kill people. It is time to change that. It is time to invest in the security of life on this planet.

Never mind alien invasions – it is time for Russia, America, China, India, Japan and the rest of us to put aside their differences and tackle these challenges here and now. With the Ukraine in flames and Russia pilloried with sanctions from the West, the prospects of a united East and West seems forlorn. Moreover, the threat of a third world war turning nuclear the stakes could not be higher. The possibility of nuclear annihilation of life on the planet was one of Professor Stephen Hawking's deep concerns for the future. We shall come to the escalation of mental ill-health in the last chapter, but for now, it never is too late for rapprochement. It is the fate of all our children that is in the balance.

## The population crisis

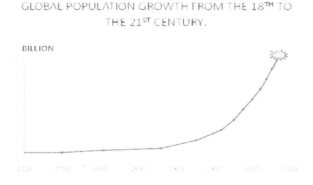

GLOBAL POPULATION GROWTH FROM THE 18TH TO THE 21ST CENTURY.

Population growth is the elephant in the room in any debate about the future. On a planet of finite resources, the rate of growth is unsustainable. To pretend that we can somehow accommodate ever-growing numbers, no matter how high they rise, is collective idiocy.

The global population was 1 billion in 1804. It took 123 years to reach 2 billion in 1927 and another 33 years to reach 3 billion in the 1960s. David Attenborough wrote about his concern in 1976.

*"It cannot continue indefinitely without ending in disaster"*[2]

By 2000 the world population had reached 6 billion and it then took only 11 years to add another billion. Although increased wealth is usually associated with reduction in population growth, nothing will change in the next 20 years. Human population growth is exponential and is built on the previous accumulation of people. The already stretched food and freshwater resources present a major global challenge.

In 2011, The UK think tank Foresight, in *global future of food and agriculture*[3], claimed we had reached the limit of land available for arable use. The report was based on input from 400 experts across the world and was two years in preparation.

While protein was discussed, there was no mention of DHA and the other brain-specific nutrients required for brain structure, growth and function – a gap in knowledge and understanding that will be all too familiar to readers by this stage of the book. The oceans as a potential saviour was not discussed.

Some 70% of your brain cells were created before you were born. The supreme importance of the mother, even before conception,[4] should be at the very centre of health policies. A joint expert consultation of the Food and Agriculture Organization of the United Nations (FAO) and the World Health Organization (WHO) held in Geneva in 2008 recommended 200 mg DHA per day during pregnancy or 250mg per day of a DHA and EPA mix. This was to support pre-natal brain growth and fetal health. Get maternal nutrition and health right at the start of life, and much of the worst of the non-communicable disorders will be dealt with. In World War Two in the UK, every pregnant or nursing mother was given milk, orange juice and cod liver oil, delivered free to her front door by the milkman. Whether or not this would be considered the best approach today is immaterial. It shows that people had a thoughtful approach. Today, we have much more knowledge but no action. The lack of active driven interest shows up in the health inequalities we have today. The highest prevalence of low birthweight and preterm birth, which carry the highest risk of children being born with brain damage, mental ill-health and behavioural and learning disabilities, is amongst the Black and Asian minority ethnic groups (BAME).[5] At the time of writing, the media is regularly reporting on the disproportionately higher levels of BAME mortality from Covid-19. Moreover, the prevalence of low birthweight and preterm birth is the same, if not worse in the UK and USA as in 1950.

## Why is the brain neglected?

The brain is what makes us different from apes and other animals. You would have thought the brain and mental health would have been prioritised by health, food production and nutrition policies. DHA is the principle structural component of the membranes of the brain's signalling systems and neurons. There is nothing more essential to our mental health than DHA; and yet there is no government food and agricultural policy *anywhere in the world* that prioritises the provision of the specific nutrients and trace elements needed for the brain. And if the world *did* suddenly digest and act upon the importance of this lipid, what then? There is not enough food containing DHA to provide for the now 8 billion mouths to feed equably.

Moreover, a recent report provides evidence that with global warming and the temperature rise in the oceans, the capacity for the production of DHA-rich foods will shrink,[6] as they require low temperatures. The significance to the brain of DHA and other lipids is not a new revelation – it was first explained in the FAO's Nutrition Report number 3, which described the proceedings and recommendations of a joint, international, expert consultation by FAO and WHO in 1976.

The lack of attention to these requirements for the brain has led to the worldwide mental ill-health epidemic and decline in intelligence, which has grave consequences for the future of humanity unless we act to plug the already existing and widening gap. But this is where the problems all feed into each other. Some commentators claim there *is* more than enough food to go around. If that is so, it is not being managed very well, as there are 925 million undernourished people in the world. That figure means that 1 in 7 people do not get enough food to lead an active and healthy life. Hunger and malnutrition are in fact the number one risk to health worldwide — greater than AIDS, malaria and tuberculosis combined (UNICEF[7]). Some 2 billion people are malnourished and are suffering from nutrient deficiencies, (especially iodine, lack of which retards brain development). Some 600,000 children died in 2015 in Africa from malnutrition. A little-recognised form of malnutrition that manifests as obesity affects more than 3 million people in the UK, with associated health costs exceeding £13 billion annually (BAPEN have 2009[8]).

The type II diabetes is another consequence of malnutrition. People are eating lots – but lots of the wrong stuff.[9] To make matters worse, the child born to a woman with type 2 diabetes carries the risk of lowered mental abilities, chronic ill-health and dementia. It is not just about money. The Gulf States have the highest prevalence of diabetes II world-wide.

Examples from across the globe over the past two centuries show how nutrition impacts entire populations. Nutritional deficiencies present in the parents will be passed down and exacerbated in the next generation. This history of malnourishment has a wide range of outward manifestations, from goitre, blindness, deformed jaws and rickets, to extremes of muscle loss and obesity and disadvantaged children. Less visible, but with tragic consequences for whole generations, are the 'hidden' diet- related ailments of type 2 diabetes, heart disease, sterility, dementia and a wide range of other mental health problems.

The runaway population expansion needs to be addressed urgently and equable nutrition set for all. We can feed a couple of billion with the correct brain safe food – but not 10 billion-plus, and not on a planet facing the calamities of human-induced climate change and war. In 2016, the late Professor Stephen Hawking gave us a deadline of 100 years to get off the increasingly spoilt Earth and find somewhere else to live[10], while accepting the near impossibility of achieving this[11].

But as a plain statement encapsulating the current fate of human life on Earth, we believe Hawking was right. As we commented earlier, the pattern revealed by the number of species extinguished as a result of human activity in the last 100 years (as recorded in the IUCN Red List[12]) mirrors the collapse of the dinosaurs and the many other species that vanished with them. The *rate* of this present path to extinction, is happening in a blink of biological time.

If you seed a nutrient plate with bacteria, it reaches a logarithmic rate of growth[28] and then suddenly dies. The planet is like that bacterial plate, with limited resources. The situation is unsustainable. Some argue that a few people in remote areas will survive and continue after the Great Calamity. Perhaps the Inuit, or a tribe tucked away in what remains of the Amazon forest, or people living on an isolated landmass such as Easter Island or New Zealand? Perhaps. That assumes that Hawking was wrong, and also assumes the escalating mental ill-health epidemic does not lead to nuclear war. At the time of writing, the

---

28   Logarithmic growth is slow, with environmental pressures constraining the rate of growth. This is the inverse of exponential growth, which begins slowly but then increases rapidly over time.

war in the Ukraine and the collapse of East-West relationships, has a fearful uncomfortable feel to it. On that front it is time for negotiation, peace and reconciliation. We are at this point in time at a turning point. Waiting in the wings is the solution to the mental ill-health and preventable disease for a future of great achievements and progress.

Yet the food situation is actually worse than the one portrayed by Foresight. In any population expansion endgame, there will always be *limiting nutrient* which acts first. Despite the present obsession, it isn't protein. It is brain nutrition, such as the sea-derived DHA, the principle structural component of the membranes of the brain's signalling systems and neurons. The planet simply does not have enough food containing DHA to provide for all 7-plus billion of its people.

Moreover, intensive land-based agriculture has been depleting the soil of its trace elements,[13] impoverishing the overstretched food chain further. We are seeing a rise in mental health problems that have the gravest of consequences for the future of humanity, and their likely cause is the damage caused by these joint impoverishments. And this is just what we know about. We need to find a way to act, and with urgency. There is so much that is wonderful about humanity – art, music, creativity, exploration in the many senses of the word and love for one another. All of that is being eroded by the escalation of mental ill health, power seekers and war mongers.

## Global instability with food shortages

Adolph Hitler was motivated by lebensraum. Amongst other things he wanted more space for the people of his Third Reich to flourish. A cursory glance at current international news reveals that many nations are fomenting conflict and nourishing war right now quite apart from the Ukraine. Seemingly deranged politicians and homicidal/suicidal gunmen present ominous case studies for the mental health problems we are talking about.

Published in May 2019, a report by David Spratt[29] and Ian Dunlop[30] titled "Existential climate-related security risk: a scenario approach" found climate change to be a current and existential national security risk, one that *"threatens the premature extinction of Earth-originating intelligent life or the permanent and drastic destruction of its potential for desirable future development"*.[14]

A runaway hot house effect resulting from climate change would lead to crop failure, armed conflict, floods and conflagrations, and finally mass starvation. Before that there would be mayhem on an unprecedented scale. Today we already have vivid illustrations of global instability and ideocracy.

The recent D-Day 75th Anniversary reminded us that it took just one man to whip a nation into a frame of mind that embraced world war with its unspeakable horrors of the Holocaust. Never again, you might hope. But consider this – in 2016, the world spent a total of $1.57 trillion on weapons – i.e. on things that kill people. There is no other single sector that approaches this amount of spending. From 2013–17, the largest importer of arms was India, with Saudi Arabia second.[15] The biggest sellers include the USA and the UK (ranked, in 2019, number one and two respectively in the list of arms exporters[16]). The money involved in this trade is astounding[31] and incomprehensible when we are faced with such catastrophe-level events as increasing desertification, mass extinctions, drastic loss of bio-diversity, rampant pollution, the disappearance of pollinating insects, and the totally unsustainable exploitation and pollution of ocean and fresh water resources.

---

29    *Research director for Breakthrough National Centre for Climate Restoration, Melbourne, and co-author of Climate Code Red.*

30    *Chairman of the Australian Coal Association, chief executive of the Australian Institute of Company Directors, and chair of the Australian Greenhouse Office Experts Group on Emissions Trading 1998-2000.*

31    *£14billion for the UK alone in 2018.*

More than 1.5 trillion dollars spent on making things that kill people! What does it say for the state of humanity, when killing and destruction as in the Ukraine is the priority of world expenditure? It is like some ghastly final solution to the problems of global overpopulation. Instead of fomenting death and suffering, our economic and business ingenuity could be focused on finding solutions to save ourselves and the planet. But it will require an unprecedented era of mutual concern, intelligence and cooperation such as Regan and Gorbachev envisaged in their slightly surreal conversation about alien invaders at the Geneva summit in 1985.

Meanwhile, somewhat amusingly, certain extraordinarily rich businessmen are pouring millions of dollars into making *humans* the alien invaders, by sending rockets and then-loads of us on trips to Mars and then colonising it. What will we do when we get there? Mars is no party, as the old joke goes, – it has no atmosphere. Its atmosphere is 95.3% carbon dioxide, 2.6% nitrogen and a bit of argon, and the surface pressure is less than 1% of what we have here on Earth. Nonetheless, one must praise the spirit of adventure and the undoubted technical success thus far. When the brave new worlders start their colony, they will need to solve the problem of how to grow brain food. Otherwise, the future generations will be a lost cause. It is all possible of course.

## The modern intensification of food production

Back here on Earth, Sir John Beddington, the UK government's chief scientist, commenting on the Foresight report at a 2012 meeting at the Royal Society in London, claimed that the challenge of maintaining the world's food supply can only be met by more intensification of agriculture and genetic modification. There was no word about a sustainable provision of the brain-specific nutrients, nothing about the potential of the oceans.

Intensification is *not* the answer. Since 1950, this approach has led to the increasing prevalence of super- processed food, which happens to be one of the causes of the decline in the nutritional value of food in the so-called Western diet. Intensification of land based food production with the power of advertising has encouraged the consumption of land based foods and the intensive production of food ends with little if any DHA and may well be poor in trace elements as witnessed by the return of iodine deficiency mentioned previously.

We have moved further and further from the wild food system which powered the development of our brain from the 350g chimpanzee size to the 1.45 Kg of the Herto people who lived before agriculture. Society has come to accept hyper-food processing where chicken skins, proteins, flavours, unhealthy fats, sugars and salts are mushed up into a TV dinner, a tin of soup or chicken masala, and other dubious confections. And where is the mass of surplus fat from the beef, pork and chicken industries going? How many calories do you have to eat to get your vitamins and minerals (sometimes added afterwards, due to the lack of nutrients in the original ingredients)? For some bizarre reason, no one seems to have digested the consequences of the fact that intensively-reared chickens and cattle are producing several times the energy from fat as compared to protein.[17,18] This stuff is getting into the consumer's stomach, whether in sandwiches, prepared meals, TV dinners, fast foods or any of the other processed stuff which we are surrounded by in the average supermarket or takeaway.

Some of the common human ailments that plague us and drain our health services – including heart disease, diabetes, tooth decay, obesity, bowel cancer and mental illness – were rare 150 years ago. They are modern phenomena, symptoms of the 'western' diet. Many illnesses are geographic, linked directly to dietary deficiencies. This can involve too little food, too much food, or a paradoxical combination of the two (i.e.

loads of unhealthy stuff and none of the good stuff – the junk food diet associated originally with America and the West, but spreading alarmingly).

The processed foods are not by any means *all* bad, but with the decline in nutrient density of modern mass-produced food and the increase in caloric value, is there little wonder that obesity, and a whole spectrum of other health issues is escalating? And yet no one in a decision-making position seems willing to address the role of food. Diabetes II is high amongst the many hazards of obesity, and with it goes the risk of heart disease and dementia, and disadvantaged children born to mothers with diabetes II. Moreover, the issue is not due to poverty, as some claim. The Gulf States currently have the greatest prevalence of diabetes II, an unenviable position that has come about in just two generations. Dementias will follow. We provide an answer in the final chapter.

## The disadvantaged child

The low socio-economic groups and ethnic minorities have the highest risk of low birthweight and poor health issues, including heart disease, hypertension, strokes, learning disabilities, obesity, diabetes II, motor dysfunction, behavioural pathology and more, along with a higher chance of mortality from Covid-19.

These groups have a higher prevalence of preterm birth, with its many complications and developmental disorders of the brain, and have a generally poor nutritional status.[19,20] For full-term births at normal birthweights, the prevalence of cerebral palsy is about 1 or 2 per 1,000 live births. However, that escalates as birthweight falls and with preterm births. Below 1,500g, the risk of cerebral palsy is 200 per 1,000 live births (these babies being born around 28 weeks or earlier). Cerebral palsy is the tip of an iceberg of neurodevelopmental and other disorders linked to low birthweight and maternal malnutrition, sentencing the child to a lifetime of physical and mental health limitations.[32]

As we have said before, there is nothing new in this story. A beautiful and well researched book titled "The Disadvantaged Child: health, nutrition and school failure", by Herbert Birch (an obstetrician) and Joan Gussow (a nutritionist), was published in 1970,[21] with a comprehensive 33 pages of scientific references. *"What we hope for"*, said the authors, *"is a programme that will break the continuous inter-generational chain of poverty … We began this book because we feared that attempts to remedy the school failure of disadvantaged children exclusively through educational intervention might well fail and, failing, revive the ancient claim that these children were genetically inferior."*

The authors set out the simple argument that poor nutrition of the mother both before and during pregnancy has a lasting effect prenatally on learning ability, which is irreparable later. This view has been proven by scientific studies many times since; and yet the prevalence of low birthweight[33] and prematurity has not changed since the 1950s in the UK, and has, if anything, increased. Money has been poured into schemes of remedial education. Although well intentioned and clearly beneficial, such schemes do not address the fundamental problem[34]. The brain, as we have repeatedly stated, has very specific nutrient requirements that are simply not being addressed in nutrition and health policies. The early development and growth of the brain sets it for life with little scope for change in pater life. Remedial education of grown children is like closing the stable

32    *Paraphrased from the opening remarks by Josette Sheeran, then Executive Director of the World Food Programme, Executive Board meeting 7 June, 2010. See also her Ted talk "Ending hunger now" 2011:*
https://www.platinumessays.com/essays/Ending-Hunger-Now-by-Josette-Sheeran/21821.html

33    *Paraphrased from the opening remarks by Josette Sheeran, then Executive Director of the World Food Programme, Executive Board meeting 7 June, 2010. See also her Ted talk "Ending hunger now" 2011:*

34    *https://www.platinumessays.com/essays/Ending-Hunger-Now-by-Josette-Sheeran/21821.htmlwell*

door after the horse has bolted. Nonetheless it is important to endeavour to help including those with early dementia.

## A London case study

In the early 1990s, Wendy Doyle compared 7-day weighed food diaries compiled by pregnant women in two areas of London – the prosperous borough of Hampstead (Royal Free Hospital) and a poorer region in the city's East-end (Homerton Hospital E9). The calorie intake of both groups was similar; but the nutrient density was poor in the East-end compared to Hampstead.[22,23] Mothers in the East End were eating much more processed food. Doyle commented at the time on the strangeness of this in such a poor community, given that bought processed foods tend to cost more than healthier food prepared at home. She taught mothers at the Well Street Mother and Baby Clinic how to buy, prepare and cook food that was cheaper and more nutritional than the processed stuff.

Subsequent research showed that nutrition correlated with low birthweight, independent of smoking, economic status and ethnicity. It did not matter if you were rich or poor – if you had a bad diet, defined by the assessment of a battery of daily intake recommendations from WHO, then you were likely to have a disadvantaged, low birthweight baby, rich or poor.[24]

Some have claimed that there is no relationship between birthweight and maternal nutrition. However, Doyle's study of 533 women reported that the relationship with birthweight was up to a weight of 3,250g. Above that, there was no relationship. Just comparing average birthweights can conceal the issue, as the largest sector is above 3,250g where there is no relationship.

That a broad range of nutrients were at stake was confirmed in a randomised controlled trial of micronutrient supplements from early in pregnancy. When the data was analysed on the basis of *intention to treat,* which is the classical method, there was no effect. If, however, the data was assessed on the basis of *those who complied* (those who took a placebo or micronutrient supplement as confirmed by blood analysis), then the micronutrient supplement[35] resulted in a better than two-fold reduction in the proportion of babies born small for gestational age.[25] Being born small for gestational age is the strongest risk factor for adverse outcomes.

## A new paradigm is needed in food production

While we cannot turn the clock back, we can at least recognise some blindingly obvious facts. First, that the brain evolved in the sea. Second, that the human genome separated from the great apes just 5–7 million years ago and today differs from theirs by only 1.5%. *That means human physiology is adapted to wild, natural foods.* There are no ifs or buts.

Any detraction from that, in the form of processed junk, spells problems. This salient conclusion reminds us of Sir Robert McCarrison's principle that good health depends on natural foods: what he called the "*unsophisticated foods of Nature*". Diets are changing and are being changed the world over. For example, in a recent conversation with us, Professor Junshi Chen , Chief Adviser of the China National Centre for Food Safety Risk Assessment, lamented the rise in colon cancer in Beijing.

The food and agriculture intensification introduced post-World War Two has changed the nature of food shockingly, from something that for thousands of years has fed the creation of music, literature, art, science and endless ingenuity, to a toxic force that is dismantling everything gained so far from our genetic heritage and evolution.

---

35  *Designed on the basis of WHO recommendations for pregnancy*

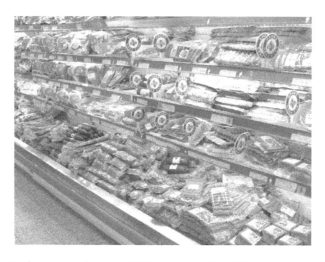

The photo above was taken in a Beijing supermarket. The shelves are piled with European, high fat, high salt and high sugar products.

There are three parallel starting points to our new paradigm for world food production: shifting the balance of fats; focusing on the mother; and farming the land and seas sustainably.

## Fat of the land – and that's the problem

First, the fats. We must reduce the burden of linoleic acid (LA). It competes with other fatty acids for biological use, including DHA. Its reduction would make the limited resources for DHA more available. As with business, two companies with similar products will be in competition with each other. Not quite the same, but close enough, the omega-6 HQ is similar to the omega-3 HQ, both being in the polyunsaturated fatty acids business but – to extend the metaphor – with different CEOs. So, the businesses of omega-6 and omega-3 compete. The brain consistently uses the same proportions of the two, arachidonic and DHA, in all species so far studied with a 2 or 1 to 1 ratio. The present dietary balance is 15 or 20 to1.

When working at the NIH in Bethesda, Maryland, USA, Captain Joseph Hibbeln pointed out the risk of the linoleic acid

(LA omega 6) explosion, competing with the omega-3 and so precipitating much mental ill-health. At the end of World War Two, LA was not a prominent feature of the diet. Cooking was done with olive oil, lard or beef fat. After the war, the LA content of the diet boomed with the idea that saturated fatty acids should be replaced by polyunsaturated ones with the hope of preventing atherosclerosis and heart disease, the number 1 killer. While LA is an essential fatty acid, too much of it is not a good thing, as it competes with the omega-3 fatty acids[26] that we need for our brains.

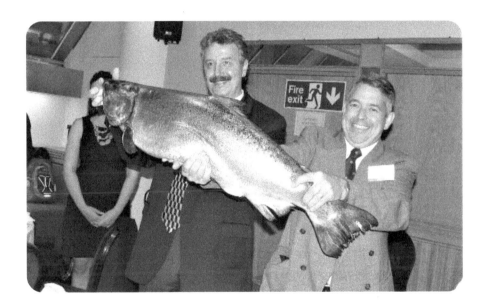

*For the 2010 DHA celebratory conference and Michael's 80th birthday at the Royal Society of Medicine, London, UK. , Randy Hartnell (left) had sent from his fishing operation in Alaska, freshly caught wild salmon flown into Heathrow arriving the morning of the conference. There was enough for over 150 guests. The salmon was cooked by Rick Stein of Padstow, the celebrity TV chef who specialised in fish and sea foods. It was delicious beyond words. Crisp, white French wine was provided by Thierry Lerond of Nutrilysdelmar to add to a stunning dinner. Joe Hibbeln who has published extensively on the cognitive benefits fish and sea food, especially on pregnancy and behavioural disorders is on the right. (see Hibbeln JR et al; Maternal seafood consumption in pregnancy and neurodevelopmental outcomes in childhood (ALSPAC study): Lancet. 2007;369(9561):578-85. doi: 10.1016/S0140-6736(07)60277-3.)*

Joe tells a lovely story:

*I gave a lecture in West Virginia to the school staff, teachers, custodians, cafeteria workers, grounds keepers, etc. After the lecture Gary McDaniels (Social Worker of the year, 2010) came up to me and said 'We really appreciate you coming out here, we don't see many from Washington. But I have to tell you, the audience nearly got up and left when you started talking about evolution. You did bring them back when you started talking about Jesus being a fisherman, and the symbol of fish. So listen here doc, you have to make your advice simpler: "up with threes, that is the number of the Lord, and down with sixes, that's the number of the devil" – that's all ya need to tell 'em, doc!'*

Take, for example, India. It has the highest prevalence of preterm births. It is being encouraged to developing corn, soya oil and other Western omega-6-linoleic acid rich oils. Instead, it should be encouraged to develop local crops already embedded in the dietary culture. One such is mustard seed oil, traditionally used in the north of India. It is rich in omega-3 alpha-linolenic acid (ALA), the parent of the omega-3 family that gives rise to long-chain DHA. Although poorly converted to DHA, ALA is nonetheless the omega-3 parent fatty acid, and by using this and similar omega-3-rich oils, you are not swamping your biology with linoleic acid omega 6. Moreover, although poorly researched, a study involving Capuchin monkeys found that an ALA omega 3 deficiency leads to poor skin condition, loss of hair and, indeed, severe behavioural pathology including self-harm.[27]

It is well known that if you want to make a horse's coat beautiful and shiny before a show, linseed cake does the trick. Linseed contains about 60% ALA. It is also true that women are better converters than men. Cutting the amount of linoleic in the diet and the food system would be a useful and achievable short-term option allowing better synthesis and utilisation of the omega 3 DHA so important for brain health..[28] Indeed, several of the big companies, including Monsanto, are now producing cooking and salad oils with less LA and more oleic acid or ALA: hope perhaps..

Populations that have been dependent for centuries on diets containing little or no fish have developed a better ability to convert short-chain omega-3s to DHA. Even so, we still find the lowest levels of DHA in Sudanese women's milk, in a region where there is little or no access to fish, and very few land sources of DHA.[29] There was also a high prevalence of preterm births, low birth weights, perinatal and maternal mortality. As we have seen, these populations are at greatest risk of iodine deficiency, and it is likely that DHA and iodine deficiencies co-exist with consequences in mental retardation.

The problem of the mother's low milk DHA status was described by one of our Sudanese students, Dr Kot Nyuar from Juba[30], while Dr Izzedin Hussein has described the incidence and effects of iodine deficiency in the Sudan.[31] It is also interesting that, having lamented the fate of our chickens, it is a fact that those chickens brought up in open spaces with access to insects and grubs that eat green foods, and green foods themselves, get a good amount of ALA in their diet, which they readily convert to DHA: an important answer.

Various green vegetables, including green cabbage, dark green lettuce, spinach and shard, are primary sources of omega-3 ALA. Although the amounts are small, they nonetheless come with a package of beta-carotene and vitamins C and E, certain minerals, a beneficial alkalinity and good dose of fibre. It has to be 'green' vegetables, though, and the darker the green, the better. The humble leguminous beans such as one uses for chilli con carne or bean stews, soups or even tins of beans in tomato sauce are all good sources.

The point here is that a proper balance of the basic forms of the two essential fatty acids (omega-3 and omega-6) can and should be obtained from the food system. The gap here is education – people need to be taught about nutrients. But then, as we are often at pains to point out, the UK Government 40-50 years ago. shut down home economics and the teacher training colleges such as the Athol Crescent College in Edinburgh which taught teachers how to teach cooking and nutritional skills to school children. Consequently, even the CEOs of food companies, and government ministers, will have had no teaching of even the basics unless they have taken a degree in nutritional science at university.

## Is the high prevalence of obesity due to the increase in energy (calories) in the foods: if so, is it reversible?

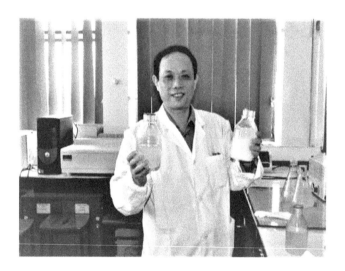

In the photo above, Dr Yiqun Wang is holding two bottles. In his left hand is a bottle with the amount of fat extracted from a single broiler chicken from a local supermarket in London. His right hand holds the fat from an allegedly free-range chicken. Even the free-range bird has many times the amount of fat that was found in chickens in the early 1970s. Whilst free-range the chickens have access to the outside world, they are also fed indoors with high energy food with added growth promoters for weight gain. We are now seeing white streaks in chicken meat.

Chickens in the UK in the 1960s and early 70s had good amounts of DHA in their meat (170mg DHA /100g), and their eggs would have been a good source as well. If they did not have any DHA, there would have been nothing to build brains in the developing chicks!. Without access to the green foods and exercise in the field, the level in intensively reared chickens, measured in 2009, was as low as 25-13mg/100g meat.[32]

Of course, the price of chickens has fallen dramatically. However, think about the price for nutrients. To get the same amount of DHA as you would have obtained from a chicken in 1970, you would need to eat around 13 times the amount of meat, and that would be accompanied by a lot of fat!

To think of the change in the DHA content of supermarket chicken in terms of value for money, if a whole 1.3kg chicken costs £5, and if you need to eat 13 times the amount of meat to obtain the same amount of DHA as you would have done in a 1970, then you would need to multiply the cost by 13, which means £65 of chicken meat, and a veritable reservoir of 3,250g fat!

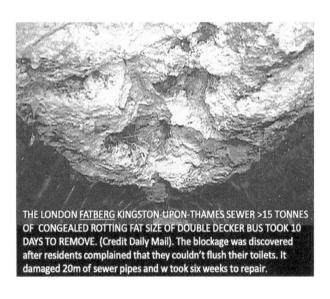

THE LONDON FATBERG KINGSTON-UPON-THAMES SEWER >15 TONNES OF CONGEALED ROTTING FAT SIZE OF DOUBLE DECKER BUS TOOK 10 DAYS TO REMOVE. (Credit Daily Mail). The blockage was discovered after residents complained that they couldn't flush their toilets. It damaged 20m of sewer pipes and w took six weeks to repair.

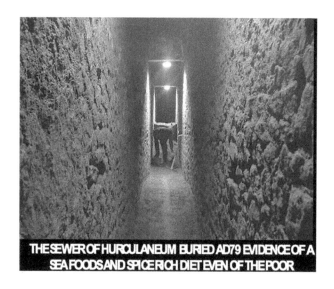

THE SEWER OF HURCULANEUM BURIED AD79 EVIDENCE OF A
SEA FOODS AND SPICE RICH DIET EVEN OF THE POOR

A 1.3 kg of chicken contains 250g fat. The chicken weighs 1,300g, so subtracting the 250g fat leaves 1,050g chicken, 40% of which is bone. That means there is 630g meat. Protein is 20% of the meat, which means 126g protein, the calorific value of which can be obtained by multiplying by four. That means there are 504 calories of protein in the carcass. However, the 250g of fat equals 2,250 calories, which means there is 4.46 times the amount of fat calories in the chicken compared to protein.

People might say that much of the fat would run out into the roasting pan. That is true, but how many people make gravy out of it? If they don't, it is a wasteful use of energy by the producers and will contribute to the 'fatbergs' that block London's sewers! It is not just chicken that is nutritionally depleted. In the 19th century, the rivers, lakes and coastlines of Britain were teeming with fish. So much so that factory workers complained that they were being fed salmon far too often – and it was wild-caught salmon, not the farmed salmon of the 21$^{st}$ century.

Prior to the fussy eating habits of the modern period, every bit of the cow, sheep or pig was eaten, and the offal was an important part of the weekly food fare. Liver is stuffed full of vital trace elements and B12. The B12 you find in the pills from the drug store is only a single variety, whereas in liver you get several forms. Of course, the variety used in the tablets has been researched and is considered to be the essential active ingredient. However, such research is limited to the known signs of deficiency. Nature may well have other uses for the different varieties of B12. Then there are the kidneys, full of B-vitamins, several related molecules, some even fluorescent, the value of which has not been exhaustively researched and of course iron. And then there's the haggis, described by Robert Burns in his 1787 *Address to A Haggis* thus:

*Fair fa' your honest, sonsie face, Great Chieftain o' the Puddin- race! Aboon them a' ye tak your place, Painch, tripe, or thairm: Weel are ye wordy o' a grace As lang's my arm.*

Still widely eaten in Scotland, and a feature of English supermarket shelves in the weeks leading up to Burns Night on 25 January, haggis is often stuffed into plastic skins these days, rather than the traditional sheep stomach.

Variety was once the spice of life. The diet featured a great array of vegetables, including wild ones gathered from the fields and forests. There was no sugary snap, crackle and pop for breakfast, but porridge, eggs, bacon, herring or kippers were commonplace. You did, of course, need money to buy the stuff; but it was not all doom and gloom and poverty. Many people were employed in manufacturing or mining, and the stories of low wages and poor working conditions are common; but there were also vast areas of land occupied by farm workers, who were able to enjoy the fruits of the land and the rivers and lakes on their borders (even if poaching was often involved). Indeed, there are stories about workmen in factories complaining about the amount of salmon they were given for lunch! At the turn of the last century, the barmen in the East-end of London provided oysters free with the purchase of a pint of beer!

## The enclosures and the emergence of the fat stock

We are not here to praise the past but to see if we can learn from it. Yes, the farm animals were very fat, and indeed they were referred to as "fat stock". Wild animals are lean, so how did the fat "stock" beast come about? It is quite simple. In the 17th century, the laws on enclosures began to bite. They had been initiated to "protect" the wild game – i.e. to monopolise it for the wealthy in the forests and on the commons, and to prevent the peasantry from nicking their venison, boar and other game.

The result was that the farmers had to enclose their livestock in fenced or walled fields. This had an immediate effect on the beef animals. Prior to the enclosures, the livestock could eat what it wished. Darwin, when discussing the long neck of the giraffe, points out that cows in a field browse the trees and level the tree growth to the exact height they can reach with their mouths. However, the luxury of browsing trees in a field disappeared after the enclosures, and bark, nuts and leaves became a luxury. The animals were no longer free to choose what they wanted to eat but were forced to eat grass. A strange thing then happened. The more animals were put into grass fields, the better their weight gain. How come?

The answer was known to Shakespeare's shepherd Corin in As You Like It, who comments "good pasture makes fat sheep" (Act 3, scene 2). If you only have a few animals in a field, the grass grows tall and spindly with low-energy stalks which will eventually develop seed heads. If you have a lot of animals in the field, they keep the grass short. That means they have continued access to the high energy young shoots. An extended, Shakespearean spring feed so to speak. So they put on weight better – i.e. they put on fat.

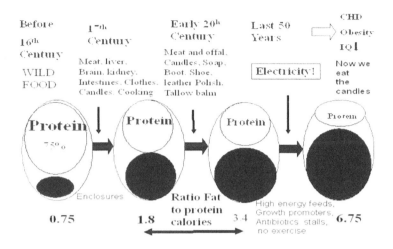

Cynical view of the rise of beef and the fat of the land

The heavier the animal, the better the price at market. The farmers would naturally select those which put on weight fastest for breeding. These would be animals genetically best suited to the conditions of the field. Moreover, the animal fat was prized. It was used for making candles, which were household essentials before electricity arrived, and for making saddle soap, leather, boot and shoe polish, lubricant, tallow balm for the skin, cooking fat including shortenings, and more. So the business of breeding fat animals thrived.

Come the industrial revolution and electricity, there was no longer a high demand for candles. What better response than to put the fat into the food chain to feed the expanding population? The table below gives a numerical comparison of the composition of beef in terms of protein versus fat in calorific terms. With muscle being around 80% water, a serving of marbled beef, with its high-calorie fat content, would deliver only 10% protein. So one arrives at a huge discrepancy between the perception of the intensive meat industry providing protein, and the reality, which is that it provides more fat calories than protein. In wild-derived meat, the opposite applies, and there is more protein than fat calories. The wild composition is taken from H,P Ledger's analysis of wild carcasses from 32 herbivore species in East Africa, published in symposium no 21 of the Zoological Society of London in 1968. The figure of 5% for the fat content is actually greater than what he found in the majority of species.

## LAND BASED FOODS 2:-
## BEEF

|  | MODERN: | WILD: |
|---|---|---|
| CARCASS LEAN | 50% | 75% |
| FAT | 30% | 5% |
| PROTEIN EQUIV. | 10 | 15 |
| PROTEIN CALORIES | 40 | 60 |
| FAT CALORIES | 270 | 45 |
| | | |
| FAT PROTEIN RATIO | 6.75 | 0.75 |
| INTENSIFICATION = | 9 FOLD FAT | |

### Rochefort-Sur-Mer and a Paleolithic Banquet

In 2007, Dr Guy-André Pelouze, a cardio-vascular surgeon, invited David and Michael to give two lectures to GRAIN, a French society of medical people interested in nutrition and health. It was held in Rochefort-sur-Mer, a town renowned for its oysters. On the final day, the morning began with David giving a talk about Lamarck, Cuvier and Darwin and his "conditions of existence". The French doctors loved David's presentation, which was in line with much of their thinking. David's talk was followed by Michael's presentation on human evolution.

These two presentations occupied the whole morning's proceedings, with a break for tea and coffee in the middle. It was not your ordinary tea break, as the tables were festooned with piles of oysters, and a crisp, cold wine from Bordeaux to wash them down. In the evening there was a Palaeolithic banquet organised by Guy-Andre.

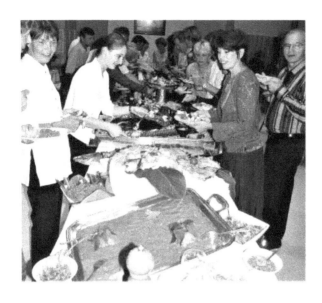

The banquet offered winkles, mussels, oysters, crabs, and several types of fish, meat, wild tubers, fruits and nuts from the forest. Whilst the great variety of sea foods was to be expected, and indeed the meat also, but the *type* of meat was not. Beef had been thinly sliced and laid on a silver tray. The trays were covered with cloths. When the cloths were removed, there was a gasp from those present. The scent of herbs in the meat and the sight of thin slices of very red meat with not a hint of visible fat to be seen was astounding (see photos).

The meat had come from Jean François Casteix, a farmer in the South of France. His animals lived in the forest and open bush land, with never a trace of artificial feed used, even in winter – which, of course, would be mild in the south of France, with plants still growing, as happens in the birthplace of H. sapiens in Africa. Some of our species' birthplace is 4,000 feet above sea level  in East Africa. The discovery of East Africa by our ancestors, with its lakes and rivers stuffed with fish and other freshwater goods would have been heaven on earth.33 In 1907, Winston Churchill described Uganda as the "Pearl of Africa".)

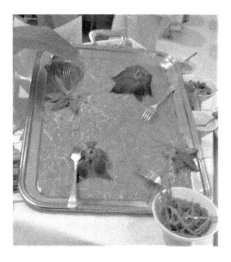

The message from the Rochefort spread is that this is what meat *should* be and *can* be – we know that, because the proof was there in front of our eyes. Although there was an indoor barbecue, most people ate the meat raw.

Compare the marbled beef below with the meat in the photographs above.

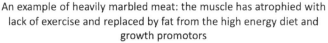

An example of heavily marbled meat: the muscle has atrophied with lack of exercise and replaced by fat from the high energy diet and growth promotors

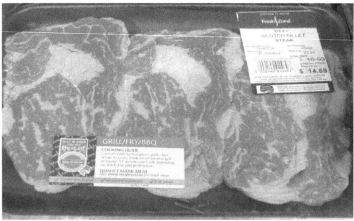

**It is not the meat that is at fault, it is what we have done to it**

To back up this story, we can say with conviction that it is not meat itself that has the adverse health connotations. The top carnivores eat a great deal of offal and meat. Take a look at the artery of a 25-year-old lion, and take a look at the artery (aorta) of a 32-year-old young man killed in a car accident (see the photographs below). Both aortas have been stained with Sudan Red, (used to show infiltrated fat deposits). You can see the stain has been used on the lion's aorta because the fat on the back of the blood vessel is stained. There is, however, no stain to be seen on the face of the aorta – unlike that of the unfortunate 32-year-old London man. Very little else needs to be said.

Aorta of a full grown, 25 year old African lion stained with sudan red for arterial atherosclerotic fatty lesions. Note staining taken up by fat depots on the back outside but not on the surface.

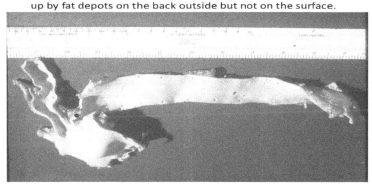

Aorta of a 35 year old London male killed in a car accident. Note extensive raised staining lipid deposits on the surface.

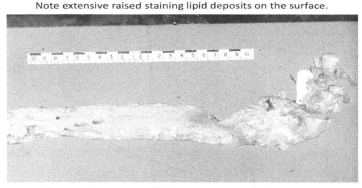

These pictures tell the story on their own.

There are several books now detailing problems with the modern food system.. If the reader is interested in delving deeper, there are three recent books reviewed in an article by Olivia Potts *"Is there anything safe left to eat?"* in The Spectator Magazine issue: https://www.spectator.co.uk/ magazines/lead-book-review/ magazine issue 22nd April 2023.

She writes: "The chapter headings alone are enough to induce a panic attack"

## Our genome is based on wild foods.

Remember, our genome is only 1.5% different to our chimpanzee ancestors. Whether or not the reader has been convinced by our story of Darwin and his conditions of existence and the evidence of the brain evolving in the sea 500 million years ago and the relevance that has to our origins as a species making the best use of the aquatic and land-based food resources, there is an inescapable fact. Our genome was shaped based on wild foods.

In evolutionary terms, the time that has elapsed between today and the first emergence of Homo sapiens is the blink of an eye. Nothing much changes in the blink of an eye. Our physiology is the same now as it was then. The foods we evolved to eat are the foods we still require, if we are to maintain optimum mental and physical fitness.

Sir Robert McCarrison, the great pioneer of the principles of nutrition and health, recognised this principle in his statement that good health depended on the "Unsophisticated foods of Nature". Straying from this principle invites ill health.

As we have seen, there is abundant evidence. Straying from the common baseline of our evolutionary heritage, populations have expanded in different regions of the globe, developing different food patterns to suit the local conditions. The story of different nutritional profiles is the story of the USA vs Japan;

the differences in the various regions of China; India versus Europe; Northern France versus the South of France; our own experience of Uganda versus the UK; or the Maldives versus the Gulf States, with their high prevalence of obesity and type II diabetes. Nutrition is the prime mover in health and non-communicable disease. Moreover, the inequality of nutrition and health across the globe, and across individual nations, is now showing up with the mortality rates from covid-19. The BAME population is suffering high mortality rates compared to white Anglo-Saxon Protestants (otherwise known as WASPS). The evidence is staring us in the face.

The question now is "what can be done about it?" We offer some solutions in the next chapter.

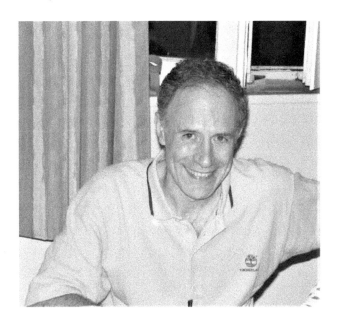

Dr Guy-André Pelouze, at the Paleolithic banquet in Rochefort-sur-mer

# CHAPTER 10
# A Solution In Africa:
# Greening The Desert

*Carbon storage in forests is a cornerstone of policy making to prevent global warming from exceeding 1,5°C (Science 19 May 2023)* [36]

*"These observations lead to the conclusion that current forests have only a limited additional carbon storage potential to substantially mitigate the increase in atmospheric CO2 without major reductions in fossil emissions."*

E lon Musk and others want to green Mars at a cost of billions if not trillions of dollars and a time span of some 100 years. So why not green the desert here at home? Extend the activity to the many semi-arid parts of Africa where plant life is sadly loosing its grip on survival. The literature on the history of Africa has that human activity was much to blame for the erosion and desertification[1,2]. That can be reversed[3]. Turn big areas of Africa into a hot bed of food production with an abundance of productive jobs and condemning poverty to past history. Help solve the increasing food insecurity. Why not?

## The semi-arid adaptations

Africa still holds evidence of Nature's last great experiment in mammalian evolution. Not disputing the role of natural

---

36   Caspar T. J. Roebroek, Gregory Duveiller, SoniaI. Senevirante, , Edward L. Davin, Alessandro, Cascati Caebon Sequestration,Science, 380, 6646. 749-753.

selection, we might argue that environment and food played a role in the evolution of various characteristics of the animals. In hot dry environments, this role is a matter of relevance to conservation and plausibly to food for tomorrow.

For example, could the moisture-retaining plants of the hot dry environments have encouraged the animals' ability to retain moisture by developing the integrity and function of surface areas? If that were so then the skin would lose less water; the lungs would develop their surface areas more efficiently, extracting more oxygen and losing less water. And the intestines too would lose less water.

This is not a wild suggestion, because we know that plants from hot dry regions must be able to control water loss more efficiently than plants from wet areas, so they must have a better range of chemicals and mechanisms for achieving this. Could those chemicals also be involved in the mechanism by which animals retain water?

As it happens, there is an extensive body of scientific evidence showing that a deficiency of linoleic acid, the essential fatty acid found in plants, increases the rate of water loss through an animal's skin.[4] Whilst, in the last chapter, linoleic acid was seen as a dampener to the utilisation of DHA, here we are talking about its value at the level of physiological needs, not the over blown excesses of the Western diet. The correction of a relative deficiency of linoleic acid improves water retention. Indeed, the effect of linoleic acid upon skin water loss continues to be felt at a range of intakes which are far above what one would call deficiency. Long before we knew this question existed, the Nuffield Institute of Comparative Medicine, at the Zoological Society of London, published several scientific papers showing that tissues from semi-arid adapted species such as eland and giraffe have significantly higher levels of linoleic, arachidonic and other essential fats than the same tissues from wet species like buffalo, zebra or cows.[5,6]

In particular, the comparison between the giraffe and zebra

is especially telling because although the zebra has plenty of linoleic acid in its tissue, the presence of arachidonic in the giraffe is many times that seen in the zebra[7]. It so happens that arachidonic is the major fatty acid component of the cell membranes which line the arteries. Indeed, the arachidonic in the arteries produce prostacyclin which protects arteries from blockage, encourages blood flow and regulates blood pressure. Moreover, there is a greater abundance of the long chain omega 3 including EPA, which are known to be supportive of the cardiovascular system in the giraffe tissues: better than the grass eating zebra[8]. It all fits with a food system supporting the greater development of the blood vessels and heart to serve the long neck as we have discussed before.

Moreover, plants of semi-arid regions such as the desert date *Balanites aegyptiaca,* a favourite food of the giraffes, and the many acacia species have oil rich seeds. These seeds are massively large compared to grass seeds and can therefore be assumed to provide the browsing animals with higher amounts of linoleic and alpha-linolenic acids in their diet. Our analysis of the kernel from the Balanites told us it was 60% oil and the oil was just over 70% linoleic acid, with a warm yellow colour and a touch of orange hinting at its high carotenoid content.

Arachidonic acid is the principle metabolic product of linoleic acid and is a major constituent of the vascular endothelium cell membrane which lines the arteries. The acacias exist in hundreds of varieties, but the seeds of one common in Karamoja in Uganda, where we carried out our study, had about 35% oil which was 40% alpha-linolenic acid and 30% linoleic. Others like the Balanites have about 70% linoleic acid in the nut oil. The leaves only contain a little oil but there again, they are alpha-linolenic acid rich, This essential fatty acid is the parent of the omega 3 family. Everyone seems to know about these days that omega 3 is cardio-protective. Hence this kind of browse material is not only good for building arteries but also for the regulation of blood pressure and for the heart. However, it is not linoleic acid but the arachidonic made from it which is important both structurally for building the endothelial cells that line the arteries and for the production of prostacyclin,[9] the topic of Sir John Vane's 1992 Nobel Prize. As we discussed previously, prostacyclin is an oxidative product of arachidonic acid made from linoleic acid and its job is to help regulate blood pressure and keep the blood flowing. With its high blood pressure, the giraffe needs that support.

In addition, the long chain omega-3 such as EPA are derived from alpha-linolenic acid and are good for the health of the heart and blood flow.[10,11,12] The giraffe needs a lot of building materials for the very long artery that goes up its neck to feed the brain. A comparison of the amounts of arachidonic acid and long chain omega 3 in the tissues of the zebra and giraffe make the point that the giraffe is much more richly endowed with arachidonic acid and indeed EPA. The zebra has lots of linoleic acid but little arachidonic.[13]

The tissue is the issue, in showing the effects of the different diets of the giraffe and the zebra or wet, grassland buffalo. One has to ask the question from these examples: did the favourable biochemistry resulting from the food selection pattern allow the extension of the long neck: or did it stimulate it through gene expression and epigenetics? Regardless of the answer, the evidence does point to a role for food selection in the shaping of species as for example of previously discussed difference between the night vision and peripheral nervous systems of the carnivores and herbivores. Food is doing that today. Humans have changed in shape, size and disease pattern in just one century. Just look at us today and the images seen in pictures and films in the1930s, 40s, and 50s.

## "The tallest of tales"

Jean-Baptist Lamarck, wrote about his idea how the giraffe obtained its long neck in 1809. "It is interesting to observe the result of habit in the peculiar shape and size of the giraffe: this animal, the tallest of the mammals, is known to live in the interior of Africa in places where the soil is nearly always arid and barren, so that it is obliged to browse on the leaves of trees and to make constant efforts to reach them. From this habit long maintained in all its race, it has resulted that the animal's forelegs have become longer than its hind-legs, and that its neck is lengthened to such a degree that the giraffe, without standing up on its hind-legs, attains a height of six meters."[14]

Funnily enough, he is wrong about the semi-arid being barren at ground level. The trees provide shade and moisture from evaporation of water drawn from the deep-water table, during the day. With a healthy tree and bush cover, there is a microclimate in which the sedges, herbs and edible grasses flourish. This multiple layer provides at the top for the giraffe, half way for the eland, lower down for the gerenuk and at ground level, several antelope species including the little Dik-Dik eating fruits, berries, flowers, leaves, and shoots and preferably not grass. At the same time there are the wart hogs and forest pigs digging for roots, with oryx out in the dryer plains. It is a stunning example of complementary species adapted to complimenting diets in all of which we have not mentioned the bees, other pollinating insects and the nesting birds all of which contribute to sustainability, replanting and natural extension.

However, where there has been tree cutting and burning and where the desert follows then everything is barren. Nature did not count on the destructive behaviour of humans. It is time to reverse the destruction.

Back to the evolution story, the long neck of the giraffe has been in constant debate since Darwin used it to support natural selection. In times of drought and scarcity, by reaching higher and higher into the trees, the present representative of the species survived when others, less able died out.

Stephen Jay Gould who we refer to in chapter 3, published an essay in 1996 "The Tallest of Tales" in which he comments "Is the textbook version of the giraffe evolution a bit of a stretch". He wrote about the biology text books for schools: "Every single one – no exceptions – began its chapter on evolution by first discussing Lamarck's theory of inheritance of acquired characteristics, and then presenting Darwin's theory of natural selection as a preferred alternative. All texts then use the same example to illustrate Darwinian superiority – the giraffe's neck.".

He further commented the "current use of the giraffe's neck as the classic case of Darwinian evolution... is both fatuous and unsupported."

This, and what we write about the chemistry, in no way diminishes Darwin's true concept of evolution. In the evolution of the long neck there must be a genetic component. Could be direct mutation but because so many alterations are required (heart, blood vessels, kidneys, rete mirabile[37], long front legs, etc) we favour epigenetics working in conjunction with the chemistry. In the same way that you cannot build your muscle without protein and cannot build a brain without specific essential fatty acids, so the giraffe needs a source of food rich in the needs for building a strong, large heart and long blood vessels strong enough to withstand the high ambient blood pressure needed to pump the blood up to the brain. So we have again, Darwin's "conditions of existence".

The adult, male giraffe's heart can weigh10 kg and serves the animal with twice the blood pressure seen in other large mammals. The Rete mirabile is a vascular network

---

37   *The adult, male giraffe's heart can weigh10 kg and serves the animal with twice the blood pressure seen in other large mammals. The Rete mirabile is a vascular network which controls the blood pressure to the brain. And is highly developed in the giraffe. If the giraffe did not have this blood pressure controlling mechanism, then when it bends its neck down to drink, the rise in blood pressure would risk a stroke. On raising its head, the sudden drop in blood pressure would cause it to black out as it swung its head upwards to six meters tall! In practice, it does not drink much at all. It gets its water needs from eating tree leaves at night when they swell with water from their root in the deep water tables..*

which controls the blood pressure to the brain. And is highly developed in the giraffe. If the giraffe did not have this blood pressure controlling mechanism, then when it bends its neck down to drink, the rise in blood pressure would risk a stroke. On raising its head, the sudden drop in blood pressure would cause it to black out as it swung its head upwards to six meters tall! In practice, it does not drink much at all. It gets its water needs, most of the time, from eating tree leaves at night when they swell with water from their root in the deep-water tables.

## Body temperature

When homeothermic animals evolved, they did not all attempt to keep their temperatures constant all the time. The most extreme example of this is hibernation. In the strict sense of the word this means letting the body temperature fall to the level of the animal's surroundings, but in practice this is rare. Of the mammals, the dormouse comes closest; but most, like the hedgehog and the grizzly bear, find a hole or a cave to shelter in and maintain enough metabolic activity to hold their temperatures at a level at which the system will keep ticking over.

Aside from hibernation, several mammals, faced with extreme conditions, have opted not to keep their temperatures constant all the time. Those that allow it to vary are known as poikilotherms , and this variation has enabled some of them to increase their efficiency in dealing with a harsh, hot dry climate. An interesting comparison has been made between the European cow and the African oryx and eland, two species of antelope similar in size to cows.

The comparison is a very revealing one, in the light of various European attempts to help African agriculture by introducing European cattle. In many places this has been a disastrous failure. The native species clearly have survival mechanisms adapted to hot, dry climates that European cattle lack; so much so that during the severe drought in northern Kenya in 1962 and 1963, European cattle died in thousands and those who depended on them became famine-stricken refugees. The eland, oryx and giraffe, however, continued to reproduce and rear their young throughout the eighteen-month period when no surface water was available.

Dr Charles Taylor of the East African Veterinary Research Organisation Muguga, Kenya, and also of the Museum of Comparative Zoology, Harvard, USA, had closely studied the work of Schmidt-Nielsen who was one of the first to explore the mechanisms for survival of desert animals.[15] Taylor worked in Kenya and was impressed by the way in which a large biomass of certain large antelopes thrived in hot dry conditions. He captured a number of oryx and eland, built a room in which he could control the temperature and humidity, and studied the mechanisms whereby they were able to live in a hot semi-arid environment.

How did the animals deal with the absence of a water supply and survive during droughts when cattle died? The first point to emerge was that the antelopes needed to hold the same amount of water in their bodies as the cows. They had no advantage there.

The next thing to look at was their kidneys. Some animals, like the desert rat, have developed super-efficient kidneys that can get rid of all the waste products passed through them by using a tiny amount of water to dissolve them and flush them out. Dr Taylor found that although the eland and oryx had quite efficient kidneys they were not in the class of the desert rat, so that could not be the answer although a partial contributor to it..

What he discovered was that there was not one answer but many.[16] Cows, like humans, maintain a constant body temperature and when it gets too hot they lose a lot of water by evaporation. The eland and oryx at some stage abandoned this approach and so their body temperature rises to over 43°C at midday and falls at night to 33°C. The loss of water through perspiration is thus avoided. The Eland (*Taurotragus oryx pictured below*) provides outstanding meat and a rich milk. Semi-arid adapted herbivores such as this are better than cows for Africa and the future need for food.

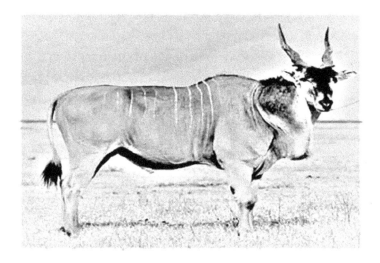

Next there is the water that we lose through our lungs, which can be seen when we breathe on a glass surface and watch it mist up. The eland and oryx have highly efficient lungs which extract more of the oxygen from the air than do the cow's lungs: so, needing to pump less air in and out of their bodies, they lose less water for the gain of the same amount of oxygen.

Then there is the animals' dung. The oryx and eland produce dung as dry, hard pellets, which means that their digestive processes extract water from their food far more efficiently than cattle, which produce wet cow pats.

The semi-arid adapted browsers like eland and giraffe also have the good sense to stay in the shade during the heat of the day and to eat at night. There is a less obvious reason for this than simply keeping cool. The semi-arid browsers eat leaves from trees rather than grass. The logic of night-time browsing can be witnessed even in Britain, where the leaves of a tomato plant will visibly shrink when the sun is burning down on them and fill out again with water in the cool of the evening. The leaves of Balanites and Acacia trees, on which the kudu, eland and giraffe browse provide food and water. At midday their water content is around 20 to 30 per cent but at midnight it rises to 60 or 80 per cent. So, by feeding at night the leaf-eating eland remains independent of surface water: it gets all the water it needs from the plants whose tap roots bring it up from the water table deep underground.

During the heat of the day the leaves transpire water and so create a local ecosystem: moisture in the air encourages herbs and sedges to grow in the shade of the tree and food for the smaller animals.

## A NEW AGRICULTURE USING THE SEMI-ARID ECOSYSTEM

This story has a bearing on agricultural policy. The potential of the plant and animal species adapted to hot, dry climates and resistant to indigenous disease has for some curious reason been consistently ignored by those who have tried to bring aid and practical solutions to Africa. For example, the physiological adaptations of giraffe, eland and oryx, to mention but a few, are so remarkable, and the meat of the young animals so splendid and their milks so rich, that one wonders why they have been ignored as possible livestock. Are the people responsible for aid in land-use unable to think outside the box?

The biomass of the pristine semi-arid regions of Uganda was the equal of the best Norfolk pasture. This massive unused potential is rapidly dwindling in terms of both plant and animal species, with desert encroachment and the threat of extinction through human misuse.[17] According to Wikipedia, the Gobi

Desert swallows up over 1,300 square miles (3,370 km²) of land annually.[18] The Southern edge of the Sahel is marching south at about 2 -4 kilometres a year.

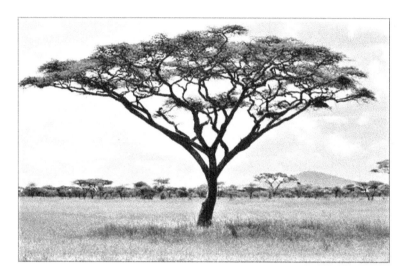

*Acacia: note the green plant growth in the shade of the umbrella. Not a typical habitat where it would be a part of densely tree and bush area but the greenness makes the point of the microclimate created by the trees of the semi-arids.*

In addition to the physiological adaptations of the semi- arid adapted mammals, the trees, bushes, special grasses, herbs, sedges and tubers exercise their unique economy with water and nutrients with a track record amounting to millions of years. They have also been a part of African traditional food ever since humans first occupied these areas. In Uganda some of the Karamajong run eland with their cattle simply because the *nyarna* (meat) is so good. They say the animals are easy to tame if caught young and that the eland have a calming effect on the cattle, somehow keeping them together. The Russians have (or had) been milking eland in Askania Nova for some years.[19] The milk, as might be expected, is richer than cow's milk and simply delicious.

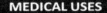

**Balanites aegyptiaca**

Found in the arid Sahel-Savannah in deep sands & sandy clay loams. Fruit is mixed into porridge and eaten by nursing mothers & oil is consumed for headache and to improve lactation

**MEDICAL USES**

Treatment of stomach pain, the emulsion of the fruits is lethal to fresh water snails that carry the bilharzia micro-organism, and to water-fleas that carry guninea (worm disease).

Note green under tree

## WHY DID INTELLIGENT PEOPLE NOT REALISE THE CONDITIONS OF EQUATORIAL AFRICA WERE DIFFERENT TO ENGLISH PASTURE?

When the Europeans brought their cattle into Africa, they cleared the trees and bushes, killed the eland and other wildlife and then dug bore holes to spill the precious underground water on to the surface, where it was exposed to the direct rays of the sun and quickly evaporated. The water tables sank and trees and bushes for some distance around were deprived of deep water and died. This destroyed the microclimate under their canopy, which was not only cooler but was also kept moist by the gentle transpiration of water through the leaves. As a result, the sedges, herbs and edible grasses also died.

Flying over Botswana for example, you can look down and see the luxurious bushveld peppered with circular dark areas devoid of vegetation which is where the cattle assembled to drink water from the deep bore holes. One day these dark patches will join up and the once rich area will become a desert. In Uganda in the 1960s, in a region the size of Wales, wild animals were shot and burnt or left to rot in the sun to make way for English cattle. Enough meat to feed several townships for a year was burnt or given to flies and vultures. Pairs of bulldozers connected by huge chains then marched across the once rich region, tearing out the deep-rooted trees and bushes. The idea was to produce grass pasture for cattle south of Mbarara where Michael Pirkis, a great friend ours, worked with the ministry of agriculture. He reported on the decimation of a massive area.

Even here, with Lake Victoria close by and a favourable rainfall, the environmental response was devastating. The uprooted shade now exposed the succulent grasses and herbs to the full radiation of the equatorial sun. The Game Department was up in arms about it. The Chief Game Warden wrote letters of protest to the Governor General, Sir Walter Coutts and the UN.

Nothing stopped the bulldozers. One could only watch as the heat-resistant and unpalatable lemon grasses took over. The cattle had little to eat, became sick and began to die. An interesting example of how fast a change in conditions of existence can change the dominant species.

The disaster would have been total had it not been for the inefficiency of the operation, which paralleled its stupidity. Many of the trees regenerated from branches trampled into the ground by the bulldozer caterpillar tracks. Sadly, the wildlife, with its unique physiological adaptation to hot dry climate and diseases to which the cattle were susceptible, did not come back.

One wonders why later, in the 1970s, the World Bank and the EEC, at a cost of several million dollars, set up an International Livestock Centre in Africa for more cattle development – in Ethiopia! Are people so blinded by their own experience?

What the eland, giraffe and oryx showed is that the evolutionary response to hot dry climates was multi-factorial. It involved the mechanism for regulating temperature, the surface areas of the lungs, the absorption of water in the intestines, the permeability of the skin preventing water loss through perspiration, the efficiency of the kidneys, a metabolic response to produce a fat-rich milk, nervous system sensor modifications, and an appropriate behaviour pattern even involving the shape of the mouth and tongue. The giraffe, for example, has a tongue which is almost prehensile. It can strip the leaves off an acacia branch between the "wait-a-bit" thorns without a scratch. These thorns are large and viciously sharp. They can puncture Land Rover tyres. The leaves transpire water from the deep-water tables, and as we commented, at night they are swollen with liquid to satisfy the thirst of these semi-arid adapted animals.

## AGRO -FORESTRY

In the late 1960s a plan was put forward by Makerere University College, Kampala, the Uganda Game Department and the Zoological Society of London to the then Overseas Development Administration of the UK. The plan envisaged developing the semi-arid adapted plants such as the *acacias* and *Balanites species* to re-forest a large region of mid- Karamoja north of Mbale and between Soroti and Moroto.

THREE-DIMENSIONAL, SELF SUSTAINABLE

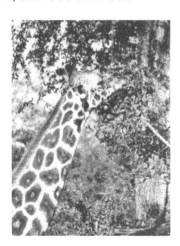

The deep roots of these trees and bushes reach the water tables 30 or more meters below. The Balanites in particular have fleshy leaves which evaporate water in the daytime and as we discussed, replenish at night. This cycle maintains a sufficient degree of humidity for the sedges, herbs, grasses and small bushes to grow under their shade. As we said earlier, the diversity of such plants, provides food and even water for a whole range of animals.

So the plan was to basically re-create the wealth of the plant and animal species adapted to these semi-dry conditions and use it as a new form of food production. Not the single layer of grass as in Norfolk, but the three layers of this wonderful diverse ecosystem, harnessed for its and our benefit. And incidentally a means of conservation through utilisation.

## The beauty about this ecosystem is five-fold

- First the animals can seek shade in the heat of the day and, being poikilothermic, rather like the camel, conserve water, allowing their temperature to rise instead of losing water to maintain temperature, as cows do.
- Second, by eating at night when the leaves are full of water they do not need surface water, which is largely non-existent in these regions.
- Third, the system is potentially self-expanding by pollinating insects and natural seed dispersal by birds and animals.
- Fourthly, during the destruction of the woodland Mbarara region to make way for the cattle, the workmen driving the tractors, were beset by attacks from bees whose homes they were destroying. It was a major problem bringing the action to a halt whilst protective measures were put in place. Pollinating insects are an integral part of the diverse plant life we are talking about, critical for self- replication and expansion. In a managed programme such as was planned, the bees would have been an important component of pollination, food production and wax.

- Fifthly, there would be hard wood timber for buildings and furniture from the management.

The basic plan was to first re-forest and establish the three dimensions of the semi-arid plant system (tree, bush and ground/root plants). Honeybees would also be introduced to ensure pollination and to provide honey. This would result in the development of wild bird populations. Birds are natural seed dispersal agents – that, in turn, would provide food while extending the boundaries and so helping to reverse desertification[20].

The project then aimed to introduce tamed animals, as the Russians had done in breeding eland in Askania-Nova for meat and milk. The local Karamajong welcomed the idea as we mentioned. Initially the test area of several square miles was to be fenced to keep the top carnivores out.

Sadly, the programme had to be abandoned when the notorious Idi Amin came into power and the country descended into brutality. Michael, when on a tour with the Game Department in 1972, witnessed first-hand the sickening catastrophe of children given guns as though they were toys and laughing at the site of an elder looking for his cows amongst a herd being taken by the soldiers, twisting and almost dancing in response to a hail of bullets.

Solar energy would have been the chief provider of power for workshop housing developments in remote areas. Such schemes do of course require large investment in practical applications and research; but the semi-arid has the prospect of both protecting present arable land, which is being eroded, and massively extending the boundaries of land-based food production in Africa and other regions where desert encroachment is depleting the potential for feeding people.

Here's some food for thought. We remind the reader that the late Professor Stephen Hawking warned before he died that with the rate of overpopulation and habitat destruction occurring on Earth, we would need to leave the planet within a 100 years.

Whilst a decade ago Elon Musk's idea of building rockets to take people to Mars might have been a laugh, it is now within his grasp. He has to green Mars. OK lets go!! Adventure is at the heart of human spirit. However, why not before Mars, first spend the money on greening the desert on *this* planet? Why not get experience first by greening the desert here. Not only might he learn a trick or too but may also be able to build and operate research plants which might become adaptable to Mars?

Leaving aside any relevance to Mars, the plan above proposes a new system of agriculture for Africa and other semi-arid regions of the world. It would provide, milk, meat, eggs, honey, wax, vegetable oils, nuts, herbal medicines, timber, climate change and desertification reversal. Not the wet stuff of contemporary Northern Europe etc, but the seemingly harsh, semi-arid stuff of Africa. It would solve the tragic and repetitive famines, and the death of several million children from malnutrition and infection: several will have died in the time taken to read this paragraph. It would have applications to India, China, Australia and Russia. If only peace would descend, the killing and war stopped and the massive financial investment in death delivering armaments turned to rescuing the productivity of the planet in a sustainable manner – if only.

## END PIECE

We conclude here with some remarks by Darwin that show how he would have argued against those who deny the influences of conditions or food, and who see no need to find any evolutionary mechanism other than random mutation and the survival of the fittest. The quotations come from *The Origin of Species:*

*'Several writers have misapprehended or objected to the term natural selection. Some have even imagined that natural selection*

*induces variability, whereas it implies only the preservation of such variations as arise and are beneficial to the being under its conditions of life.*

*In looking at many small points of difference between species, which, as far as our ignorance permits us to judge, seem quite unimportant, we must not forget that climate, food etc., have no doubt produced some direct effect.*

*Changed conditions of life are of the highest importance in causing variability, both by acting directly on the organisation, and indirectly by affecting the reproductive system.*

*Our ignorance of the laws of variation is profound. Not in one case out of a hundred can we pretend to assign any reason why this or that part has varied . . . Changed conditions generally induce mere fluctuating variability, but sometimes they cause direct and definite effects; and these may become strongly marked in the course of time.*

*To sum up on the origin of our Domestic Races of animals and plants. I believe that the conditions of life, from their action on the reproductive system, are so far of the highest importance as causing variability [21].*

If the greatest events in evolution history were actually determined by physics and chemistry which is synonymous with the environment, then it is indeed most likely that the smaller events will have been similarly fashioned. How some of those "direct and definite effects" came about, and how they and the Giraffe's neck became not only "strongly marked" but irrevocably built into various species and our own has been the topic of this book so far.

Image below from a paper by Treus and Kravchenko in *Comparative nutrition of wild animals.* Ed. M A Crawford, Symposium No. 21 Zoological Society of London 1968.

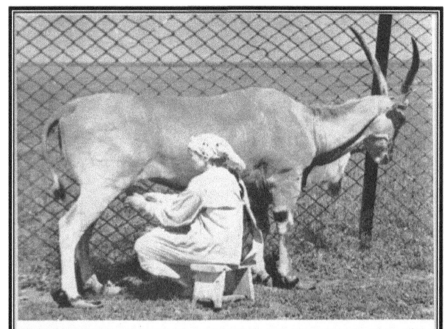

Milking a young eland cow at Askaniya Nova in the Ukraine. The milk is more concentrated than cows' milk and is in fact natures 'long-life milk'. This is the answer to those who believe that wild animals cannot be domesticated.

**THE TREE BROWSING GIRAFFE HAS MORE ARACHDONIC ACID (ARA) THAN THE GRASS EATING ZEBRA BETTER TO BUILD A STRONG ARTERY AND BLOOD PRESSURE CONTROL FOR THE LONG NECK..**

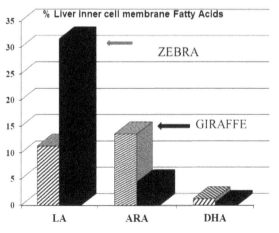

Genetics, epigenetics, nutritional differences from the tops of the trees compared to the grasses conspired with prostacylin to support the long neck. A competitive advantage is suspect as the female has a shorter neck.

Data from: Williams G, Crawford M 1987 J Zool. Lond. 213: 673 - 684.

# CHAPTER 11
# Mental Health

## The Past

*"Life began in the oceans, we have to save the oceans to save ourselves"* (South Korean Pavilion and theme for EXPO 2012)

The International Expo 2012, "The Living Ocean and Coast", was held in Yeosu, a port city in South Korea. The theme was "life began in the oceans, we have to save the oceans to save ourselves". Michael was invited to open the UN-FAO conference at the EXPO which reflected that theme. A highlight of the EXPO was a video shown on a wall-to-wall IMAX-like screen. It was introduced by a young boy. The beginning of life 3.5+ billion years ago, and then the evolution of air-breathing, multicellular life over the last 600 million years resulting in the present diversity and sheer magnificence of marine life.

Then came the modern chapter featuring human pollution, rubbish dumping, destruction of the estuaries and ripping-up of the seafloor and its delicate ecosystem, creating swathes of marine deserts. The young boy who had invited us to watch the video has disappeared and was now seen riding on a dolphin underwater, showing the harsh reality of what we are now doing to such an exquisite product of Nature and highlighting the sheer beauty of that marine creature. At the end of the video, the young boy appeared as if by magic from the back of the theatre, floating through the air on the back of a seal. He prompted us to act.[38]

---

38    (An FAO colleague sitting next to Michael said "They are showing your book"!).

Despite this vivid clarion call from EXPO 2012[39],[1] matters have, if anything, worsened since then. We have now added microplastics to the list of human excreta being mindlessly thrown into lakes, rivers and seas.

Life began in the sea and the brain evolved in the sea. The only substances available for fashioning its remarkable signalling systems came from the sea. For a long time, there was nothing else. The evidence today justifies us in describing marine food as brain food. During the evolution of the mammals, almost at the earliest opportunity, many returned to the sea. The seals, dolphins and whales have the largest brain size relative to their body size of any mammals apart from humans. Our ancestors, since diverging from the great apes, would have used the best of land and aquatic foods, ensuring sufficient brain food to power the evolution of our large brain. It could not have been otherwise. With the rise of cheap, intensively reared land foods, that positive pattern has changed in recent times, and we are paying the cost in terms of mental health.

We need to clean the estuaries and coastlines and restore the oceans and their productivity to save the oceans and save ourselves. With the decline in mental health and the escalation of climate change, time is running out. Nature is in the wings waiting for the day of the Dolphins[40].

---

39    Expo 2012 concluded on 12 August 2012 with the adoption of the Yeosu Declaration for the Living Ocean and Coasts. The Expo was "intended not only to enhance the awareness of dangers faced by the sea but also to promote the necessity of international cooperation for turning these challenges into hopes for the future." More information on the Declaration can be found on UNESCO's website or the Expo 2012 website. See: http://eng.expo2012.kr/is/ps/unitybbs/bbs/selectBbsDetail.html

40    All the bones of the human hand are inside its flippers. It has vestigial legs during transition from and embryo to a fetus.

## The Present

On 12 December 2020, MSN issued the following headline:

UN SECRETARY GENERAL URGES ALL COUNTRIES TO DECLARE CLIMATE EMERGENCIES: António Guterres tells Climate Ambition Summit more must be done to hit net zero emissions.

In 1992, Severn Cullis-Suzuki, the 12-year-old daughter of an environmental scientist in Vancouver, Canada, traveled with three friends to the United Nations climate conference in Rio de Janeiro. Now perhaps forgotten, she became known at the time as "the girl who silenced the world for six minutes".[2]

She drew attention to the looming crisis of climate change. Twenty-seven years later, in September 2019, the 17-year-old Swedish girl Greta Thunberg stood in the forum of the United Nations in New York City castigating the political and business leaders of the world for lack of action.

Thunberg said, "All you can talk about is the money and the …. economic growth. How dare you!" She stressed the scientific evidence for global warming, saying "For more than 30 years the science has been crystal clear. All you can do is look away – how dare you!" She referred to the tipping point where climate change goes beyond human control and becomes a runaway disaster. It is we, she said, we children "who have to live with the consequences".[3,4]

When you consider the pace of change compared to the time taken to fashion our species, it is painfully clear , it is painfully clear to quote Vice Admiral Carmona that "we do not have time"[5] to sort both the mental ill-health crisis and climate change. Yet, as we have discussed, the mental ill-health crisis is largely being brushed under the carpet.

A year after Thunberg's speech, António Guterres, UN Secretary General, called for a global effort. Will it happen? Do people know how to deal with the already present tonnage of excess carbon dioxide, oceanic acidification and other pollutants defecated by human activities?

We will offer a realistic means of addressing and halting the Catastrophe.

## 2021 And Climate Change

In the first week of January 2021, Kelly-Ann Mills wrote an article in the UK Mirror newspaper based on a series of more than 500 aerial photographs from NASA that paint a stark picture of the reality of climate change.[6] The photographs were taken over a period of 40 years, graphically illustrating the shrinking ice cap. The Arctic Sea ice is declining by 13.1% per decade, relative to the 1981 to 2010 average[7]. The OK Glacier in Iceland has simply vanished. These images must surely convince the most hardened sceptics of the reality of global warming.

According to the International Energy Agency, global energy-related $CO_2$ emissions flattened in 2019 at around 33 gigatonnes (Gt), following two years of increases. This was primarily the result of a sharp decline in $CO_2$ emissions from the power sector in advanced economies,[8] thanks to the expanding role of renewable sources (mainly wind and solar PV), fuel switching from coal to natural gas, and the higher nuclear power output.[9] It is an encouraging development and shows we can make a difference, but our efforts are still far too small.

Moreover, this hint of the possible so often overlooks the pollution of the rivers, oceans and estuaries and its implications for the provision of 'brain food'. Therein lies a hidden crisis: the threat from escalating mental ill-health and a fall in IQ, which, if left unchecked, will lead to the degradation of the brain, and with it the attrition of our essential humanity. "*We do not have time*" to mess about. Action is needed now, on a global scale.

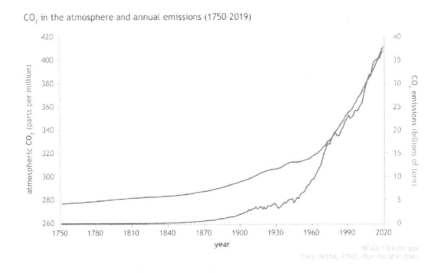

CO$_2$ in the atmosphere and annual emissions (1750-2019)

Remember, the brain evolved in the seas at the beginning of vertebrate evolution, and it still uses marine nutrients for form and function. The 2012 Joesu EXPO theme from South Korea was "Life began in the oceans; we have to save the oceans to save ourselves". Their theme video highlighted the toxic impact of marine pollution, with the seas being used as a dumping ground for our trash. That trash includes the microplastics that now inhabit the marine food web including the sea foods we eat. And yet it was the seas which first brought life to the planet, giving birth to the plants, animals and ourselves.

On the 14th January 2020, The Blue Planet Society commented on human actions in EU waters, saying "The slaughter of common dolphins by fishing vessels may be the largest non-cull slaughter of a large mammal species on Earth. The cetacean carnage witnessed recently on the south coast of England is just the tip of the iceberg."[10]

The same story was taken up by Ciaran McGrath in the Daily Express on the 9th December 2020, under the headline "EU super trawler hell as dolphins killed".[11] These super trawlers have been referred to as the Death Stars of the oceans. The dolphins are just one casualty of a trawling practice which scours the seabed, killing delicate marine flora and with it the beginning of the food web on which the fish depend.

This book is not about global warming or the ecologically toxic treatment of our rivers, estuaries and oceans, relevant as they are. But our theme of mental health is inextricably linked with environment, and these factors connive to produce a world antagonistic to mental health, and indeed to physical health. Global warming and ocean acidification are changing the flora and fauna of oceans which we are still exploiting in a reckless manner.

The pleas by Severn Cullis-Suzuki, and Greta Thunberg were about protecting humanity from a runaway global climate change that threatens extinction. But there is another terrible threat – the main theme of this book – which to us and many of our colleagues is an even graver one: the escalation of mental ill-health.

Some people find it possible to be complacent about climate change, claiming that we will simply adapt to changing circumstances as we have done before, but there is no room for complacency regarding the rise in mental ill-health, the fall in human intelligence and our species' diminishing brain size. If allowed to continue, the continued increase in mental ill-health and diminishing intelligence has only one logical conclusion. It means the loss of that which makes us human.

Make no mistake, the epigenetic susceptibility that transformed *Homo sapiens* in terms of health, height and body size in a single century is a visible example in living memory of how fast environmental and nutritional misadventure can shape our species, and these factors are now wreaking havoc with our mental health. The shift in shape, size and physical health happened quickly; and drastic changes are now reshaping our species' mental health and intelligence. The reduction in our brain size has been ongoing for quite some time, some say since the establishment of land-based agriculture. The present deterioration in mental health can have only one logical and unthinkable conclusion.

The nutritional needs of the brain have been bypassed in recent times in favour of protein for body size. We need an amplification of António Guterres' call for the declaration of a worldwide climate emergency applied to mental health: the UN must spearhead global action before it is too late and our politicians and business leaders become too dumbed-down to understand and take action. The wonderful fact is that actions to reverse the deterioration in mental health and arrest climate change shake hands, as we shall discuss in this chapter.

## The Inequality Of Food Security

We are not alone in getting anxious about food security. Ricardo Salvador, director of the Food and Environment Program at the Union of Concerned Scientists, expressed deep concern regarding the state of food in relation to the escalating human population and the lack of political will to address even the present crisis of hunger and malnutrition. While many starve, 73% of the US population is overweight or obese,[12] and the obesity rate there has doubled since the beginning of the century.

Nor is it just the USA – obesity levels in Scotland are among the highest of the OECD countries with 65% of adults being overweight, which includes 28% obese (2018).[13] Worryingly, 22.4% of primary one pupils in Scotland are at risk of being overweight or obese. This gross over-consumption of food, whether through greed or the search for missing nutrients in high-energy, low-quality foods from intensive production,[14,15] is a matter of debate, even though the certainty of the conclusion is staring us in the face. Either way, obese people are often malnourished due to the nutritionally poor junk foods they consume[16]. The reality is a gross inequality in food security. With political will, this inequality – which causes sickness and death from hunger and malnutrition on the one hand and diabetes and chronic disease on the other – could be remedied.

The World Food Programme accepted the 2019 Nobel Peace Prize, a well-deserved acknowledgement of the wonderful work done by this organisation. Ricardo Salvador commented in response, on the growing global hunger crisis amid the pandemic. Concerning the present state of food insecurity, he made the point that there still is enough food to go round. "It's important to remember that hunger does not always happen because of natural disasters." He added wistfully that there could be a world in which there was no longer a need for the WFP.

**Two images of the conditions of our world**

**that speak for themselves.**

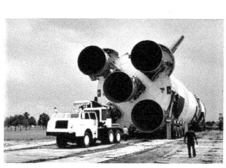 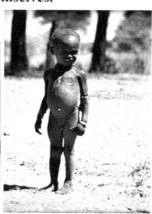

In the picture above the rocket is to be used for peaceful space exploration. Who knows what the USA, China and Russia are developing in secret? President Putin has been unabashedly trumpeting the success of new hypersonic nuclear missiles so fast that no defence system could intercept them. Just one of his missiles has enough warheads to destroy an area the size of France. What madness is this? With these kinds of weapons to hand, there can be no doubt that their use will be terminal for much of the life on this planet. The combination of nuclear proliferation and the mental ill-health pandemic brings to mind Stanley Kubrick's 1964 black comedy Dr Strangelove,[17]

starring Peter Sellers. The plot involves a mentally ill general who attempts to start a nuclear war. The film culminates in the automatic activation of the USSR's retaliatory doomsday cobalt bomb.

Whatever one thinks about the causes of the strange events of 6 January 2021, when US democracy was stormed, the point is that we cannot afford to continue the downward spiral of mental ill-health. If there has to be a 'finger on the button', it has to belong to someone with peak mental health! Even without the doomsday bomb, the several thousand thermo-nuclear warheads in readiness today across the world are enough to wipe out life on the planet seven times over, a scenario at the forefront of the extraordinary brain of Professor Stephen Hawking when he said humanity would need to leave the planet in a 100 years' time.[20] That is far too generous a time slot. Once again - *"We do not have time".*

## The Supreme Importance Of The Mother

The first call to action concerns the immediate need to focus on the lack of awareness of the supreme importance of the mother. Let's get things right at the start rather than focusing on trying to patch them up later. The second call is about sorting out the food system (which we will come to later).

The most critical period of brain development is before birth, when the brain soaks up 70% of the energy received from the mother, all to fuel the astonishing velocity of brain growth. Poverty cannot be eradicated without attention to the health and nutrition of the mother, before, during, and after pregnancy, so that the next generation is functioning at full physical and mental capacity and capable of taking on the colossal challenges of life in an over-heated, over-populated world.

Even after birth, the mother donates essential brain growth-supporting nutrients via her milk. This means she herself is losing these nutrients. Human milk is a rich soup of micronutrients and hormones vital for the development of the gut, the biome, gut and nerve growth. The principle of first choice should be to feed the mother so that she can feed her baby, not persuade her to bottle feed. And if for some reason the mother is unable to feed her newborn, then as the 1976 FAO/WHO meeting on fats in human nutrition recommended, the formula to be used should mimic human milk as closely as possible.

The pivotal role of the mother is constantly ignored or sidelined. When director general of the WHO Dr Gro Harlem Brundtland opened the XVIII European Congress of Perinatal Medicine, Oslo, in 2002, she said:

*"In most countries in Europe, women can receive the news of a pregnancy confident that it will be a period of attention, support, and assistance. But for pregnancies in our world, the reality is very different. A young woman in Ethiopia, for example, goes into the reproductive phase of her life with a one-in-ten chance that she will die as a result of pregnancy or delivery. That is not only shocking – it is totally unacceptable."*

Sir Kenneth Stuart, a previous medical adviser to the Commonwealth and trustee of the Mother and Child Foundation, saw grounds for optimism in the past support for developing countries, if that support can be galvanised to address the pivotal issue of poverty. This effort must start with the mother and extend to children at school and during puberty (in but a few years' the future parents of the world).

Recent evidence shows us that much of the outcome of pregnancy is decided before conception. Nature prepares in advance for critical events. Focusing our attention here is basic logic and common sense. It is like the parable of the seed sown on poor soil versus one sown on rich soil. The importance of maternal nutrition and health prior to conception is a matter of supreme importance.

On day 7 after conception, the fertilised egg implants into the *milieu intérieur* of the mother. Cells have a long turnover time. The red cell, for example, has a life of 120 days. If one takes the membrane lipids of the cell, its composition on day 7 after conception will be an integration of the maternal diet, behaviour, absorption efficiency, metabolomics and genomics over the last several months. So on day 7, the *milieu intérieur* of the site of implantation will have been determined by the diet and behaviour of the mother around the time of conception and well before. The period preconception will be and has been shown to be a principle determinant of outcome. People will recognise this fact from the need for folic acid prior to and around the time of conception to prevent neural tube defects which result in spina bifida or an infant being born anencephalic – that is, without a brain and unsurvivable.

And yet at the Chelsea and Westminster Hospital in London, Professor Mark Johnson, who heads obstetrics and gynaecology, tells us that some 50% of the pregnancies he sees are unplanned. Where it is planned, much of the planning has to do with provision for the birth of the child, its cot and postnatal care.

Professor Johnson's aim is to see the creation of a centre for women that addresses the importance of maternal health and nutrition prior to conception, and which works for women to ensure the physical and mental health of the mother and her newborn child. He wants a centre that focuses on women in the same way the many Institutes of Child Health focus on children.

We repeat the words of Dr Mark Belsey, Director of Maternal and Child Health at WHO, spoken in 1993 at a meeting at the Royal Society of Medicine organised by the Mother and Child Foundation.

"Wherever you look, the interests of the child are served with UNICEF, Save the Children Fund, the ubiquitous Institutes of Child Health and many other organisations.

But – there is no voice for the mother!"

Those words were spoken 30 years ago, but there is the same apparent lack of interest today. If you are interested in the health and ability of the child, you need to get things right at the start of life. That means the mother, and that means her health and nutrition before conception and throughout the pregnancy and the nursing of her infant. The supreme importance of the mother cannot be overestimated. She is the answer to breaking the cycle of deprivation and poverty.

Sadly, in the UK and the US the prevalence of preterm birth and low birthweight has remained stoically unchanged since the 1950s. These principle causes of brain damage and mental ill-health have not budged, despite the notable advances of medicine and science. Knowing what we have known since the 1960s, about the irreversible impact of being born before the growth spurt of the brain is finished, this fact is a scandal. At the same time, mental ill-health carries a stigma that has a long and vicious history. All the more extraordinary that its causes have not been the focus of any national health or food policy.

Good brain health is not just about ensuring a child has a good diet. Preconception, prenatal and post-natal nutrition alike are vital, and it is the mother who does lots of the nutritional legwork. Seventy percent of our brain forms early in pregnancy, making the mother's health and wellbeing the most important of the various factors which go towards a child's mental fitness.

During the Nuremberg trials of the Nazis for war crimes after World War II, four psychiatrists were condemned to death for killing 167,000 of their patients in Germany. After the war, the practice of lobotomy was much publicised but eventually brought to shame by One Flew Over the Cuckoo's Nest, a 1962 novel set in a psychiatric hospital, written by Ken Kesey. [21] Lobotomy had been widely practiced for more than two decades as a treatment for schizophrenia, manic depression and bipolar disorder, among other mental illnesses. One surgeon alone carried out 50,000 lobotomies. Astonishingly, the Portuguese neurologist Egas Moniz, the initiator of the technique, was awarded the Nobel Prize in 1949 – for developing surgery that cuts the connections to the frontal cortex of the brain, resulting in an individual being unable to care for themselves and left largely in a vegetative state.

One Flew Over the Cuckoo's Nest exposed the abuse of authority and the unquestioning connivance of those involved. Much the same would have applied to many of the Nuremburg psychiatrists, acting under the spell of those pursuing the concept of a purified race. It was made into a film starring Jack Nicholson as a mental patient. It was the second film to win all 5 Academy awards.

## The Cost Of Mental Ill-Health

Today we have a better understanding of the causes of poor mental health than ever before; and yet we struggle to help those afflicted. The stigma attached to mental health problems and the lack of attention given to the issue has led to a rise in mental ill-health since 1950.

The EU called for an audit of the cost of ill-health in 2004. Published in 2005, disorders of the brain was top of the list, at a cost of €386 billion. Some people, in disbelief, said this figure was simply due to clever advances in diagnosis. Even if that were proven to be the case, you would have thought that if brain disorders unexpectedly headed an official list of health costs, someone would have said "Let's do something about this!" But no.

In 2006, Michael and the late Rev Paul Nicholson of the charity Z2K approached Lord Morris of Manchester, previously active in the Labour movement (he had introduced the Chronically Sick and Disabled Persons Act 1970). Their request was to ascertain the cost of mental ill-health in the UK following the EU's audit. When asked about this in the House of Lords, Lord Warner, the Minister for Health, did not know the answer. But he knew the cost of drugs used for the mentally ill in hospital. This had risen five-fold between 1990 and 2002.

To give the Department of Health and Social Care (DHSC) its due, it did the numbers. Dr Jo Nurse of the Mental Health division of the Department reported that in 2007 the cost for mental ill-health, was £77 billion. [22] That was a cost, she said, greater than heart disease and cancer combined! In other words, it was now the costliest burden of ill-health in the country.

You would expect such a response to make the government swing into action, demand answers and introduce solutions. But no. Once again, it was all said to be due to new, improved diagnostics.

The EU and DHSC crunched the numbers again, using the same criteria. There would now be no question of new diagnostics. The EU's figure came out at €789 billion – over double the cost in six years. Admittedly, Bulgaria joined in 2017, but the country only had a population of just over 6 million, so that was hardly going to have any major bearing on the statistics. The DHSC figure was £105 billion – a 36% increase in five years. The Wellcome Trust then did their own sums and published the numbers on their web site in 2013: £113 billion.

The late Simon House, a trustee of the Mother and Child Foundation, considers these numbers to be underestimates. Violence was not included in the definition of mental ill-health, nor were severe neurodevelopmental disorders such as cerebral palsy. If these were to be included, the numbers would increase dramatically.

There is evidence that whereas at the beginning of the 20th century IQ increased with the passing years, it has declined since 1950. Borderline mental retardation is associated with a child with an IQ between 70 and 90. If the trend continues, then by 2080 between a third and half of the world's population will be borderline mentally retarded.

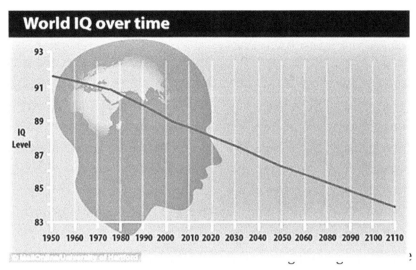

**World IQ over time**

greatest threat to the sustainability of humanity, ever. It is a graver threat to survival than global warming, as critical as that is. The two together, unchecked, lead to the sixth extinction in the middle of the next century if not before. It is Nature's way of testing her evolutionary products that come to dominance and then seeing to their end. The five main extinctions of the past have been environmentally triggered, one way or another. This coming one is rather unique: it is self-inflicted. It is a form of environmental destruction with no thought for the needs to support the very specific nutrition of the brain which made us human in the first place. It is a form of self-inflicted lobotomy.

## The Covid-19 and mental ill-health

There can be absolutely no doubt about mental ill-health now being the costliest burden of ill-health in the EU, UK and USA. The only doubt that remains is that those figures may be underestimates. The problem is being globalised in the wake of the spread of Western-style diets. And now along comes Covid-19 into the bargain, with its impact on mental health. As Natalie Tronson, Associate Professor of Psychology, University of Michigan, wrote for *The Conversation* in August 2020:

"It is now clear that many patients suffering from Covid-19 exhibit neurological symptoms, from loss of smell, to delirium, to an increased risk of stroke. There are also longer-lasting consequences for the brain, including myalgic encephalomyelitis/chronic fatigue syndrome and Guillain-Barre syndrome. These effects may be caused by direct viral infection of brain tissue. But growing evidence suggests additional indirect actions triggered via the virus's infection of epithelial cells and the cardiovascular system, or through the immune system and inflammation, contribute to lasting neurological changes after Covid-19." [23]

In this book we have been critical of the overemphasis on protein in nutrition education and government recommendations and the lack of attention given to lipids and the brain. The lipids were pivotal to the evolution of multicellular species [24], so it is perhaps relevant that the Covid-19 virus has a lipid coating. Coronavirus infection involves the fusion of the virus envelope and the host cell's outer (plasma) membrane, which house certain receptors. This enables the virus to penetrate the interior of the cell. Corona-type viruses remodel cellular membranes to form viral replication compartments (VRCs), which are the sites where viral RNA genome replication takes place. Recent research has provided evidence that "To induce VRC formation, these viruses extensively rewire lipid metabolism ... membrane contact sites and lipid transfer proteins are hijacked by the virus and play pivotal roles in VRC formation."[25]

Several studies complement this evidence. A rapid response review discussed the possibility of vitamin D involvement[26], and selenium deficiency has also been identified as an amplifier of risk.[27] Although sunlight is a major source of vitamin D, both vitamin D and selenium occur at their richest in the marine food web, which we have identified in this book as being of critical importance to the immune system, the brain and its integrity.

While DNA, RNA and protein compositions are not affected by diet, the lipid membrane is susceptible in a way that is thought to affect health and play a causative role in inflammatory disorders and non-communicable diseases. The evidence from hospital admission rates for Covid-19 being "synonymous with an elevated risk of non-communicable disease"[28] mirrors the disproportionate coronavirus mortality rates amongst Black, Asian and Minority Ethnic (BAME) groups, highlighting the longstanding inequalities of health in which lipids are particularly relevant.[29]

The synthesis of lipids for the viral coat is essential for its replication, as shown in studies on dengue virus replication. The influence of the membrane lipids of our cells cannot be overestimated. The cells outer, plasma membrane is the guardian and protector, housing lipid molecules that maintain cell health, blood flow and blood pressure. They also provide immune surveillance, responding to trauma and infections acting to resolve any damage caused. The 1982 Nobel Prize awarded to Sune Bergstrom, Bengt Samuelsson and Sir John Vane was for discovering the previously unknown molecules responsible for these behaviours.

With the diagnostic early sign of Covid-19 infection being loss of smell (a neurological attack), with long-term impacts on the brain, here we have yet another good reason for being concerned about the deficiency of lipids in our diets and the need to re-shape the food system to prioritise the needs of the brain, which shares common ground with the immune, vascular and reproductive systems. The heightened risk of the BAME fits with the studies by Wendy Doyle, mentioned previously, namely a poor diet before and during pregnancy leading preterm birth and low birthweights which carry the highest risk of brain defects and stunting.

The extraordinary evolution of the human brain could only have happened if it was fuelled by nutrition specific to brain growth and function and hence healthy pregnancy outcomes followed by lengthy periods of breast feeding. It is Darwin's conditions of existence again. But what goes up can also come down.

This new burden of mental ill-health is another bit of evidence that we have missed out on Sir Robert McCarrison's 'unsophisticated foodstuffs of nature'.[30]

## Fishing For Answers

Up to now, we have painted a sorry state of the food system. There will be a knee jerk reaction against our telling of this story, but the facts are evidence-based and cannot be denied. With Foresight claiming we have reached the limit of arable land,[31] the ocean's resources having reached a sustainable limit at the turn of the century, and with the escalation in mental ill-health putting the sustainability of humanity under threat, solutions are urgently needed. Previously we mentioned that at a conference in Washington DC, organised by Capt Joe Hibbeln and Military colleagues in 2013[41] to discuss post-traumatic stress disorder (PTSD) and mental health, Vice Admiral Richard Carmona, the seventeenth Surgeon General of the United States, he commented on the urgency for action in response to the crisis in mental ill-health. He twice said: " *We do not have time.*"[32]

Nearly a decade since then there still has been no action.

To do the maths, let's say the population is 7 billion, and the recommended daily intake of DHA is 200 mg. That equals a requirement for 1.4 billion grams (or 1.4 million kilograms) of DHA a day. However, you need to eat on average around 200 grams of fish to get 1 gram of DHA; so if we multiply the figure by 200 to convert it to fish, that gives us a requirement of

41   Published in Military Medicine, 2014, volume 179

280 million kilos of fish every day. If we then multiply that by 365, we get a requirement for 102 million tons of fish needed per annum. That number approximates to the total fish catch. However, nearly a third of the fish catch is fed to animals. Moreover, our initial figure of 7 billion is already history and we are knocking on 8 billion and will soon be anticipating 9 billion.

The nutritional requirements of the brain are not being met in today's world, rife as it is with such gross inequalities of food, never mind fish or sea foods. In 2013, 6.3 million children died before the age of five.[33] 44% died in the first month of life, with preterm birth being a prime cause of mortality and poor brain development. Pneumonia and diarrhoea are the next most common causes. According to UNICEF, "Nearly half of all deaths in children under five are attributable to undernutrition, translating into the loss of about 3 million young lives a year".[34] A further huge number live in hunger.

Seventy-one per cent of the planet is covered with water. Of the remainder, only about a third is suitable for use as arable land; and nearly all this is already occupied. In the 1960s, it was thought that the oceans would continue to supply us with enough food to feed everyone. However, the FAO reported that the annual wild fish catch stopped rising in 2000. Since then it has levelled, with increasing concern being expressed about over-fishing, destructive fishing practices, and unsustainability. Some species having reached the tipping point, including perennial staples such as cod and haddock. Where measures have been taken, welcome recovery of stocks has been seen. The establishment of marine conservation zones is one answer, but of limited long-term functionality if the hunting-and-gathering mentality continues unchecked, decimating marine populations and tearing up the flora and fauna residing on the seabed.

In 1961 in Siglufjörður, northern Iceland, 17,000 barrels of herring were salted in one day. The herring have now gone, documented in a beautiful historical account by Mike Smylie,

*Herring: A History of the Silver Darlings.*[35] The cod was also a commonly caught fish, once so bountiful that 19th century Newfoundland fisherman used buckets to scoop them from the sea – one of the many tales told in the excellent *Cod: A Biography of the Fish That Changed the World* by Mark Kurlansky.[36] Both books remind us of just how important fishing was. It is the most significant factor in our evolutionary history, despite the protestations of the admirers of the Savannah theory of origins (a habitat in which all brains shrank as the various species grew bigger, protein fueled bodies).

But, leaving the evidence of the origin of our big brain behind, even recent history is telling. Daniel Defoe, on his visit to Scotland in the 18th century, could hardly believe the richness of the Firth of Forth. In writing about the description of his visit he marvelled that the method of catching fish was difficult to believe, as all they had to do was lift them from the water.

We also have modern data relating to the fishing catch.

At the outbreak of World War One, the UK's fish landings stood at 1.2 million tons. During the periods covering both World Wars, they collapsed to about 350,000 tons, and no one knows how many fishing boats were sunk by enemy torpedoes. However, post-World War Two there was a recovery, and in 1950 the landing reached 1.1 million tons. The final collapse began in 1973, with a steady decline down to 400,000 tons in 2015 but made a bit of a recovery when it was 6000,000 tons in 2019. Importantly, the population of the UK in 1914 was 43 million. In 2019 it stood at 67.5 million. The UK's fish landing has declined to a third of its pre-First World War level, but the population has increased by over a third. The biggest decline in fish landings in the UK has occurred from the 70s onwards, which is consistent with the increase in mental ill-health and the downward trend seen in statistics taken from various measures of intelligence. The EU subsidised the burning of boats. With the decline in fisheries, whole fishing communities have vanished. Small fishing boats have been replaced by giant, death-star trawlers scouring the seabed, to the detriment of marine life.

Roger Harrabin, environment analyst for the BBC, claimed that long-line fishery for Mahi Mahi in Costa Rica had a tally of collateral damage over a decade that included 402 silky sharks, 625 stingrays and 1,348 turtles. "Globally about 85% of stocks are said to be fully exploited, over-exploited, depleted or slowly recovering", the BBC reported. "Using data from 1889, researchers assessed catches of bottom-feeding fish like cod, plaice and sole in England and Wales. They calculated that over 118 years of industrial fishing, the productivity of this fishery dropped by 94%. Not to 94% but by 94%".[37] The practice of fishing with great dredging nets that scour the ocean floor is a thoughtless and irresponsible destruction of life on the ocean floor: a rape-and-pillage approach that leads to the creation of man-made deserts in the ocean. Little wonder the fish have no food themselves.

Having 'fished down' the cod size, the reproductive age boundary has now been reached. That is, young fish entering the breeding phase are being fished out. In 1992, Canada issued a moratorium on the Northern Cod Fishery, catches having fallen to 1% of previous levels.[38] In 2012 the US Commerce Department issued a formal disaster declaration for the entire north-eastern commercial ground fishery of the North Atlantic.[39] That includes the decimated cod banks that supplied 50% of the English treasury's income in the reign of the first Queen Elizabeth. Admittedly, there have been some notable recoveries; however, the bottom line is a resource hovering on sustainability or disaster.

We have been destroying the wealth that gave birth to life and ultimately to *H sapiens*. Remember, the brain evolved in the sea and still requires marine n nutrients. You can once again hear Greta Thunberg saying, "How dare you!"[40]

There is *some* good news in this fishy saga, however. In 2013, the EU voted for sweeping reforms of the controversial EU Common Fisheries Policy. Following restrictions on fishing imposed in 2000 on the Pacific West Coast of the USA, there has been a good recovery of groundfish including rockfish, sole, flounder and sablefish. Randy Hartnell of Vital Choice[41] has told us of great stocks of Alaskan wild salmon. Hence, it is not *all* bad news. But the point remains. Population is growing logarithmically and we are going to have to agriculturalise the oceans.

# CHAPTER 12
# Solutions:
# Let's Fix The Food Crisis, Mental Ill- Health And Global Warming: All At The Same Time

## Food security

The solution to the present food insecurity is to first recognise that while there is malnutrition in Africa and other poor part so the world, there is also malnutrition in the European and USA cultures which includes brain malnutrition. To solve the mental health crisis we have to change the food paradigm to care for the brain. The brain evolved in the sea, so the third prong on the trident of our new food paradigm takes us back to the sea once again – to marine environments both ancient and modern. As we have underlined throughout this book, the evolution of the brain was fuelled by marine nutrients over millions and millions of years. Unfortunately, those nutrients are in finite supply from the land food web. They are almost non-existent in the intensively reared food sector. They are found abundant still in aquatic resources with a few remaining pockets of wild-based land foods.

Blundering along, ignoring the increasing need to feed an expanding population with little foreseeable increment in land-based agriculture to meet the present demand, is the present name of the game. So where is the next chunk of arable land coming from? People learnt to farm the land some

10,000 years ago; but our approach to aquatic resources still follows the pattern of our earliest human ancestors: hunting and gathering. 10,000 years ago this method of hand-to-mouth existence was recognised as unstainable and the challenge was met with action, in the form of agriculture, animal husbandry and community-based living. We now face the same challenge of unsustainability, and save for a precious few, those people in positions of power and influence seem paralysed, with minds in a closed box. We have to 'think outside the box'.[1]

The solution has to involve farming the sea. Food and nutrition policy needs to prioritise the requirements of the brain. For Heaven's sake, it is the brain which makes us human. To ignore the brain as in current practice, is mind boggling unacceptable.

A new paradigm is needed and it will require support from education in nutritional science and health, including primary secondary and medical education. In all this, the importance of the mother needs to come into focus and remain at the forefront. The supreme importance of prioritising maternal nutrition and health, even before conception, needs to be understood and put into practice to reverse the rise in mental ill-health and create new generations of children able to enjoy optimum intelligence and health they deserve from their genetic heritage as being human. The alternative is unthinkable.

Aquatic resource development will bring incredible bounty through restoring jobs and fishing communities, new research, and educational, health and industrial developments. It would also assist aquaculture as there would be ample fish offal for feeding fish instead of grinding up chickens and using vegetable oils better used as human food. Most crucially, it will lead to an abundance of health foods and nutrition for the brain and will also challenge climate change. How?

## We cannot create new rainforests. We can, however, grow the equivalent in the sea: kelp farms.

Both rain forests and kelp forests are oxygen-pumping carbon traps. We can also grow sea grass, which, similarly, is a powerful $CO_2$ guzzler. Hence farming in the sea will:

1. Provide for food-security for centuries to come.
2. Provide brain food to reverse the escalation of mental ill-health, decline in IQ and lead to healthier and more intelligent children.
3. Address oceanic acidification and contribute to the control of global warming by fixing $CO_2$.
4. Provide fertiliser to replenish soils depleted of trace elements and iodine so addressing the 2 billion mentally retarded from iodine deficiency and improve the productivity of conventional farming.

In Japan, Dr Takehiro Tanaka has been developing marine agriculture between two islands off the coast of Okayama. He calls it Shiraishijima Island's Marine Ranching Project in Okayama. [2] Tanaka's team started their work in 1991 and spent 15 years in research to define the local ecology with the aim of restoring marine deserts, enhancing the marine ecology and natural food web with regional and artificial reefs. They used *Zostera marina* – a species of sea grass known as common eel grass – to create marine pastures. These are pastures for fish, parallel to land-based grass pastures created for cows and sheep. Tanaka's team sank artificial reefs into the water designed for different species of fish (e.g. for gilt-head bream) both to enhance the natural productivity of their feeding areas and to allow for differences in fish behaviour. The kelp and grasses, along with other algae and phytoplankton, fix $CO_2$ in the same way as rainforests and help counteract ocean acidification. [3] (To put this into perspective, if atmospheric $CO_2$ concentrations continue to grow at their existing rate, the current figure of around 400 ppm will rise to around 480 ppm by 2035.)

Moreover, the scheme created new jobs for local people, fisher families and people with new skills and new manufacturing, skills and continuing research to monitor and improve performance. This is a self- sustaining model. It relies on an ecological and sustainable harnessing of the natural productivity of the seas and sunlight – tapping into something the sea has been doing for the last billion years. Kelp, sea grasses and mangroves provide cover and food for juvenile fish, and other marine life, enhancing natural productivity. In reducing ocean acidification, kelp helps create marine conditions that favour the farming of oysters, mussels, scallops and cockles, which all lock away $CO_2$ in their shells. Shellfish are a paradox, as they produce $CO_2$ during their lives, but sequester large quantities of it in their shells, which are principally calcium carbonate. The White Cliffs of Dover date back to the oceans of over 136 million years ago and are essentially a $CO_2$ dump from tiny, dead marine life, including the skeletons of planktonic green algae. Furthermore, kelp also feeds us directly, being a rich source of iodine and other nutrients. It is a traditional, rich fertiliser for land use. The Okayama scheme has created a sustainable system which led to a trebling the local fish harvest, while catches fell in adjacent regions.

The Okayama scheme with its artificial reefs could be a model for the oil companies. The legs of extinct marine oil rigs can provide extra millions of hectares of surface area for the marine food web to latch onto and do its magic.

LAND - GREEN PASTURE

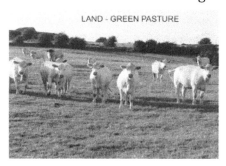

Marine pastures- Zostera marina

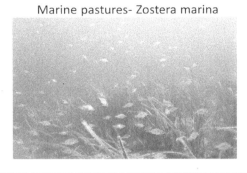

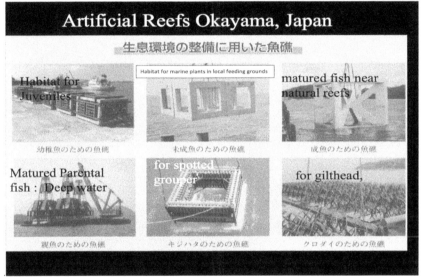

In 1993 the Indonesian government started kelp farming to help counter the high prevalence of iodine deficiency. The kelp farmers are now making more money than the inland farmers. China has been farming kelp for 5,000 years.

On the Island of North Ronaldsay, which is the northernmost island in the Orkney archipelago of Scotland, the sheep eat seaweed. Consequently, their liver and meat provide a good helping of omega-3 fatty acids and are also likely to be rich in trace elements and fat-soluble vitamins such as vitamins A and D. Kelp is the key ingredient of lava bread in Wales, which, like so many traditional foods, has been swept away by the tide of intensive food production and its persuasive advertising. There is an increasing interest in sea grass, kelp, mangroves and marine farming, but this is largely confined to individual initiatives.

The farming of the seabed and subsequent development of oceanic resources will answer the even bigger question of 'where are we going?

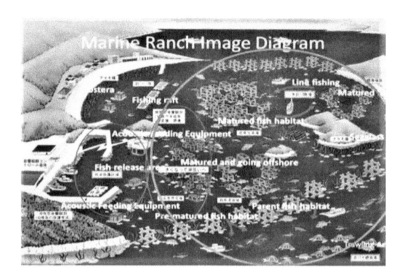

There will be technological spin-offs to meet the need for infrastructure, workshops, breeding and laboratories for marine health and reproduction research. Tools are required for farming the seabed and for underwater communication, artificial reef construction, underwater laboratories, and marine plant and animal husbandry.

There would also be the potential use of trained marine mammals such as dolphins to corral fish – something the Romans are thought to have done, and something still practiced in some Brazilian fishing communities.[4] It's a skill we take for granted in our trained sheep dogs – clever animals. Dolphins are also clever and can be trained to coral fish like the sheep dogs, as was done in Roman times. It might even be possible to tame whales in order to access their omega-3 rich milk (there being no such riches in the milk of cows, sheep or goats, and certainly not in vegetable-derived 'milk substitutes'). Research facilities will be needed along the lines of the Moredun Research Institute in Scotland, which carries out studies to improve livestock health and welfare.

There are also many marine research organisation as in Woods Hole and Scripps in San Diego USA, The Institute of Marine Research in Bergen, Plymouth in England and the legendary work of the late Jacques Cousteau and his children, and in many other part of the world such as Bermuda, Australia, South Korea where knowledge of the marine system has been developed to a high degree and can be brought to bear.

## Sea Bed Kelp Farming –Bali, Indonesia

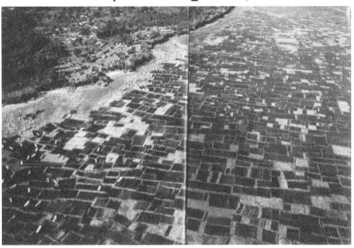

*Photograph from National Geographic Magazine. The Indonesian Government responded to evidence led by Dr Darwin Karyadi of the Ministry of health, Bogor, 1990-1993. The data showed 60% of the school children had palpable goitre, i.e. a sign of iodine deficiency. There were none in the fishing villages. There was something like 1.5 million severely mentally retarded children and 800,000 cretins. Iodised salt had drawbacks as iodine is volatile and so in the heat and humidity, the iodine diminished. The farming of kelp to provide iodine was recommended by Darwin and Michael as it was a transportable food resource, rich in iodine and other trace elements and also contained some omega 3 fatty acids. It can be eaten, fed to animals and used as fertiliser to replenish the soils which were badly depleted due to the incessant rain fall. We are told the kelp farmers are now making more money than the inland farmers.*

Like CERN, the marine research industry will develop useful spin-offs, the most important of which will be foods both new and old. Part of the answer to the question 'where are we going?' would then be 'towards populations of healthier and more intelligent people', with ocean acidification and atmospheric CO2 excesses tamed, an outcome that might just foster friendship and peace, and an intelligent, unified response to existential issues such as climate change and the impacts of unchecked population growth and the killing fields.

## Once-upon-a-time in Maryland USA

**Once-upon-a-time:** Oyster catch in Maryland
Pollution - Ocean acidification

- 1889: 616.000 tons
- 2002: 12,000 tons

Apart from the loss of health giving food:
1889: 270,000 tons of solid CO2 was removed - permanently.

- 2002: Only 7,000 tons CO2 removed. #

- Difference: 263,000 tons CO2 not removed.

New York also was a hot bed of oyster production at one time as of course was the Thames estuary.

# Maryland is now actively restoring the oyster beds.

870 estuarine oyster beds working like Maryland in 1889 would dump an amount of fixed CO2 equivalent to the annual human production of CO2

**A special note about oysters:** When the oyster dies, the shell with its crinkly surface acts as a haven for microscopic marine flora which soak up $CO_2$ for many years afterwards. Oyster farmers knew this and used to put the shells not used for roads or other human utilitarian purposes back into the water. So, yes – the oyster *does* produce $CO_2$, being an animal that breathes; but in the long run the equation favours $CO_2$ sequestration. Moreover, to help keep the waters free from acidification and favour the aquatic climate for oysters, kelp can be grown nearby, providing an added commercial product, for food and fertiliser for land farming, while reducing the burden of atmospheric $CO_2$ and ocean acidification.

## Iodine and DHA: nutritional treasures of the marine food web

Another issue that impacts on mental health is iodine, of which 2 billion people in the world are at risk. Iodine deficiency has been mentioned before as being long known to cause mental retardation. The vast majority of people suffering iodine deficiency live inland, distant from the coast or even freshwater food resources. While carrying out work for the Indonesian Ministry of Health and the WHO in 1990-93, Michael found that 60% of school children in Indonesia had palpable goitre, a clear sign of iodine deficiency. There were no such problems in the country's fishing villages. The same situation prevailed in Kerala, a beautiful state in the southwest of India. The 60% goitre rate was reported to a conference on Nutrition and the Brain in New Delhi, organised in 1998 by the late Coluthur Gopalan FRCP, FRS, FAMS, FASc, President of the Indian Nutrition Foundation (pictured).

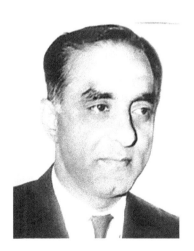

Possibly because iodine deficiency was once a subject so well known, it has, ironically, been overlooked again until recently. People are now returning to the subject with an extra impetus generated by recommendations from departments of health to reduce salt intake to avoid hypertension. Reducing salt can have unforeseen consequences. Iodised salt used to be an important source of iodine; and in a 2012 study in the UK, for example, a worrying proportion of schoolgirls were found to be borderline or deficient in iodine status. [5]

The marine food web is rich in both DHA and iodine. Drs Izzeldin Hussain and Kot Nyuar, two postgraduate students working in the Sudan 2006–2010, described severe iodine deficiency in their study. At the same time, Kot recorded the lowest levels of DHA in mother's milk that we have ever seen in over 6,000 samples across the planet. He reported levels as low as 0.036% DHA.[6] The multi-ethnic mothers in our 1980s East-end of London studies had more than ten times that amount. [7] With the co-existence of DHA and iodine in the marine food web, the likelihood is that the 2 billion people at risk of iodine deficiency are also at risk of DHA deficiency. Both lead to mental retardation. Consequently, DHA deficiency may be of much greater prevalence than is being currently considered.

With not enough DHA today for all 8 billion people, things can only get worse tomorrow. In effect, last century the intensification of land-based agriculture was commercially and, in some sense, nutritionally very successful. The mind boggles at the logistics of feeding people daily in and around the major cities of the world. New York has about 8.3 million people, London 10 million and Tokyo 9 million, while greater Tokyo has over 35.6 million men, women and children to feed. In China, there are several cities with more than 30 million. The logistics of feeding these vast numbers every day, is a colossal undertaking. And yet it happens every day, which is entirely to the credit of the food industry. We just need to do better in terms of not just "full cups" but that what is in the cup is appropriate for brain health.

Note that the Indonesian women in our 1990s' study appeared well fed but were still iodine and iron deficient, is central to the case put forward in this book – that the upward thrust of human evolution could not have happened without the nutrients present in aquatic foods, and that a lack of these foods in our diets impoverishes us mentally, However, external appearance may be just fine. Whilst land foods were also critical DHA, is the all-important brain-specific requirement, and it would have been present in practically every meal eaten by young girls and pregnant and lactating women during our evolution as they wandered around, at that time, unbelievably rich coastline.

The DHA in sea foods would have been accompanied by an ample supply of iodine and critically important, accessory trace elements, from those same foods. Moreover, the prodigious energy requirements of the brain would also have been met from this resource [8]. With the ability of DHA to switch-on gene expression in the brain, epigenetics would have ensured the enhancement of brain development. Generation after generation, before and after birth, an evolutionary path that led to *H. sapiens.*

The brain has a wish list. It consists of omega-3 DHA, iodine, and an array of trace elements. These were the ingredients with which it was able to develop in the first place, and without them its development is a no go. The human brain has reached a remarkable level of complexity fed on this basic wild diet, but it does not emerge with all the hardware and software fully functioning every time a child is born. It needs teaching and sustaining. Like anything else, if you take way that sustenance, it will fail.

Today, the recent takeover of our diets by intensive land-based agriculture, animal production, and the powerful lobbies behind them, is a poor provider of DHA. Replacing herring at breakfast with sugar-stuffed processed cereals has been a nutritional disaster. Even the humble egg from hens properly fed in the old days would have been a good source of DHA and trace elements, otherwise how would the chicken be able to make a brain (or, indeed, cross the road)? In part the problem is one of diminishing availability – in our pre- history, and until relatively recent times, almost every meal would have included DHA. Today, however, there is simply not enough to go around. As predicted in 1972 by Michael, [9] failure to respect the requirements of the brain has resulted in the current crisis in mental ill-health.

## The prediction 1972: take no action we will become a race of morons

Michael and his wife Sheilagh wrote a book "What We Eat Today Published in 1972 based on their science of declining value of food and the importance of DHA for the brain. In the book they wrote that unless the food system provides for the brain, then brain disorders will follow. . It was reviewed by Graham Rose in the Sunday Times, 5th November 1972. He wrote that unless action was taken to heed the message, we would become "a race of morons"!

This prediction has now been proved correct. There is no longer an 'if'' – it has happened. It is getting worse, and is being rapidly globalised. The endgame logically is the end of humanity in all the meanings of that word i.e. extinction. Considering the atrocities by mindless people last and this century, the path to mindlessness is the unthinkable. "We do not have time".

The worse the loss of intelligence and increase in mental ill-health gets, the less chance people have of understanding and put in place the necessary measures to reverse this trend. Our brains truly are under siege, and thought-leaders are being denuded of the ability to think, robbed of the understanding that would help them put in place the necessary measures to reverse this sinister trend.

There is no reason why every child should not be born what

we call today gifted. We have been guiding human evolution in reverse. It is in our power to stop the decline and continue the upward thrust of humanity with all that word means.

## A solution to the food system, mental ill-health and climate change

The answer to our food conundrum lies in the oceans and the development of marine agriculture, of the kind currently being developed in China, Japan, South Korea, Indonesia, and Oman. We are sure the idea is stirring elsewhere, especially in the USA.

71% of the planet is covered in water, and an island nation like the UK has huge potential for marine agriculture. The country has approximately 18.3 million hectares (according to 2010 DEFRA figures) of arable land for animals and crops. Its coastline is estimated at 9,128 miles. Sustainably farming the sea bed could nearly double the UK's food production, create a new natural resource and generate new industries. Just as some land is unusable for agriculture, some of it being used for urbanisation and some for leisure, the same would apply to the coastline – not all of it could be used for marine agriculture. But that would not matter – there are many islands in the UK waters, several of them uninhabited, particularly in Scotland. Even Boris Johnson's planned expansion of marine wind farms could play their part by designing their feet as artificial reefs. Canada has the largest coast line and in Australia, most people live close to the coast line. In India with its high prevalence of preterm births and low birthweight, its large coastline could be put an end to that by the harvest from farming their coastal waters. Healthier and more intelligent children would be the reward all round.

Capture fisheries reached their limit 20 years ago. Aquaculture [10] will also reach a limit where it depends on by-products of the wild catch. Salmon farmers are already having to use chicken feathers and meat and vegetable oils to feed their fish, so that DHA levels are falling and linoleic acid levels rising in their products. There is only one solution: fresh water, coastal, estuarine and oceanic agriculture.[11] Marine agriculture does not require input of pellet-feed and fresh water. The sun and the natural mineral wealth of the oceans, gathered since the beginnings of the planet, do it all.

Maybe we could go deep too. It is always a surprise to see a giant squid dredged up from deep water. To reach these enormous sizes in the very deep ocean demonstrates that there is a good food chain down there. The hydrothermal vents, at colossal depths, feed an ecosystem that gives rise to worms of more than two metres in length. The oceans are packed full of nutritional riches about which too little is known. The sperm whale knows about this food resource.

In looking in the far away direction, perhaps we have lost respect for the riches on our doorstep. Do the Mars thing as well but lets do the obvious in our home planet. Why not instead aim those billions at greening Earth's deserts as we suggested earlier. Deserts occupy nearly one- third of the planet's land surface? [12]

The naive notion of never-ending riches, married to a lack of foresight, has led to almost every estuary and much of the world's coastlines being seriously polluted. Lakes, rivers and oceans have been used as rubbish tips for centuries. The reality is, settlements and civilisations have always arisen beside rivers, estuaries, lakes and coasts. Consequently, we have now built industries, oil refineries, harbours and towns beside our water sources, and where these things go, pollution follows, destroying the once rich resource of oyster and mussel beds, crab, lobster, scallops and crayfish havens in New York harbour and the Rhine. Our starting point has to be cleaning the rivers and estuaries, to detox, stabilise and then manage their ecosystems. The natural process is that rain washes trace elements such as iodine, zinc, selenium and copper from the land into the sea. At the estuaries the sunlight penetrates the shallow water to the seabed, which is fertilised from these river-borne nutrients, and marine life flourishes. Allowing these natural processes to flourish is the first step in feeding the marine flora and fauna. The once salmon rich river flowing through Basel has been decimated. Although efforts are being made to clean the Rhine, its recent history as a conduit for pollution washed down to the industrial laden estuary is repeated across the planet.

## Pollution of the rivers, estuaries and oceans from the land must be reversed

In 2009, of the 777 UK beaches tested, only 370 were declared Marine Conservation Society (MCS) 'recommended' – the first time since 2002 that fewer than half made the grade. Thomas Bell, the MCS coastal pollution officer, said: "Today's results reflect last summer's heavy rain which swept waterborne pollutants like raw sewage, petro-chemicals and farm waste into rivers and the sea."[13]

Surfers Against Sewage (SAS) alerted people in 2009 to the fact that certain English water companies were clandestinely letting raw sewage out into the oceans. One surfer reported recovering his head above water after a being caught by a big wave, he was greeted by floating human faeces. SAS complained bitterly about ear infections linked to the practice of releasing raw sewage.[14]

Bergen, Norway. A lovely picture but one which portrays how a once rich coastal resource has been built on. The same is true in many parts of the world. In Norway, the pollution is minimal, and the government has made a bit of an effort to control marine destruction. In many places in Europe, the pollution and destruction of the estuarine coastal habitat is appalling. Practically every estuary across the planet, from the Rhine to the Ganges, Yellow River and Manila Bay, has been destroyed by pollution in the last two centuries, to the detriment of the marine food web.

The early settlers on the coast of what is now Manhattan, commented on the abundance of fish "striped bass, sturgeon, shad, drum fish perch, pike and trout" in the Hudson and other rivers entering the ocean. They were so abundant you could catch them by hand. The coastline was the home of oyster beds.

**Bergen! The cost:** Human building as well as sewage has destroyed estuaries world wide.

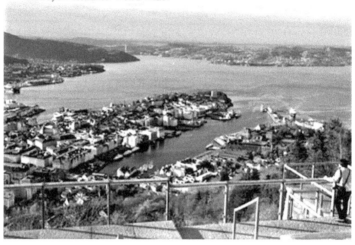

New York was surrounded by immense natural oyster reefs. By 1880 New York was the undisputed capital of history's greatest oyster boom. By 1880 steam power increased the oyster haul 12-fold compared to the previous sail-powered vessels. People thought there was no end to their productivity and New Yorkers simply loved their large oysters, raw, fried, stewed or any way described in the cookbooks which sprouted[42].

As New York grew, oyster stands became as common as hot dog stands today. A story goes that an English Earl on returning to England arrived at New York harbour too early. "What shall we do?" his American traveling friend asked. His lordship replied "Return to Broadway and have some more oysters!". In the UK, by 1990 the East-London public house owners were

---

42     Information from The Big Oyster: A Molluscular History of New York Paperback – 5 April 2007  By Mark Kurlansky, Vintage Books, London, ISBN 9780099477594

still placing oysters on the bar for people to have free with their beer. In New York as with London, the pollution and overfishing was starting to set the rot in progress.

In Edinburgh, in Michael's youth, fish and sea foods were in plentiful supply from the great estuary of the Firth of Forth. Nearly every day, a lady would walk from the harbour of Leith with a huge wicker basket strapped to her forehead and back, to bring fresh fish to sell to the people in the centre of Edinburgh. She put her son through university with the money.

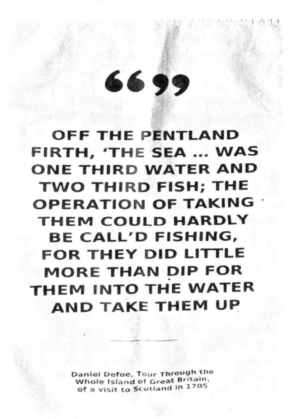

**OFF THE PENTLAND FIRTH, 'THE SEA ... WAS ONE THIRD WATER AND TWO THIRD FISH; THE OPERATION OF TAKING THEM COULD HARDLY BE CALL'D FISHING, FOR THEY DID LITTLE MORE THAN DIP FOR THEM INTO THE WATER AND TAKE THEM UP**

Daniel Defoe, Tour Through the Whole Island of Great Britain, of a visit to Scotland in 1705

On the outskirts of Edinburgh, stood Crammond Inn. Located at the mouth of the River Almond it was spectacularly known for its sea food. The proprietor would collect the sea foods from the shore early in the morning, so it was fresh.

The picture below is of Crammond Inn, just outside Edinburgh on the shore of the Firth of Forth. As a child Michael was regularly taken here to celebrate whatever his father felt needed celebrating and somehow a celebration was often in order.

Returning from five years teaching at Makerere, Medical College, in Uganda in 1965, Michael proposed a family trip to Crammond Inn to go down memory lane and enjoy its renowned sea food of his early years. It was a sunny evening in July, so a visit to the foreshore to see the wonderful iron railway bridge across the Firth of Forth, was planned before calling at the inn for dinner.

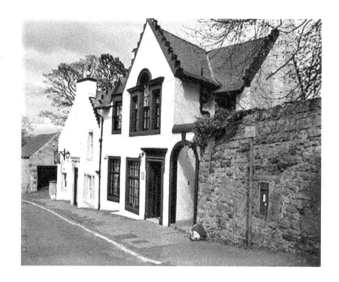

*Cramond Inn – once famous for its sea food gathered from the local shore. The great estuary of the Firth of Forth has been killed in the latter half of our lifetime.*

They had arrived early so parked the cars at the back of the Inn and walked to the shore to see the wonderful view. They were greeted by the notice below. The wealth of the Firth of Forth had been destroyed in his lifetime.

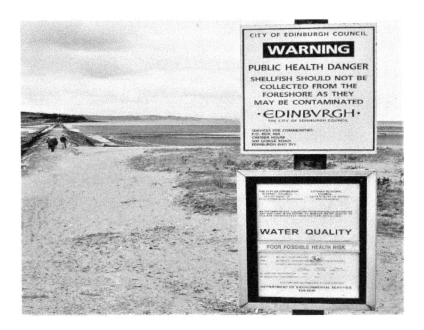

Visiting Edinburgh in April 2007, Michael was greeted with the news that Edinburgh's Seafield Wastewater Treatment Plant had failed and was ejecting a thousand litres of raw sewage every second into the Firth of Forth. Residents in Leith had been campaigning for years about the smell from the plant, saying it was not fit for purpose. Rob Kirkwood, the chairman of Leith Links Residents' Association, said: "*It has an infrastructure that is basically Third World technology.*" Local vets, Michael was told, instructed people walking their dogs along the foreshore to keep their pets on a leash in case they ate the poisonous sea food.

The original image of this warning signpost was published in "The Earth in Danger" by Ian Breach who wrote the first section on POLLUTION and the second by Michael on CONSERVATION. David Attenborough wrote the Foreword[15].

Now Sir David, he was in 2022 named as **Champion of the Earth** by the UN's Environment Programme (UNEP). Sir David has spent his life travelling the world bringing to people's attention the wonders of Nature in animal and plant life for some 60 years. In a quiet, unassuming and brilliant way he communicated with people about the richness and wonders of the planet in which we live.

## Champion of the Earth

Sir David's concern over our destruction of our planet is not new. In his foreword of Earth in Danger he commented that "this book urged us to change our ways". "Whereas once the effluents from our homes and factories were easily swept away by tides and winds, now there are so many of us, the seas and the skies are not big enough to cope with the overwhelming quantities of waste and we are choking in our own filth".

He then expresses his concern about the exponential growth of the human population as he did a decade ago on the Wellcome Trust's website. Population growth "cannot continue indefinitely without ending in disaster. ... questions raised in this book must be tackled and answered ..... by us all". This was by no means the only cry for help last century.

But who is listening? 1976 was before the present horrors of plastics and microplastics. The richest Nation has put a man on the Moon but, in the poorest countries two children will have died from malnutrition or infection whilst you read this sentence. Sir David was writing before the soul was torn out of the Middle East and at the time of writing, the present escalation of maiming, death and destruction of homes in the Ukraine.

Sir David, at 96, has been for the last 60 years a worldwide champion of the world in which we live. It is said that if it were not for the fact we have a Monarchy in the United Kingdom, he would have been appointed President by popular acclaim. In recent time he has used his energy to speak on behalf of our world "warning of climate change and mass extinction"

Sir David's voice as far back as 1976 was by no means the only person demanding action. Indeed, concern over the relationship between humans and nature goes back a long way and Buddhism is an example. Even before that, the original Australian Aboriginals recognised the need for population control and had a deep respect for the conservation of the land and sea resources on which they depended before the English arrived and took over their costal habitats.

Edinburgh is by no means unique. This pollution of rivers, estuaries and coastlines is a pattern repeated across the globe, and it cannot but impact upon the marine resources of the planet, their productivity and carbon sequestration.

Somehow people will not accept that the conditions were any different in the past. Indeed it is often claimed how terrible conditions were. Leaders of the world are too young to remember what it was like other than in recent past and with a smugness think of the past as a period of privation with poor food availability. Let us look at the physique of the people jumping into the deep end of the outdoor swimming pool in Portobello just outside Edinburgh in 1936. (David Hepburn, Edinburgh Evening News). Think of their physique compared to today with the prevalence of obesity in the USA at 42.4% in 2017 – 2018. Compared to today, these people look emaciated but far from it they were fit and healthy as Michael can testify – he was one of them.

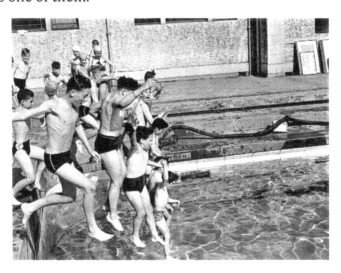

Then we hear influential people, chastising Sir David Attenborough for chairing a meeting to present scientific evidence for the use of marine and fresh water resources during the evolution of our large brain! (See chapters 6 and 9). Then they claim that water resources were not part of our history and the early settlement around estuaries, rivers, lakes and coastlines were only because of trade. They did not think the brain evolved in the sea and still needs marine foods. The rise from a 340g chimpanzee sized brain to the 1,45 Kg of the Herto people 160.000 years ago, could not have happened without the required building nutrients of which DHA and sea foods are essential providers. Perhaps they don't realize they already would needed to be pretty smart to start a village or indeed to trade in the first place. Those attitudes contribute to sorting the problem that today where we are struggling to keep what we had and for the most part are losing it with the fall in IQ and mental health. They do not seem to realize how rich these resources were. Michael was evacuated form Edinburgh at the beginning of WWII to Fort Augustus Abbey when the Government sent the children out of the cities to the country so they might be protected from the expected bombing of the cities by Hitler. He recalls that on Fridays, the monks at the Abbey would take a rowing boat out into Loch Ness to catch salmon for dinner for the boys and themselves. They would put anything below 25 lbs back in the water, they were so plentiful. "They even taught us to fish."

Aldus Huxley's Brave New World of 1932 was a broadside against environmental destruction. Then Sir Frank Fraser-Darling wrote about the devastation of the Scottish Highlands with deforestation. In In 1949, he was invited to be one of UNESCO's representatives at the United Nations conference on conservation at Lake Success on Long Island. His 1969 BBC Reith Lectures "Wilderness and Plenty" stirred the growing public concern on our responsibility for our natural environment with the threat to sustainability on the planet from misuse. His lectures were a statement of the dependence of all living things on one and another.

Then we had Rachel Carson with her 1962 publication of "Silent Spring" and now "The Sixth Extinction: An Unnatural History" by Elizabeth Kolbert, in 2014 and Greta Thurnberg, the 19 year old Swedish activist, hammering at the politicians and leaders of industry on their inactivity and demanding immediate action on climate change. Her speech to the UN is everywhere in the Web "How Dare You". Tere have been many more people – to many to mention. But who is listening?

Finally we have Professor Stephen Hawking's claim shortly before he died, March 2018, that we need to have left the planet by 100 years' time. There have been plenty of warnings over a long time yet the hugest investments are still in things that destroy, kill and maine.

## We Must Clean The Rivers And Protect the Estuaries

The important point needed to understand the solution to our escalating survival issues, is that the estuaries of the planet are the places where the marine food chain takes off in earnest. The trace elements washed down from the mountains provide a rich nutritional environment in the shallow waters, where sunlight can reach to the floor of the sea, providing the perfect habitat for the small marine flora and fauna that provide safe areas for egg laying, and safe cover for the emergence of fry.

Known since for ever, the rain, melting snow and ice in the mountains washes nutrients down to the sea. We have recklessly polluted the lakes and rivers and so destroyed the most important estuaries where, in days gone by, the marine food web started in earnest.

In 2012, the Declaration of Manila, and before that, in 2008, the Declaration of Muscat, called for an end to the pollution of estuaries and coastlines, which had contributed to the collapse of the inshore marine food web and may also be responsible for the decline of the phytoplankton at the beginning of the food web.

The reason for optimism is enhanced by recent actions from the FAO fisheries department, and by the action taken by New Zealand in 2012 when it passed an Act on Exclusive Economic Zone and Continental Shelf (Environmental Effects) to protect its marine ecology.

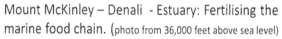

Mount McKinley – Denali - Estuary: Fertilising the marine food chain. (photo from 36,000 feet above sea level)

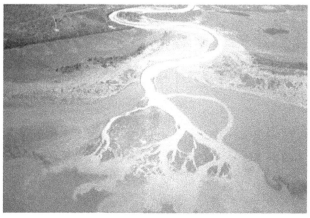

Melting ice takes nutrients to the estuary

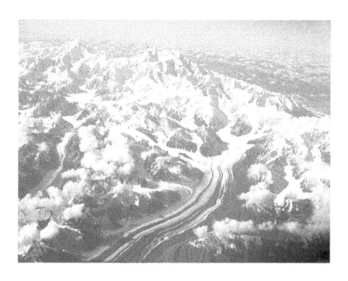

As an island nation, New Zealand has also been engaged in a serious expansion of marine protected areas (MPAs). It has the largest MPA in the planet. There are many other encouraging examples. In England, the River Otter in Devon is being restored. Its habitats – including the estuary, so vital for the marine food web –are being regenerated for birds and other wildlife. This should form a template for every river on the planet.

Reniel Cabral and colleagues at the University of California have claimed that the expansion of MPAs by a mere 5% could increase future fish catches by 20% through 'spillover' of fish from MPAs into wild fisheries. The spillover from the development of mariculture, marine agriculture, or whatever you want to call it, would be huge. The Food and Agriculture Organisation (FAO) of the United Nations has estimated that the total fish production would expand from 179 million tonnes in 2018 to 204 million tonnes in 2030. This is not just wild-caught fish – aquaculture will play a large part in the expansion.

A team of 22 global experts has claimed that reform of fish stocks management could sustainably increase beyond even that. According to Stefan Gelcich, associate professor at Pontifical Catholic University of Chile and one of the authors of the report, seafoods currently provide "3.3 billion people with roughly 20% of their average intake of animal protein. Seafood hasn't really been an integral part of the future food system narrative though ... We wanted to ask whether the seas have a more sustainable potential."

Our answer to this is yes, they do, but not through a hunting-and-gathering model or the increased use of land-derived food products to sustain aquaculture. And not by referring to it primarily as a source of protein either! This is the 2020s, so let's recognise seafood's proper value as a source of the lipids and trace elements needed for a healthy human brain. The brain is the priority in early human development so get the brain right and the rest will follow

In-depth knowledge of the ocean floor is vital to the next chapter in humanity's use of marine resources. We know more about the surface of Mars than we do about the ocean floor – to date, only one-fifth of the sea floor has been mapped, compared with 90% of the Martian surface.

There needs to be a global cooperation on agriculturalisation of the oceans. Rival nations need to get together to save the planet rather than building self-destructive doomsday weapons. Cleaning freshwater resources, eliminating ocean pollution, designating extensive marine protection areas, and undertaking sustainable marine agriculture can solve the food conundrum for generations, reverse the world's escalating mental ill-health problem and address global warming.

## Time For Global Action

The message from the past is that nutrition is a determinant of evolution. We will repeat this one last time: the increase from a 340 cc chimpanzee brain size to 1.450 cc by the time of Herto could only have happened if the nutrients required for building a brain were available. Again, the brain evolved in the sea some 500–600 million years ago using the marine food web and especially DHA, iodine, selenium, zinc and other trace elements, to form the agents of brain structure, function and protection. While people are trying to genetically modify land plants to make DHA, helpful as that maybe, plants cannot make iodine, selenium or the other trace elements that are being progressively depleted from our soils. Moreover, with a billion more people to feed in a few years' time, and Foresight estimating that there is little room for expanding conventional land-based agriculture. Plant production of phospholipid-DHA, would face the challenge that there would not be land enough to produce it in the amounts required globally. Although every little helps, the sea actually does it in abundance for free. The challenge now is to make use of that resource to reverse the escalating mental ill-health and declining measures of intelligence.

It is time for recognition of the challenge, and for the global action necessary to meet that challenge. The scale of the requirement to maintain the sustainability of human intellect is here and now. We cannot today meet the requirement for a uniform distribution of brain-specific foods and nutrients and give all children born an equal chance and the joy of enjoying the full potential of this wonderful organ that makes us human. The stunting of the brain – which must be happening in millions of children who will grow up to be adults, denied their full genetic heritage in intelligence, and be in charge of our world – is unacceptable.

We have been caught out by a trick of nature, hiding the very essence of what made us human. The driving force of our taste for sea foods and consequent brain development was probably DHA and its link to feelings of happiness, as we discussed before and as Captain Joseph Hibbeln has stated, EPA and DHA leads to happiness and calm.[16] But, deprived of DHA, we are coming close to Robert Ardrey's "killer ape" of the DHA-poor savannah. Last century was the bloodiest in human history, and the many recent atrocities of this century and current wars, show that things are no better.

The most obvious precedent for the current mass nutritional distortion of brain development was the mental retardation associated with iodine deficiency, prevalent in the mountainous regions of Europe a century ago. It is also seen today on a large scale in developing, low income regions of the world, along with such issues as vitamin A deficiency, and in the large-scale impact of poor maternal nutrition and children born prematurely and/or at low birth weights. Babies born of malnourished mothers, and often premature, remain at nutritional risk even after birth and are "...sentenced to a lifetime of physical and mental limitations". These are the descriptive words of Josette Sheeran, when she was executive director of the UN World

Food Programme. She is now Vice Chair of the World Economic Forum, and President of the Asia Society. In her TED talk she complains about the death of children every ten seconds from malnutrition, and about malnutrition's lasting impact on the brains of the survivors. And this is despite there being enough food to go around, and the fact that "we know how to fix it".[17]

But we don't make the fix. And "we don't have time".

More generally, the fundamental error of food policy last century, with its focus on protein and omitting the needs of the brain, is leading to concerns about the dumbing down of humans. People who commit such acts as shooting school children and teachers or bombing a crowd of onlookers at a public event must have had deficits in brain development. There is a Gaussian curve (the well-known bell-curve pattern) of the intelligence and humanity of any population, reflected in behaviour and the ability or efficiency of doing things. There will always be people at the bottom of the curve and others at the top. But the Gaussian curve is slipping, and that means more at the bottom and less at the top. One grim observation is that many perpetrators of today's crimes against humanity come from populations that have little access to fish and sea foods and have a high prevalence of preterm, low-birthweight births.

What is a "good balanced diet"? Different nations define it differently. Too often, the experts behind the recommendations have put too much emphasis on protein. Protein is important, of course; but, as this book has described in some detail, the brain, neural network, vascular network, and indeed every cell membrane in our bodies, require unsaturated fats such as omega-3 DHA. But the brain is still being ignored in most quarters, and the intensification of land-based foods – good for the brawn but not for the brain – continues.

Of course, there are beautiful and wonderful things being done in art, music, literature, medicine and science. It is not necessary to enumerate these as they make up the rich culture of the societies that today live in peace with democratic governments. Even if you deny the evidence that brain size started to shrink with the beginning of land-based agriculture, or that intelligence is now lower than it was in the 1950s, maintaining the status quo of whatever we have is not good enough.

We need to enhance brain power, just as happened during our long evolution. The international crises, wars, and genocides of late testify to the need to reverse the slide into mental ill-health and oblivion. We need to seek conditions to restore the upward evolution and majesty of our brain power. Hence, for a solution in agriculture, fisheries and food production we must heed the messages of Sir Jack Drummond in WWII, and Caroline Hurford (UN-WFP): who commented "...it is not just a full cup of food that matters, *it is what is in the cup.*" With the focus on calories and protein, combined with ignorance on issues of brain-specific fatty acids, the contents of the cup are what it is all about – even more important than whether the cup is half empty or half full! The continuing rise in mental ill-health this century is an undeniable threat to peace and, finally, to the survival of humankind.

## The Seventh Extinction

In 2015, Elizabeth Kolbert's book *The Sixth Extinction* was published,[18] its title referring to the extinction of humankind. The title of the book reflects the belief that there have been five previous extinctions. However, David Bond of the University of Hull has pointed out that there were two extinctions in the Permian, not one. That means that we are threatened with the *seventh* extinction.

It might be nice to think there was a time when humans lived in harmony with the biosphere; but, as Kolbert writes "it is not clear that they ever did"! Maybe the Australian Aborigines were the exception, until they were displaced by European invaders and pushed from their coastal resources onto poor land. This time round the driving force for extinction is not a volcano or an asteroid, but us. We are doing it to ourselves out of culpable ignorance: it is self inflicted injury! Kolbert is not alone: many authors, ecologists and biologists have written in a similar vein.

## Some sobering points:

- "About 29,000 children under the age of five – 21 each minute – die every day, mainly from preventable causes" (Unicef).[20]
- "Hunger kills more people each year than AIDS, malaria and tuberculosis combined" (FAO, The State of Food Insecurity in the World).[21]
- "One in four of the world's children are stunted — an indicator of chronic malnutrition and calculated by comparing the height-for-age of a child with a reference population of well-nourished and healthy children. In developing countries, the proportion rises to one in three" (UNICEF).[22]
- "One study showed that women's education contributed 43% of the reduction in child malnutrition over time, while food availability accounted for 26%". (FAO, Women in Agriculture: Closing the Gender Gap for Development).[23]
- The United Nations claimed in 2019 that world food security is increasingly at risk due to climate change: "More than 500 million people today live in areas affected by erosion linked to climate change, the UN warned on Thursday, before urging all countries to commit to sustainable landuse to help limit greenhouse gas emissions before it is too late."[24]

How will the dramatic increase in population impact on the above points and on global food security?

Today, in the high-income countries, obesity, diabetes and dementia are now of grave concern. Obesity and diabetes type II go hand in hand. Those countries with the highest rates of diabetes type II are some of the richest: the Gulf States – Saudi Arabia, Qatar, Kuwait, UAE and Oman. Diabetes itself leads to dementia and Alzheimer's, which some call type III diabetes. Worse still is the fact that the child of a diabetic pregnant mother will give birth to a child with a high risk of compromised mental ability, and a high risk of diabetes II and hence dementia. This means that the rich Gulf States are facing an epidemic of dementia.

The reason is blindingly obvious when you consider that these people were originally fishing and seafaring communities. The desert did not have much food to offer, but what was there was good and the coastlines and seas were bountiful. Traders from the Gulf area were sailing to Indonesia and China before Columbus crossed the Atlantic. In some regions, including Oman, attention is again being returned to the sea and its foods – let's hope it is not too late.

However, unlike many parts of the world, Oman and Dubai are surrounded by pristine seas that could again become a support for health and intelligence and indeed provide a solution for 'what comes next' after the oil revenues run out. Oman has taken up the challenge, and as of 2018 had 350 hectares of artificial reefs constructed and seeding a flourishing bio-diversity. A good start!

Little of our concern is new. Paul Ehrlich wrote his comments in the 1960s. In June 2013, during the global summit of the G8, *The Guardian* newspaper reported: *Malnutrition is the underlying cause of death for at least 3.1 million children, accounting for 45% of all deaths among children under the age of five and stunting growth among a further 165 million, according to a set of reports released ahead of a nutrition summit in London.*[25]

The shocking figures, published in *The Lancet* at the same time, emerged as world leaders prepared to meet on Saturday to pledge extra money for nutrition, ahead of the G8 summit of industrialised countries on 17th June 2014.

In 2015 Elizabeth Kolbert[26] wrote:

Humans have altered the composition of the atmosphere, acidified the oceans, hunted and fished large species to their brink, and destroyed ecosystems. Right now, we are deciding without quite meaning to, which evolutionary pathways will remain open and which will be closed. No other creature has ever managed this, and it will unfortunately be our most enduring legacy.

The threat, as Greta Thunberg declared to the assembly of the UN, is to our children and their children. It is real and very sinister.

We have a global war on our hands. But it is not about enemies and guns – the war is with ourselves and the weapon is selfishness. It is an economic, ecological and biological food war, and it is our intelligence and survival which is at stake. We need to listen to those voices whispering to us from the past. We need to learn from the past to enlighten the future. With the evidence of shrinking brain size and diminishing cognition, together with the frightening rise in mental ill-health, the present and future health and survival of our children depends on what we do *right now*. "We do not have time".

We have used the brain size of the Herto people who lived 160,000 years ago throughout this book. Their brain capacity of 1,450 cc seemed to us to be a conservative and easily acceptable number. . Homo superior is a name coined by Robert John Langdon a writer, historian and social philosopher. Homo Superior ranged from 1,500-1,700cc, 28,000-32,000 y.a.

## The Status Quo Is Not Good Enough

We have quoted JFK before and will do so one last time: "We celebrate the past to awaken the future."

The beauty of this quote is that it is a message of hope. It does not envisage the dumbing down into 'idiocracy' or the predictable collapse of civil society. Even if Dr Marta Lahr of Cambridge University[27] is wrong and our brains have not shrunk, and IQ has not diminished since the 1950s, and the Finns are wrong about mental decline, and our data on brain fatty acids and grey matter development and nutrition pre-conception is all wrong too, it simply will not do for the status quo in brain power to remain the same.

The increasing necessity for everyone to reach a higher level of intelligence is obvious when you consider the challenges faced by society today, including the colossal hurdles of climate change and the rising human population. *Homo sapiens* arose because of increasing brain power. Today we seem bent on reversal. Reversal of brain power simply means the end of humankind.

It is unacceptable that over 2 billion people are mentally below their genetic potential; and that figure is almost certainly a serious underestimate. Perhaps the reality is that except for the few gifted children, we are all below our genetic potential. Some 26% – which is just over a quarter of all children worldwide – are stunted,[28] which means the brain did not form properly before birth and during early infancy. The astounding rise in mental ill-health shows that adverse development of the brain is global. The reason we have this problem is that people have taken the brain for granted. There is always an average, and it seems that the average is slipping downwards, with the bottom end expanding. At the opposite end, some are born gifted; but all children need to be born 'gifted' if we are to awaken the future. The potential is all there, in our brains. It just needs feeding. All it will take is the recognition that the brain is different biochemically from the body and has different requirements. Food and agricultural policies prioritise body growth, we need to prioritise the brain.

The issue also requires recognition of the singular importance of the mother, her health and nutrition, even before conception. One has to recognise that the emancipation of women is still a very recent turning point in history; and in many cultures, women are still subjugated. As we said earlier in this chapter, we need Dr Kenneth Stuart's call from the Mother and Child Foundation for a World Charter for Mothers as a vital new step. Human milk has less protein than the milk of other large mammals, and yet is rich in the essential lipids required for the postnatal phase of brain development. We need to listen to nature.

The energy of the mother during lactation devoted to providing ARA and DHA for the development of the brain, blood vessels and immune system, is greater than that which she invests in all the essential amino acids for protein.

We have seen previously, that before birth the placenta magnifies the content of ARA and DHA, as well as the saturated fatty acids specifically require to build the membranes and signalling systems developing in the foetal brain and elsewhere in the developing nervous, vascular and immune system. Linoleic acid is deselected in that proportions in fetal blood are less than half that of the mother. DHA is not just required for the growth and development of the functional structures of the brain, it is also required for its maintenance and, critically, for the protection of the brain against peroxidative damage. There is good evidence that the lack of such protection makes a significant contribution to the development of strokes,[29] pre-senile dementia and Alzheimer's Disease.[30]

DHA is about the building of the functionality of the very system that makes us different from the apes, and indeed from any other animal that has ever lived on this planet. Any distortion of that development before birth has lifelong consequences. Any damage is irreparable. The inadequate nutrition that distorts prenatal brain development is exactly what Josette Sheeran, (cited earlier), referred to as "sentencing the child to a lifetime of physical and mental limitations".

We must listen to nature and change our priorities. Vast sums of money are spent by well-intentioned governments and organisations to help children and save babies. We saw earlier how the crucial note was struck by Dr. Mark Belsey, then Director of Maternal and Child Health at WHO, Geneva. In his talk at the conference for the launch of the Mother and Child Foundation at the Royal Society for Medicine in 1993. He said: Everywhere the interest of the child is served from UNICEF, Save the Children Fund, the ubiquitous Institutes of Child health and many child supportive NGOs. But ..... *"There is no voice for the mother".*

The Gates Foundation, one of the richest philanthropic organisations (funded by Bill and Melinda Gates) put out a call, repeated several times, to "save babies". But the mother must come first. Of course, let's help the children too; but let's also read the scientific literature on saving babies and note the critical importance of health *before* birth, and even before conception. And that means mothers. Saving babies is right and proper but it is the same story of closing the stable door after the horse has bolted. Maternal nutrition and health must come first. Despite being so firmly based in physiology, science and folklore, the mother is so often neglected.

Post-World War II, there was a strong movement to reduce infant mortality. It worked. Perinatal (around the time of birth) mortality fell. However, Peter Pharoah of the University Medical School of Liverpool followed events in the counties of Merseyside and Cheshire in the years 1966 to 1989, and he and his colleagues found that while perinatal mortality fell (babies saved!), the prevalence of cerebral palsy amongst low-birthweight infants rose three-fold.[31] The same rise was recorded by Karen Nelson[32] at the National Institutes of Health of the USA, and Fiona Stanley in Western Australia.[33] Just saving babies may be emotionally attractive but it is not the answer. The prenatal developmental process is all important which tells us of the supreme importance of the mother. This fact is so blindingly obvious yet "there is no voice for the mother".

We hope we have by now explained clearly why and how

biological considerations centred on the brain ought to direct food and agricultural policies worldwide. If we get the brain right, the rest will follow. To do that we not only need the right nutrients, we also need to understand the value of the mother, and the overriding importance of maternal health and nutrition before conception.[34] The brain and the miracle of pregnancy have been taken for granted for too long. This statement is evidenced by the fact that in the UK and US the prevalence of preterm birth as we have said before, is the same as in 1950. Its prevalence is frighteningly high in many developing countries, especially South Asia.

The brain, as we have said many times, is the biological priority of *H. sapiens*. The aim of 'agricultural development' and food policy usually ignores this fact, and that simply has to change. At the same time, the story is far from being one of doom and misery. The advances in science and technology in this century alone leave one with no alternative view other than that man has the ability to find solutions and do the right thing. The danger lies in the rise in mental ill-health reaching the point of no return. In that case, the Gaussian curve will have slipped so much that our leaders will no longer have the intelligence to understand the challenges and work out solutions.

This decline in mental health and its allied disorders are preventable. Sadly, the investment in preventive research in the UK and elsewhere is at an all-time low.

If society responds to the WHO's call for 'Health for All',[35] and if we do accept the fact – and the challenge – that the shape of future human development is in our own hands, then our hopes of a world of peace and humanity for our children and grandchildren will be attainable. However, the WHO call was in 1998 and based on aspirations for the coming new century. During the first 20 years of this century, we have failed. But it is not too late. All we need do is to unlock our knowledge and technology to open a new approach to food production based on our biological priorities, of which the brain has to be foremost – that is non-negotiable. Continued decline in mental ability and escalation of climate change lead to extinction. We are not alone in this concern. In addition to the views of the late Professor Steven Hawking, a science gathering reported by Alexa Phillips for Sky News on 30 July 2021 concluded that a worldwide breakdown could happen "within a few decades" and identified the five countries most likely to withstand future threats[36]. That is, unless someone starts a nuclear war first and finish it all. The situation in the Ukraine at the time of writing is not encouraging. None of us can afford to sit idly by.

Our achievements since the turn of the last century, when Marconi flew a box kite above Signal Hill in Newfoundland and the first transatlantic radio message was heard in the form of three faint dots, are extraordinary. In this short space of time man has gone from the box kite to satellites. A hundred years ago we would not have known how to save humanity. Today we do. With land-based agriculture reaching its limits but population expanding by the billion, there are many who have proved and are developing the feasibility of marine farming to complement advances in land based farming and the arrest of desertification. The effort now needs to become global. If that happens, we solve the issues of food for all and mental and physical health for all, we arrest and reverse global warming and very likely send the obesity and type 2 diabetes epidemic into history. With the brain being prioritised, and preconception care taken for granted, it is likely that epigenetic changes will remove the automatic fear of dementia and Alzheimer's as we approach old age.[37]

## CONCLUSION

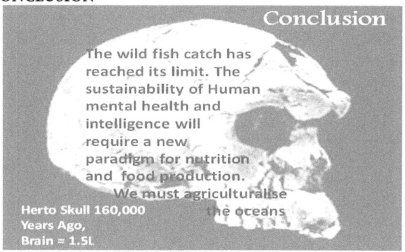

Conclusion

The wild fish catch has reached its limit. The sustainability of Human mental health and intelligence will require a new paradigm for nutrition and food production. We must agriculturalise the oceans

Herto Skull 160,000 Years Ago, Brain = 1.5L

*Fossilised skulls of two adults and one child were discovered[38] in the Afar region of eastern Ethiopia. Carbon dating estimates that they lived the 160,000 years ago. The so-called Herto skull is the earliest known fossil that is anatomically identical to modern humans, Homo sapiens; apart from the fact the Herto brain is significantly larger. The well preserved skull, belonging to an adult male, was estimated to have a brain capacity[39] of 1,450 cm³. Present day estimates of average brain capacity are 1,336 cm³ and falling. Needless to say, these early humans were living close to the sea and also hunting. They lived in an area which is now a salt mine. They would have lived like the Pinnacle Point people, on sea food and land-based animal and plant diets, enjoying the best of both worlds. The brain capacity of the more recent time of 28,000-32,000 y.a. has been found to range from 1,500 to 1,700 ccs. The average today is of the order of 1,336 ccs.*

In this book, Darwin's voice rings out again with his complete thesis, no longer silenced by self-interested curtailment. We explained in chapters 2 and 3 how Darwin stated that all species, both animal and plant, were influenced by the environment, and that those 'best fitted' to it would survive. He called this the 'conditions of existence', or 'conditions of life'.

In 1890 Weismann cut off the tails of many generations of mice, and because they did not start begetting tailless mice, he claimed he had proved that the conditions of existence

– environment – were irrelevant. This was crass and mind-blowingly unscientific, but had broad implications: it was clearly mutilation, not environmentally induced modification. Yet, astonishingly, it was accepted by English speaking (not French) academics, and very extensive deductions were made from this ideocratic result.

From that day until now, abetted by UK philosopher Herbert Spencer's distortion of Darwin's phrase 'best fitted' to 'fittest' (in 1864) the environment has been abused, because humans dominate the planet, they have regarded themselves as the fittest to do so. This distortion has led to the rape of the planet, leading to the potential of wholesale destruction of life itself.

The discovery of DNA as the information chemistry of genetics in the 1950's re-affirmed the genome as the centre for scientific, commercial and popular thought. Any suggestion that the environment could influence the gene was ridiculed.

Despite the undeniable importance of the DNA, we have challenged this dogma as the sole arbiter of life. After 150 years Darwin's voice can again be heard. British embryologist, C. H. Waddington, a medical researcher, came up with the term epigenetics in 1942 when he described environmental influences on the genome. His views were countered by evolutionary biologists including Theodosius Dobzhansky and Ernst Mayr as too Lamarkian. Resistance to his ideas were fierce but as Professor of Human Genetics at Edinburgh University he persevered. He died in 1975[83].

This gave birth to a new paradigm, that of epigenetics, which has proved that somatoplasm (body cells) phenotype can be altered through environmental influence. Likewise, cells of the germplasm (gametes -sperm and ova) can experience epigenetic effects which are heritable. The exact mechanism of the epigenetic effects varies but may be reversible. DNA in the cells is modified in ways that affect expression of a given gene with consequences that range from inactivation to enhancement.

This in turn vindicates Darwin's original, undistorted thesis that the 'conditions of life' – the environment – influences what is 'best fitted' to survive therein, so we need urgently to ensure that the planet, our environment, remains 'best fitted' for life, ours included.[40]

> We can and must save humanity from its present mental health decline. We can and must address inadequate maternal nutrition. We can and must enhance the intelligence, abilities, and prospects of future generations. Children are the future, and with the present challenges and stresses of population expansion, we need children with more intelligence, not less. That will depend primarily on healthy mothers. To do all of this we have to clean the rivers, lakes, estuaries, coastlines and oceans, and we need to farm the seas.[41,42,43]

We need Molly Malone with her cockles and mussels alive alive-ho! We need fishmongers like Whitechapel's celebrated Tubby Isaacs, famous for his jellied eels and his stall stuffed with crabs, lobsters, oysters, scallops, mackerel and herring.[44] And the fresh fish shops, huts and the Netshop shellfish bar on Rock a Nore Road, Hastings, East Sussex. We also need food from the land which is once again fit for healthy consumption.

The photo below shows the harvest of mussels being brought aboard from the farmed mussel beds in the Menai Straits, for supper at the World Oyster Society's International Symposium at Bangor University 2017. On another evening our hosts centre piece were fresh oysters from many different geographical regions to taste for comparison.

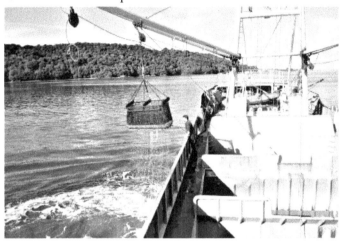

# EDUCATION, EDUCATION, EDUCATION

In particular and foremost, we need education on nutritional science brought back to the primary and secondary schools and medical colleges. In 1994, the Agriculture Food Research Council, which was closed with several research centres, including the internationally renowned Wye College. Originating in 1447, it grew from teaching children to a school specialising in how to grow food and the care of the environment. In 1891 the Earl of Winchilsea proposed the school and farms owned by the combined Thornhill Trust should form the basis of an agricultural college for Kent, Surrey and Sussex. It then became the first and only agricultural and food college founded and maintained by public money solely for the benefit of England.

At the time, it was compared favourably with the state funded agricultural institutions in France, Denmark and Germany[45]. In Edinburgh, Atholl Crescent College for Home Economics, taught the teachers the nuts and bolts of teaching children about home economics, agriculture, food and nutrition. It was closed in 1970. Indeed, the teaching of Home economics and anything proper about food and nutrition was progressively removed from the school curriculum. This deprived children of knowledge needed to make decisions about food and their health. The information they received came only from TV and Media advertisements and the dying wealth of knowledge from their mothers and grandparents.

Sir William Henderson, secretary to the Agriculture and Food Research Council (AFRC) in 1994, announced the closure of the AFRC, Wye and other related Colleges. He said "agriculture was a success story". Hence the AFRC could be closed and a new vision for research was envisaged. With Home economics already shut, the industry now had carte-blanche. Young people grew up to lead industry with little or no knowledge other than that seen in the Media. Another example of the decline was events at Unilever Research Laboratories in Vlaardingen, Holland. Run by the soft spoken, Professor Jan Boldingh it supplied the intelligence for the food production division. Previously, he had been a Professor of Organic Chemistry at Utrecht University. He led the Unilever Research Department from 1967 till he retired in 1980. He equipped the labs with state-of-the-art gear from gas chromatography, to NMR, and various forms of spectroscopy. He was ably supported by Professor David van Dorp a giant of a man, both physical and intellectual. He seemed to know most of Shakespeare's plays by heart along with a wealth of English and French literature. Van Dorp assisted Bengt Samuelsson in his research on prostaglandins, first reported by Sune Bergstrom in the 1930s. Both van Dorp and Samuelsson had determined the structures which led to the idea that the source of these highly active compounds regulating immune, vascular, blood flow and reproductive functions, was arachidonic acid. Van Dorp made radioactive arachidonic acid so that Samuelsson could prove it to be the source of these prostaglandins and other eicosanoids which earned him with Vane and Bergstrom the 1982 Nobel Prize. Many said David should have shared the prize but that would have been politics in the road. The leading research conferences on nutrition and fats would almost always have one of Boldingh's research staff presenting new data.

That was the calibre of the research being done at Unilever's top research labs which included pioneering work on essential fatty acids, fats in food and nutrition to support company development. Second to none. After David and Jan Boldingh retired it all changed.

We need to restore this once great interest in research and teaching in nutrition and health. Nutrition is a major force in prevention of non-communicable diseases. Sir David Cooksey was invited by Gordon Brown, then Chancellor of the Exchequer, to tell him how to get value from the escalating costs of bio-medical research so he could save money at the NHS. In his report on re-organisation of research administration he has an item on the investment by all Government Research Councils and the Health Service. In Sir David's report he itemises costs. Prevention was at a miserable 3% of the total investment on health research[46]. Not much has changed and Preventive Medicine gets little attention in the medical schools. If you want to save costs, then prevention is by far the best option.

The people at the Nobel Prize winning United Nations World Food Programme, know that *"it is not full cup of food that matters, it is what is in the cup that matters*[43]. A young woman thinking about bringing a new life into the world needs to know what to put in the cup. But there is no education and the messages from the media, and even from science are confused and conflicting. A paradigm change is needed which will empower children in

---

43    Josette Sheerhan's Executive Directors Report to the Board of the UN-WFP 2010.

knowledge to make their own decisions about their nutrition and health. Young doctors need an evidence based knowledge but they only get 3 hours of lectures on nutritional science in England to equip them to deal with and take a leadership in the rampant obesity non-communicable diseases and escalating mental ill health to mention but a small corner of the link between nutrition and health and the responsibilities of the general practitioner..

There is another industry where expertise can help to spread the message. Wonderfully, Ben Jackson and Kian Marshall won the 2022 Young Seafood Chef of the Year trophy at the Grimsby Institute. The judges included Rick Stein, Mark Hix, Mitch Tonks and Nathan Outlaw. These events and the people are such good communicators and teachers, there is a natural source of spreading the enthusiasm for sea foods of all kinds. Then there are the events such as the Oyster Festivals in Whitby, the south of England and Stranraer in Scotland extolling the way of life of the still vibrant fishing communities. These are mirrored across the planet all of which raise the superb products of the sea with its supporting brain foods, so recently buried in the plethora of land based intensive food production, convenience foods and chicken batteries.

## GROWING CONCERNS

There is real interest and growing recognition of the problem. But one has to look for it. The Gulf States have in two generations since turning from their traditional fishing to the supermarket has seen type II diabetes hit over 25% and is growing. Diabetes II can lead to heart disease, stroke and dementia. In pregnancy it compromises the intelligence and mental health of the next generation. Oman with one of the highest at 29% held and international conference in Muscat, March 2008. Organised by His Excellency, Dr. Hamed bin Said Al Oufi, the Undersecretary, Ministry of Fisheries and Wealth, Dr Izzeldin Hussein and his colleagues at Sultan Qaboos University and an international team a seminal conference to discuss the problem and solutions.

*"The Economic Importance of Fisheries and their Impact on Public Health"* which led to the Declaration of Oman 2008.

In 2012 EXPO in Yeosu, South Korea, the main theme at the exhibition hall was

**"Life Began in the Oceans, we have to save the Oceans to save ourselves".**

In that same year, the Declaration of Manila sought to unite all the Nations in the far east to arrest the pollution of the rivers, estuaries and coastal resources.

These are only snap shots of the good things that are happening worldwide. There are fortunately many. We hope this book can give power to these initiatives and help better understand the sheer gravity of the rise in mental ill health, disorders of the brain and the shrinking measures of intelligence. If left to continue these trends are a far greater risk to the future of our children and their families than climate change, as serious as that is. *We do not have time.* It is the fate of our children and theirs that is at stake.

We must now echo what our ancestors did 10,000 years ago in the Fertile Crescent when they domesticated plants and animals. We must agriculturalize the oceans. In so doing, we can reverse the decline in mental health and intelligence and at the same time help reverse global warming through the sequestration of $CO_2$ by the marine flora.

*The photo below was taken in 1968 by Michael at a rural health clinic in Bangalore, the capital of the Indian state of Karnataka. Notice the size of the infant's hands compared to the mother's. Then notice the size of the infant's head compared to the mother's. This photo encapsulates the essence of this book. The priority of human development is focused on the brain, not the body. It also illustrates the supreme importance of the mother and her environment[47].*

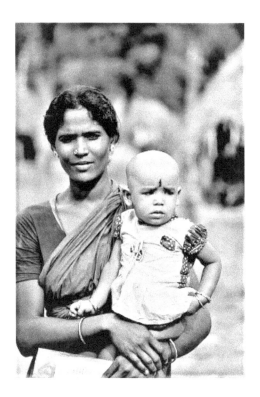

We are one of many creatures that the long progression of life on Earth has thrown up. We are not the most favoured or the best adapted in every respect, and yet our unique intelligence means that we alone can look back and see what made us, and look ahead to gauge what that knowledge implies for our future.

Among that accumulated knowledge is a fact so simple that it is strange it should be so often ignored: whatever else we may be, we are a particular structure of organic chemicals. To maintain that structure in good order, the materials from which it is built – that is to say for example, the brain-specific foods – must match the different needs of the body and the brain. Above all, the balance of nutrients must be right during that critical time when the organism is being formed in the womb, to emerge in due course as one of a new generation of that species whose actions will determine the fate of every species on Earth.

Standing at the moment of intersection between the vast gulf of the past and the dangers and promises of the future there stands a figure whose importance overwhelms all others: the figure of a human mother and her child.

MICHAEL A CRAWFORD & DAVID E MARSH

Visiting Professor Michael A Crawford, PhD, FRSB, FRCPath
The Department of Metabolism, Digestion and Reproduction. Imperial College, London, Chelsea and Westminster Hospital Campus, Room 3,34
369 Fulham Road, London SW10 9NH, UK
michael.crawford@imperial.ac.uk

David E Marsh, Dip Ag. Agronomist and Science Writer
McCarrison Society for Nutrition and Health, Retired
37 Waterhouse Close, LONDON W68DQ +44(0)20 8741 1998
www.davidmarsh.org.uk
davidmarsh.dip.ag@gmail.com

# REFERENCES

## Chapter 1

1. Bill Gates, The Next Outbreak? We're Not Ready https://www.ted.com/talks/bill_gates_the_next_outbreak_we_re_not_ ready?language=en
2. Black D, Morris J, Smith C, Townsend P. Inequalities in health: report of a Research Working Group. London: "
3. Securing Our Future Health: Taking a Long-Term View Derek Wanless, April 2002, Determent of Health."prematurity and other adverse pregnancy outcomes presenting the highest risk to developmental disorders of the brain."
4. Rees G et al (2005) The nutrient intakes of mothers of low birth weight babies – a comparison of ethnic groups in East London, UK, Maternal and Child Nutrition, 1(2), 91–99.
5. Varatharaj A, et al. Neurological and neuropsychiatric complications of COVID-19 in 153 patients: a UK-wide surveillance study Lancet Psychiatry. 2020;doi:10.1016/S2215-0366(20)30287-X
6. Kaufman HW, et al.(2020) SARS- CoV-2 positivity rates associated with circulating 25-hydroxyvitamin D levels. PLoS ONE 15(9): e0239252. https://doi.org/10.1371/journal. pone.0239252
7. Robert A Brown, Amrita Sakar, Low vitamin D, high risk COVID-19 mortality, BMJ 2020; 369 doi: https://doi.org/10.1136/bmj.m1548. (Published 20 April 2020)Cite this as: BMJ 2020;369:m1548
8. Viral rewiring of cellular lipid metabolism to create membranous replication compartments Jeroen RPM Strating and Frank JM van Kuppeveld, Current Opinion in Cell Biology, vol. 47, Aug 2017

9. Bratsberg B, Rogeberg O. Flynn effect and its reversal are both environmentally caused. Proc Natl Acad Sci U S A. 2018 Jun 26;115(26):6674-6678. doi: 10.1073/pnas.1718793115. Epub 2018 Jun

10. "Surgery and Diet", British Medical Journal, 1 (3675): 1031–1032, 13 June 1931, zoi:10.1136/bmj.1.2841.1031-a, PMC 2314713

11. *McCarrison, Sir Robert (29 February 1936), "Nutrition and National Health", British Medical Journal, Cantor Lectures by Sir Robert McCarrison, 1 (3921): 427–430, doi:10.1136/ bmj.1.3921.427, PMC 2457947*

12. https://www.ted.com/talks/josette_sheeran_ending_ hunger_ now?

13. Ghebremeskel, K., Crawford, M.A. (1994) Nutrition and health in relation to food production and processing. Nutr. Health 9: 237-253.

14. Wang Y, Lehane C, Ghebremeskel K, Crawford MA (2010) Modern organic and broiler chickens sold for human consumption provide more energy from fat than protein. Public Health Nutr;13(3):400-8

15. Ogundipe E, Johnson M, Wang Y, Crawford MA (2016) Peri-conception maternal lipid profiles predict pregnancy outcomes, PLEFA, 114, 35–43. http://dx.doi.org/10.1016/j. plefa.2016.08.012

## Chapter 2

- A, 1894 The Effect of External Influences on Development. Romanes lecture. London, Frowde.
- Crawford MA and Marsh DE, The Driving Force, Food, Evolution and the Future. 1989, 1991.
- Crawford MA and Marsh DE,1995: Nutrition and Evolution. Keats.

# Chapter 3

1. Stott R. Darwin's Ghosts: In search of the first evolutionists. Bloomsbury, UK. ISBN 978_1_4088_0908_2. 2012.
2. Crawford MA, Marsh DE. Nutrition and Evolution, Keats New Canaan, CT. USA. ISBN 06840_0876. 1995.
3. Darwin CR. On the Origin of Species by means of Natural Selection: or the Preservation of Favoured Races in the Struggle for Life. John Murray. London. 1868.
4. House SH. McCarrison Society for Nutrition and Health newsletter 43/1: Spring 2009.
5. Darwin CR. The Variation of Plants and Animals under Domestication' (1868). John Murray. London. 1868.
6. Weismann A. Translation: Germ-Plasm, a theory of Heredity Charles Scribner's Sons – Full online text 1893. Also in Reference 2.
   Weismann A. The All Sufficiency of natural selection. In Contemporary Review, 64:309-38; 596-610. 1893.
7. House SH SH House. Handbook of Epigenetics: The New Molecular and Medical Genetics. Editor: Trygve Tollefsbol, Publisher: Academic Press; 1st edition. Evolutionary Epigenetics. Chapter 26 - Epigenetics in Adaptive Evolution and Development: The interplay between evolving species and epigenetic mechanisms. ISBN-10: 0123757096, ISBN-13: 978-0123757098. 21 Oct 2010. House SH. Refs pp1-3
   Golubovsky M, Manton KG. A three-generation approach in biodemography is based on the developmental profiles and the epigenetics of female gametes. Frontiers in Bioscience 10, 187-191. (2005).
   Mill J, Tang T, Kaminsky Z, Khare T, Yazdanpanah S, Bouchard L, Jia P, Assadzadeh A, Flanagan J, Schumacher A, Wang SC, Petronis A. Epigenomic profiling reveals DNA-methylation changes associated with major psychosis. Am J Hum Genet. 82(3): 696-711. (2008)
   Gillman MW, Barker D, Bier D, Cagampang F, Challis J, Fall

C, Godfrey K, Gluckman P, Hanson M, Kuh D, Nathanielsz P, Nestel P, Thornburg KL. Meeting report on the 3rd International Congress on Developmental Origins of Health and Disease (DOHaD). Pediatr Res. 61(5 Pt 1):625-9. (2007) Pembrey ME, Bygren LO, Kaati G, Edvinsson S, Northstone K, Sjostrom M, Golding J; ALSPAC Study Team. Sex-specific, male-line transgenerational responses in humans. Eur J Hum Genet. 14.2:159-66. 2006.

Marsh DE. (2007) The Origins of Diversity. Nutrition and Health 19, No 1-2. 2007.

8.  Proceedings National Academy Sciences April 2, 2013; Time Magazine Sept 6, 2012.

9.  Science Daily July 24, 2014; PLoS Genetics July 24, 2014.

10. Aging Cell Oct 2011 onlinelibrary.wiley.com › ... › Cell Biology › Aging Cell
    Current Drug Targets Dec 2011 www.google.co.uk/webhp?sourceid=chrome-instant&ion=1&espv=2&ie=UTF-8#q=+Current+Drug+Targets+Dec+2011

11. Genetics Generation. www.google.co.uk/webhp?sourceid=chrome-instant&ion=1&espv=2&ie=UTF-8#q=genetics%20generation

12. PLoS Genetics May 2014 www.plosgenetics.org/article/browse/issue/info%3Adoi%2F10.1371%2Fissue.pgen.v10.i05

13. Clinical Chemistry July 16, 2010; Nature March 18, 2010 www.lewrockwell.com/2014/07/bill-sardi/the-human-dna-debate/

14. Knowledge of Health April 25, 2014 https://mailman.stanford.edu/pipermail/protege-user/2014-April/000373.html

15. The Journals Of Gerontology: Series A: Biological Sciences & Medical Sciences www.researchgate.net/journal/1079-5006_The_Journals_of_Gerontology_Series_A_Biological_Sciences_and_Medical_Sciences June 2014.

16. PLoS Genetics May 8, 2014 http://journals.plos.org/plosgenetics/article?id=10.1371/journal.pgen.1004351
17. Genomicron April 25, 2007 www.genomicron.evolverzone.com/2007/04/onion-test/
18. see16. PLoS Genetics May 8, 2014.
19. Genome Biology & Evolution 2013. http://gbe.oxfordjournals.org/content/by/year
20. Seminars Nephrology July 2013. www.seminarsinnephrology.org/issues
21. Nutrition & Health Jan 2012. http://nah.sagepub.com/content/19/1-2/103.abstract
22. Discover Nov 22, 2006 http://discovermagazine.com/2006/nov/cover
23. Time Magazine Jan 6, 2010 http://content.time.com/time/covers/0,16641,20100118,00.html
24. LewRockwell.com April 25, 2014. 24. The Best of Bill Sardi. July 29, 2014. www.lewrockwell.com/2014/07/bill-sardi/the-human-dna-debate/
25. Darwin, CR. Origin of Species. Chapter 5. See References 3 and 2, Nutrition and Evolution, p112.

## Chapter 4

1. Juhász-Nagy S. (2002) Albert Szent-Györgyi - biography of a free genius. Orv Hetil. 2002 Mar 24;143(12):611-4. [Article in Hungarian] PMID: 11963399
2. Hoyle F. *Evolution from Space Evolution from space (the Omni lecture) and other papers on the origin of life* (Enslow Publishers, New Jersey, 1982)
   Hoyle F. and Wickramasinghe N.C. *Evolution from Space: A Theory of Cosmic Creationism* (Simon & Schuster, London, 1984)
3. Wallis MK, Wickramasinghe NC, Hoyle F. (1992) Cometary habitats for primitive life.Adv Space Res. 1992;12(4):281-5. MID: 11538150

4. see: http://www.angelfire.com/in/hypnosonic/Parable of the Monkeys.html

5. For an overview of his life and work see *Obituary Norman Pirie (1907-97)* Nature v.387, p.560 (1997) https://www.nature.com/articles/42378

6. Waddington, C. H.: *The Strategy of the Genes.* (Allen and Unwin, London, 1957. Reprinted 2014.)

7. Dawkins R., *The Blind Watchmaker*, (Longman, Harlow, 1987)

8. Fiennes R.N.T-W., Sinclair A.J. and Crawford M.A. 1973: Essential fatty acid studies in primates: linolenic acid requirements of Capuchins. (J. Med. Prim. 2: 155-169. PMID: 4203709).

9. Gould S.J. and Eldredge N. 1977: Punctuated Equilibria: The Tempo and Mode of Evolution Reconsidered (Paleobiology v3, no.2; pp. 115-151).

10. Eldredge, Niles, and S. J. Gould (1972). "Punctuated equilibria: an alternative to phyletic gradualism." In T.J.M. Schopf, ed., Models in Paleobiology. San Francisco: Freeman, Cooper and Company,

11. Norman Maclean and Brian Keith Hall (1987) Cell Commitment and Differentiation (Cambridge University Press 1987)

12. Caroline Hurford, UN World Food Programme, in conversation.

## Chapter 5

1. https://www.space.com/11425-photos-supernovas-star-explosions.html.

2. http://www.ted.com/speakers/craig_venter

3. S.W. Fox and K. Dose, *Molecular Evolution and the Origin of Life (Revised Edition.)* (New York, Marcel Dekker, 1977)

4. Margulis, Lynn (1998). Symbiotic Planet : A New Look at

Evolution, Basic Books, ISBN 0-465-07271-2. Comment in Amazon Books.

5. Antonio Lazcano of the Universidad Nacional Autonoma de Mexico gave a conference on December 6, 2017 at 2 p.m. titled "Symbiosis and cell evolution: Lynn Margulis and the origin of eukaryotes" held in the *Muséum National d'Histoire Naturelle, Paris, France* in honour of Lynn Margolis...

6. These are phospholipids which have two hooks, one for a saturated (e.g stearic as in beef fat) or oleic (as in olive oil) and the other for a polyunsaturated fatty acid either omega 6 or 3 or occasionally 9.

7. John Serjeant (personal communication). sent a sample to Michael and Holm Holmsen (Bergen University} who were working together at the IBCHN, London Metropolitan University. They confirmed .Di-DHA phosphoglycerides..

8. Benolken RM, Anderson RE, Wheeler TG. (1973). Membrane fatty acids associated with the electrical response in visual excitation. Science. 182(118):1253-4.

9. Ryznar RJ, Phibbs L, Van Winkle LJ. Epigenetic Modifications at the Center of the Barker Hypothesis and Their Transgenerational Implications. Int J Environ Res Public Health. 2021 Dec 2;18(23):12728. doi: 10.3390/ijerph182312728. PMID: 34886453; PMCID: PMC8656758.

10. Heijmans BT, Tobi EW, Stein AD, Putter H, Blauw GJ, Susser ES, Slagboom PE, Lumey LH. Persistent epigenetic differences associated with prenatal exposure to famine in humans.
Proc Natl Acad Sci U S A. 2008 Nov 4;105(44):17046-9. doi: 10.1073/pnas.0806560105. Epub 2008 Oct 27. PMID: 18955703; PMCID: PMC2579375.

11. https://www.youtube.com/watch?v=TdNyLYE1xv8

12. Mark D. Uhen (2007) Evolution of marine mammals: Back to the sea after 300 million years. Anatomical Record, Special Issue: Anatomical Adaptations of Aquatic Mammals 290,6, pp 501-759, https://doi.org/10.1002/ar.20545

13. Hibbeln JR. From homicide to happiness--a commentary on omega-3 fatty acids in human society. Cleave Award Lecture. Nutr Health. 2007;19(1-2):9-19. doi: 10.1177/026010600701900204..

14. Eldredge, Niles and S. J. Gould (1972). "Punctuated equilibria: an alternative to phyletic gradualism" In T.J.M. Schopf, ed., Models in Paleobiology. San Francisco: Freeman Cooper. pp. 82-115

15. Thewissen, J.G.M. (14 January 1994). "Fossil Evidence for the Origin of Aquatic Locomotion in Archaeocete Whales". Science. 263 (5144): 210–212. Bibcode:1994Sci...263..210T. doi:10.1126/science.263.5144.210

16. Brown, R.E., Shaffer, R.D., Hansen, I.L., Hansen, H.B. and Crawford, M.A. (1966) Health survey of the El Molo. E. Afr. Med. J. 43: 480-488. Hansen, I.L., Brown, R.E., Shaffer, R.D. and Crawford, M.A. (1966) Biochemical findings on the El Molo tribe. E. Afr. Med. J. 43: 489-500.
Crawford, MA., Rivers, JPW., and Hassam, AG. (1978) Essential fatty acids and the vulnerability of the artery during growth. Post Grad. Med. J. 54: 149-153..

17. Blood pressure and atherogenic lipoprotein profiles of fish-diet and vegetarian villagers in Tanzania: the Lugalawa study. Pauletto P, Puato M, Caroli MG, Casiglia E, Munhambo AE, Cazzolato G, Bittolo Bon G, Angeli MT, Galli C, Pessina AC. Lancet. 1996 Sep 21: 348(9030):784-8.

18. Claudio was a great friend and highly respected scientist. He organised several wonderful conferences on essential fatty acids and prostaglandins in Italy with his Professor Rudolpho Paoletti. Claudio died 2017 and is sorely missed.

19. Brown, R.E., Shaffer, R.D., Hansen, I.L., Hansen, H.B. and Crawford,
M.A. (1966) Health survey of the El Molo. E. Afr. Med. J. 43: 480 488. Hansen, I.L., Brown, R.E., Shaffer, R.D. and Crawford, M.A. (1966) Biochemical findings on the El Molo tribe. E. Afr. Med. J. 43: 489 500

## Chapter 6

1. Gordon Rattray Taylor, The Great Evolution Mystery, Publisher Abacus, 1984 ISBN 0-349-12917-7
2. Ridley Mark (1983) New Scientist, 28 April, p233.
3. Gould, Stephen Jay, & Eldredge, Niles (1977). "Punctuated equilibria: the tempo and mode of evolution reconsidered." Paleobiology 3 (2): 115-151. (p.145)
4. https://kaiserscience.files.wordpress.com/2015/01/eyeevolution.jpg
5. Blakemore C, Van Sluyters RC, Peck CK, Hein A. (1975) Development of cat visual cortex following rotation of one eye. Nature. 1975 Oct 16;257(5527):584-6. PMID: 1165784
6. Blakemore C, Cooper GF. (1970) Development of the brain depends on the visual environment.
   Nature. 1970 Oct 31;228(5270):477-8. PMID: 5482506.
7. Grayson DS, Kroenke CD, Neuringer M, Fair DA. (2014) Dietary omega-3 fatty acids modulate large-scale systems organization in the rhesus macaque brain. J Neurosci;34(6):2065-74. doi: 10.1523/JNEUROSCI.3038-13.2014. PMID: 24501348
8. Barker FM 2nd, Snodderly DM, Johnson EJ, Schalch W, Koepcke W, Gerss J, Neuringer M.(2011) Nutritional manipulation of primate retinas, V: effects of lutein, zeaxanthin, and n-3 fatty acids on retinal sensitivity to blue-light-induced damage. Invest Ophthalmol Vis Sci;52(7):3934-42. doi: 10.1167/ iovs.10-5898. PMID: 21245404
9. Benolken RM, Anderson RE, Wheeler TG. (1973) Membrane fatty acids associated with the electrical response in visual excitation. Science. 182(4117):1144-6., PMID: 4750611.
10. Crawford, M.A. and Sinclair, A.J. (1971) Nutritional influences in the evolution of the mammalian brain. In Lipids, malnutrition and the developing brain: 267-292. Elliot, K. and Knight, J. (Eds.). A Ciba Foundation Symposium (19-21

October, 1971). Amsterdam, Elsevier. PMID: 4949878.

11. https://news.harvard.edu/gazette/story/2000/02/why-onions-have-more-dna-than-you-do/

12. Hopkins, F.G. Analyst, 1906, vol.31, p.391, DOI: 10.1039/AN906310385B

13. See Drummond J. C. and Wilbraham A. *The Englishman's Food* (London; Jonathan Cape, 1939, revised edition 1957).

14. https://en.wikipedia.org/wiki/Vitamin_B12_deficiency

15. Rivers, J.P.W., Sinclair, A.J. and Crawford, M.A. (1975). "Inability of the cat to desaturate essential fatty acids." Nature 285: 171 173.

16. Crawford MA, Schmidt WF, Broadhurst Leigh C, Wang Y. Lipids in the origin of intracellular detail and speciation in the Cambrian epoch and the significance of the last double bond of docosahexaenoic acid in cell signaling. (2020). Prostaglandins, Leukotrienes and Essential Fatty Acids 166 (2020) 102230. https://doi.org/10.1016/j.plefa.2020.102230

17. Sinclair AJ, Crawford MA, The accumulation of arachidonate and docosahexaenoate in the developing rat brain, J Neurochem. 1972, 19(7):1753-8

18. Serhan CN et al, 2008; Resolving inflammation: dual anti-inflammatory and pro-resolution lipid mediators, Nat Rev Immunol. 2008 May;8(5):349-61. doi: 10.1038/nri2294

19. Crawford MA, Wang Y, Forsyth S, Brenna JT. (2015) The European Food Safety Authority recommendation for polyunsaturated fatty acid composition of infant formulaverrules breast milk, puts infants at risk, and should be revised. Prostaglandins Leukot Essent Fatty Acids. 2015 Dec;102-103:1-3. doi: 10.1016/j.plefa.2015.07.005. Epub 2015PMID: 26432509

20. Farquharson J, Cockburn F, Patrick WA, Jamieson EC, Logan RW.(1992) Infant cerebral cortex phospholipid fatty-acid composition and diet. Lancet; 340(8823):810-3. PMID: 1357244

21. Birch EE, Carlson SE, Hoffman DR, Fitzgerald-Gustafson KM, Fu VL, Drover JR, Castañeda YS, Minns L, Wheaton DK, Mundy D, Marunycz J, Diersen-Schade DA. (2010) The DIAMOND (DHA Intake And Measurement Of Neural Development) Study: a double-masked, randomized controlled clinical trial of the maturation of infant visual acuity as a function of the dietary level of docosahexaenoic acid.Am J Clin Nutr. 91(4):848-59. doi: 10.3945/ajcn.2009.28557. PMID: 20130095

22. Drover JR, Hoffman DR, Castañeda YS, Morale SE, Garfield S, Wheaton DH, Birch EE. (2011) Cognitive function in 18-month- old term infants of the DIAMOND study: a randomized, controlled clinical trial with multiple dietary levels of docosahexaenoic acid. Early Hum Dev; 87(3):223-30. doi: 10.1016/j.earlhumdev.2010.12.047. PMID:21295417.

23. Birch EE, Garfield S, Castañeda Y, Hughbanks-Wheaton D, Uauy R, Hoffman D.(2007)
Visual acuity and cognitive outcomes at 4 years of age in a double-blind, randomized trial of long-chain polyunsaturated fatty acid-supplemented infant formula. Early Hum De; 83(5):279-84.PMID: 17240089

24. Lauritzen L, Fewtrell M, Agostoni C. Dietary arachidonic acid in perinatal nutrition: a commentary. Pediatr Res 2015;77:263–9 doi: 10.1038/pr.2014.166

25. Dobbing J, (1972) Dobbing J. Vulnerable periods of brain development. In: lipids, malnutrition & the developing brain. Ciba Found Symp. 1971:9-29. PMID: 4949882,. Elliot, K. and Knight, J. (Eds.). A Ciba Foundation Symposium (19-21 October, 1971). Amsterdam, Elsevier. PMID: 4949878

26. Galli C, Paoletti R (1971). In: lipids, malnutrition & the developing brain. Ciba Found Symp. 1971:9-29. PMID: 4949882.

27. Gould S.J., Hens' Teeth and Horses' Toes (NY -; W.W. Norton & Co, 1983)

28. Crawford MA, Leigh Broadhurst C, Guest M, Nagar A, Wang Y, Ghebremeskel K, Schmidt WF (2013) A quantum theory for the irreplaceable role of docosahexaenoic acid in neural cell signaling throughout evolution Prostaglandins Leukot Essent Fatty Acids (PLEFA); 88(1):5-13. doi: 10.1016/j.plefa.2012.08.005. PMID: 23206328

29. Crawford MA, Thabet M, Wang Y, Broadhurst C L, Schmidt WF (2018) A theory on the role of the π-electrons of docosahexaenoic acid in brain function. OCI, 24, A403. doi.org/10.1051/ocl/2018011

30. For an overview of his life and work see Obituary Norman Pirie (1907-97) Nature v.387, p.560 (1997) https://www.nature.com/articles/42378

31. FAO Nutrition paper no 3, FAO, 1977, Rome ISBN 92-5-100467-6.

32. Yavin E, Himovichi E, Eilam R. (2009) Delayed cell migration in the developing rat brain following maternal omega-3 alpha linolenic acid dietary deficiency. Neuroscience. ;162(4):1011-22. doi:10.1016/j.neuroscience.2009.05.012. PMID: 19447164

33. Kim HY, Spector AA. Synaptamide, endocannabinoid- like derivative of docosahexaenoic acid with cannabinoid-independent function. Prostaglandins Leukot Essent Fatty Acids. 2013 Jan;88(1):121-5. doi: 0.1016/j.plefa.2012.08.002. Epub 2012 PMID: 22959887

34. Yavin E, Himovichi E, Eilam R (2009) Delayed cell migration in the developing rat brain following maternal Omega-3 alpha linolenic acid dietary deficiency. Neuroscience. 2009 May 14. [Epub ahead of print]

35. Brand A, Crawford MA, Yavin E. (2010) Retailoring docosahexaenoic acid-containing phospholipid species during impaired neurogensis following omega-3 alpha-linolenic acid deprivation. J Neurochem. 114(5):1393-404

36. Kitajka K, Sinclair AJ, Weisinger RS, Weisinger HS, Mathai M, Jayasooriya AP, Halver JE, Puskás LG. Effects

of dietary omega-3 polyunsaturated fatty acids on brain gene expression. Proc Natl Acad Sci U S A. 2004 Jul 27;101(30):10931-6. doi: 10.1073/ pnas.0402342101. Epub 2004 Jul 19. PMID: 15263092; PMCID: PMC503722.

37. See LH Lumey et al 2007, Cohort Profile: The Dutch Hunger Winter Families Study; Int J Epidemiol. 2007 Dec;36(6):1196- 204

38. Hibbeln JR, Davis JM, Steer C, Emmett P, Rogers I, Williams C, Golding J. Maternal seafood consumption in pregnancy and neurodevelopmental outcomes in childhood (ALSPAC study): an observational cohort study. Lancet. 2007 Feb 17;369(9561):578-85. doi: 10.1016/S0140-6736(07)60277- 3. PMID: 17307104.

## Chapter 7

1. The Guardian, 18th April 1986

2. Chicxulub impactor en.wikipedia.org/wiki/ Chicxulub_impactor

3. Keller G, Adatte T, Stinnesbeck W, Rebolledo-Vieyra M, Fucugauchi JU, Kramar U, Stüben D. (2004) Chicxulub impact predates the K-T boundary mass extinction. Proc Natl Acad Sci U S A; 101(11):3753-8. PMID: 15004276.

4. Schulte P1, Alegret L and 36 authors (2010) The Chicxulub asteroid impact and mass extinction at the Cretaceous-Paleogene boundary. Science. 327(5970):1214-8. doi: 10.1126/science.1177265. PMID: 20203042.

5. Lowery CM, Bralower TJ and 35 authors (2018) Rapid recovery of life at ground zero of the end-Cretaceous mass extinction. Nature; 558(7709):288-291. doi: 10.1038/ s41586-018-0163- 6, PMID: 29849143.

6. https://skepticalscience.com/print.php?n=177

7. Corals of the World Vol. 1 2 3 (in Slip Cover) by J.E.N. Veron

(ISBN: 9780642322364)

8. Schoene B, Eddy MP, Samperton KM, Keller CB, Keller G, Adatte T, Khadri SFR. (2019) U-Pb constraints on pulsed eruption of the Deccan Traps across the end-Cretaceous mass extinction. Science;363(6429):862-866. doi: 10.1126/science.aau2422. PMID: 3079230

9. Condamine FL, Guinot G, Benton MJ, Currie PJ. Dinosaur biodiversity declined well before the asteroid impact, influenced by ecological and environmental pressures. Nat Commun. 2021 Jun 29;12(1):3833. doi: 10.1038/s41467-021; 23754-0. PMID: 34188028; PMCID: PMC8242047.

10. Crawford MA, Gale MM, Woodford MH. (1969) Linoleic acid and linolenic acid elongation products in muscle tissue of Syncerus caffer and other ruminant species. Biochem J.;115(1):25-7. PMID: 5346367

11. Crawford, M.A., Casperd, N.M. and Sinclair, A.J. (1976) The long chain metabolites of linoleic and linolenic acids in liver and brain in herbivores and carnivores. Comp. Biochem. Physiol. 54B: 395-401.

12. Crawford MA, Leigh Broadhurst C, Guest M, Nagar A, Wang Y, Ghebremeskel K, Schmidt WF (2013) A quantum theory for the irreplaceable role of docosahexaenoic acid in neural cell signaling throughout evolution Prostaglandins Leukot Essent Fatty Acids (PLEFA); 88(1):5-13. doi: 10.1016/j.plefa.2012.08.005. PMID: 23206328.

13. Belayev L, Mukherjee PK, Balaszczuk V, Calandria JM, Obenaus A, Khoutorova L, Hong SH, Bazan NG. (2017) Neuroprotectin D1 upregulates Iduna expression and provides protection in cellular uncompensated oxidative stress and in experimental ischemic stroke. Cell Death Differ. 24(6):1091-1099. doi: 10.1038/cdd.2017.55. PMID: 28430183

14. Crawford, M.A., Cunnane, S.C. and Harbige, L.S. (1993) A new theory of evolution: quantum theory. IIIrd International Congress on essential fatty acids and eicosanoids, Am. Oil

Chem. Soc. ed A.J. Sinclair, R. Gibson, Adelaide, 87-95.

15. Sakayori N, Maekawa M, Numayama-Tsuruta K, Katura T, Moriya T, Osumi N. (2011) Distinctive effects of arachidonic acid and docosahexaenoic acid on neural stem/progenitor cells.Genes Cells. 16(7):778-90. doi: 10.1111/j.1365-2443.2011.01527.x. PMID: 21668588

16. Bitsanis D, Crawford MA, Moodley T, Holmsen H, Ghebremeskel K, Djahanbakhch O. (2005) Arachidonic acid predominates in the membrane phosphoglycerides of the early and term human placenta. J Nutr.135(11):2566-71. PMID: 16251612.

17. Crawford, M.A. and Frankel, T. (1980) Models for the human brain. Proc. Nutr. Soc. 39: 233-240

18. Aird WC, (2005) Spatial and temporal dynamics of the endothelium. J Thromb Haemost; 3: 1392–1406

19. Crawford, M.A., Hassam, A.G., Williams, G. and Whitehouse, W.L. (1976) Essential fatty acids and fetal brain growth. LANCET (i): 452-453. PMID: 55720.

20. The role of dietary fats and oils in human nutrition, A joint report by the FAO aand WHO, Nutrition report no 3, 1977, FAO Rome.

21. ZamenhofS,EichhornHH.(1967)Studyofmicrobialevolution through loss of biosynthetic functions: establishment of "defective" mutants. Nature. 216(5114):456-8. PMID: 4964402

22. Gurdon JB, Uehlinger V. (1966) "Fertile" intestine nuclei. Nature. 210(5042):1240-1. PMID: 5967799

23. Gurdon JB. (2017) Nuclear transplantation, the conservation of the genome, and prospects for cell replacement. FEBS J. 284(2):211-217. doi: 10.1111/febs.13988. PMID: 27973726

24. Kitajka K, Sinclair AJ, Weisinger RS, Weisinger HS, Mathai M, Jayasooriya AP, Halver JE, Puskás LG. (2004) Effects of dietary omega-3 polyunsaturated fatty acids on brain gene expression. Proc Natl Acad Sci U S A.101(30):10931-6. PMID: 15263092..

25. Mangeney M1, Cardot P, Lyonnet S, Coupe C, Benarous R, Munnich A, Girard J, Chambaz J, Bereziat G (1989). Apolipoprotein-E-gene expression in rat liver during development in relation to insulin and glucagon. Eur J Biochem. 181(1):225-30. PMID: 2653821.

26. Cairns J, Overbaugh J, Millar S, The Origin of Mutants. Nature vol. 3235: pp. 142-145, 1988

27. Cairns et al., ibid

28. McCracken JA, Schramm W, Barcikowski B, Wilson L Jr (1981)
The identification of prostaglandin F2 alpha as a uterine luteolytic hormone and the hormonal control of its synthesis. Vet Scand Suppl. 1981; 77:71-88. PMID: 7030035

29. Samuelsson B. (1986) Leukotrienes and other lipoxygenase products. Prog Lipid Res. 1986;25(1-4):13-8. PMID: 2827184a

30. Ramstedt U, Ng J, Wigzell H, Serhan CN, Samuelsson B (1985) Action of novel eicosanoids lipoxin A and B on human natural killer cell cytotoxicity: effects on intracellular cAMP and target cell binding. Immunol;135(5):3434-8. PMID: 2995494

31. Serhan CN, Chiang N, Dalli J, Levy BD. (2014) Lipid mediators in the resolution of inflammation. Cold Spring Harb Perspect Biol. 7(2):a016311. doi: 10.1101/cshperspect.a016311. PMID: 25359497

32. Vane JR.(1983) Prostacyclin.JR Soc Med. 1983 Apr;76(4):245-9. PMID: 6341583

33. Samuelsson B.(1983) From studies of biochemical mechanism to novel biological mediators: prostaglandin endoperoxides, thromboxanes, and leukotrienes. Nobel Lecture, 8 December 1982. Biosci Rep. 1983 Sep;3(9):791-813. PMID: 6315101

34. Moodley T, Vella C, Djahanbakhch O, Branford-White CJ, Crawford MA (2009). Arachidonic and Docosahexaenoic Acid Deficits in Preterm Neonatal Mononuclear Cell Membranes. Nutr Health, 20: 167-185

35. McKinney, B. and Crawford, M.A. (1965) Fibrosis in the guinea pig heart produced by plantain diet. LANCET (ii): 880- 882.

36. Bitsanis D, Crawford MA, Moodley T, Holmsen H, Ghebremeskel K, Djahanbakhch O. (2005) Arachidonic acid predominates in the membrane phosphoglycerides of the early and term human placenta. J Nutr.135(11):2566-71.

37. Mandelin M, Kajanoja P (1978) Induction of second trimester abortion: comparison between vaginal 15-methyl-PGF2alpha methyl ester and intra-amniotic PGF2alpha. Prostaglandins. 1978 Dec;16(6):995-1001.

## Chapter 8

1. Broadhurst LC, Schmidt WF, Crawford MA, Wang Y, Li R. (2004) $^{13}$C Nuclear Magnetic Resonance Spectra of Natural Undiluted Lipids: Docosahexaenoic-Rich Phospholipid and Triacylglycerol from Fish J Agric Food Chem, 52(13):4250-4255.

2. Brash AR. Arachidonic acid as a bioactive molecule. J Clin Invest. 2001;107(11):1339-1345. doi:10.1172/JCI13210

3. Buckley CD, Gilroy DW, Serhan CN. Proresolving lipid mediators and mechanisms in the resolution of acute inflammation. Immunity. 2014;40(3):315-327. doi:10.1016/j. immuni.2014.02.009

4. Kitajka K, Sinclair AJ, Weisinger RS, et al. Effects of dietary omega-3 polyunsaturated fatty acids on brain gene expression. Proc Natl Acad Sci U S A. 2004;101(30):10931-10936. doi:10.1073/pnas.0402342101

5. Niemoller TD, Stark DT, Bazan NG. Omega-3 fatty acid docosahexaenoic acid is the precursor of neuroprotectin D1 in the nervous system. World Rev Nutr Diet. 2009;99:46-54. doi: 10.1159/000192994. Epub 2009 Jan 9. PMID: 19136838.

6. Belayev L, Hong SH, Menghani H, Marcell SJ, Obenaus A, Freitas RS, Khoutorova L, Balaszczuk V, Jun B, Oriá RB, Bazan NG. Docosanoids Promote Neurogenesis and Angiogenesis, Blood-Brain Barrier Integrity, Penumbra Protection, and Neurobehavioral Recovery After Experimental Ischemic Stroke. Mol Neurobiol. 2018 Aug;55(8):7090-7106. doi: 10.1007/s12035-018-1136-3. Epub 2018 Jun 1. PMID: 29858774; PMCID: PMC6054805.

7. Cunnane SC, Trushina E, Morland C, Prigione A, Casadesus G, Andrews ZB, Beal MF, Bergersen LH, Brinton RD, de la Monte S, Eckert A, Harvey J, Jeggo R, Jhamandas JH, Kann O, la Cour CM, Martin WF, Mithieux G, Moreira PI, Murphy MP, Nave KA, Nuriel T, Oliet SHR, Saudou F, Mattson MP, Swerdlow RH, Millan MJ. Brain energy rescue: an emerging therapeutic concept for neurodegenerative disorders of ageing. Nat Rev Drug Discov. 2020 Sep;19(9):609-633. doi: 10.1038/s41573-020-0072-x. Epub 2020 Jul 24. PMID: 32709961; PMCID: PMC7948516.

8. Iodized salt coverage and COVID-19 inMENA/EMR Izzeldin Hussein; IGN Regional coordinator for MENA/EMRO; Samia Al-Ghanamia, IGN national coordinator, Oman; Salima Al Mammary, Nutrition Department/Ministry of Health, Oman; Lamia Mahmoud, Public Health Specialist, WHO, Oman; Ahmed Farah Shadol, Public Health Specialist, WHO Consultant, Oman; Salwa Sorkati, Micronutrition specialist, WFP Officer, Sudan; Nawal al Hamad, IGN National Coordinator, Kuwait. Iodine Global Network,IDD Newsletter, 4 8. 2, MAY 2020,

FAO/WHO international expert consultations on the role of dietary fats in human nutrition took place in 1976, 1994 and 2008.    CHAPTER 8 REFERENCE 9 All three ISBN NUMBERS;

FAO Report no 3 1966/77  ISBN 92-5-100467 6

FAO Report no 57  1994 ISBN 92-5-103621-7

FAO Report no 91  2008-2010 ISBN 978-92-5-106733-8

9. Dart, R (1925). Australopithecus africanus: The Man-Ape of South Africa. Nature 115 (2884): 195–199 doi:10.1038/115195a0

10. Crawford MA, Sinclair AJ. Nutritional influences in the evolution of mammalian brain. In: lipids, malnutrition & the developing brain. Ciba Found Symp. 1971:267-92. doi: 10.1002/9780470719862.ch16. PMID: 4949878.

11. https://www.thearticle.com/was-basman-right-iconoclasm-ridicule-and-chess

12. Elaine Morgan ~ 100 Years Towards Origins. . Algis Kuliukas 2021.

13. Sinclair, A.J. and Crawford, M.A. (1972). The incorporation of linolenic and docosahexaenoic acid into liver and brain lipids of developing rats. FEBS Lett. 26: 127-129. PMID: 4636721 DOI: 10.1016/0014-5793(72)80557-x

14. Desaturase and elongase-limiting endogenous long-chain polyunsaturated fatty acid biosynthesis.
Zhang JY, Kothapalli KS, Brenna JT. Curr Opin Clin Nutr Metab Care. 2016 Mar;19(2):103-10. doi: 10.1097/MCO.0000000000000254. PMID: 26828581

15. Crawford MA, Schmidt WF, Broadhurst Leigh C, Wang Y. Lipids in the origin of intracellular detail and speciation in the Cambrian epoch and the significance of the last double bond of docosahexaenoic acid in cell signaling. (2020). Prostaglandins, Leukotrienes and Essential Fatty Acids 166 (2020) 102230. https://doi.org/10.1016/j.plefa.2020.102230.ttp://www.bbc.co.uk/radio4/science/scarsofevolution.shtml

16. Crawford MA, Bloom M, Broadhurst CL, Schmidt WF , Cunnane SC , Galli Ghebremeskel K, Linseisen F, Lloyd-Smith J and Parkington J (1999) Evidence for the unique function of DHA during the evolution of the modern hominid brain. Lipids 34, S39-S47

17. Nobuyuki Yamaguchi1*, Andrew C. Kitchener2, Emmanuel Gilissen3 And David W. Macdonald1 Brain size of the lion

(Panthera leo) and the tiger (P. tigris): implications for intrageneric phylogeny, intraspecific differences and the effects of captivity, Biological Journal of the Linnaean Society, 2009, 98, 85–93

18. Wang DH, Ran-Ressler R, St Leger J, Nilson E, Palmer L, Collins R, Brenna JT.(2018) "Sea Lions Develop Human-like Vernix Caseosa Delivering Branched Fats and Squalene to the GI Tract. Sci Rep. 10;8(1):7478. doi: 10.1038/s41598-018- 25871-1. PMID: 2974862

19. Gislén A, Dacke M, Kröger RH, Abrahamsson M, Nilsson DE, Warrant EJ. (2003) Superior underwater vision in a human population of sea gypsies. Curr Biol.;13(10):833-6. PMID: 12747831 Free Article

20. Gislén A, as in20.

21. Hardy, A. (1960). Was Man More Aquatic in the Past? New Scientist, 7, 642-645.

22. Dr Algis, Kuliukas, School of Anatomy Physiology and Human Biology, University of Western Australia, Perth.

23. Human Evolution: Past, Present and Future, conference, 8-10 May 2013, programme can be seen at https://calenda. org/242649

24. Attenborough under attack over theory of aquatic ape, by Hannah Devlin, The Times, 11 May 2013, (online at www. thetimes.co.uk/article/attenborough-under-attack-over-theory-of-aquatic-ape-8fltd2jwcvd)

25. Leigh Broadhurst C., Cunnane. S.C. and Crawford M.A. (1998) Rift Valley lake fish and shellfish provided brain specific nutrition for early Homo. Br J. Nutr. 79: 3-21.

26. Marsh DE, Waters-edge evolution, Nutr Health. 2001;15(1):63-7

27. https://journals.sagepub.com/doi/10.1177/ 02601060010 1500108.

28. Crawford MA, Bloom M, Broadhurst CL, Schmidt WF , Cunnane SC , Galli Ghebremeskel K, Linseisen F, Lloyd-Smith J and Parkington J (1999) Evidence for the unique function

of DHA during the evolution of the modern hominid brain. Lipids 34, S39-S47

29. Kyriacou K, Blackhurst DM, Parkington JE, Marais AD. (2016) Marine and terrestrial foods as a source of brain-selective nutrients for early modern humans in the southwestern Cape, South Africa.J Hum Evol. 2016 Aug;97:86-96. doi: 10.1016/j. jhevol.2016.04.009. PMID: 27457547

30. Jerardino A, Marean CW. (2010) Shellfish gathering, marine paleoecology and modern human behavior: perspectives from cave PP13B, Pinnacle Point, South Africa. J Hum Evol. 2010 Sep-Oct;59(3-4):412-24. doi: 10.1016/j. jhevol.2010.07.003.. PMID: 20934094

31. The shoreline of the Red Sea coast of the Buri Peninsula contains the earliest well-dated evidence of Homo sapiens in the Red Sea coastal environments, dated to 125, 000 years. This technological evidence was later followed by the Middle Stone Age and Late Stone Age stone tool technologies. Evidence of these have already been reported from sites on the coastal territories of the Red sea at the Gulf of Zula. These include, Abdur, Asfet, Gelealo NW and Misse East. These sites represent the most significant event of human evolution during the Pleistocene epoch www. http:// shabait.com/about-eritrea/history-a-culture/25675-stone-tool-technology

See also Beyin, Amanuel, and John J. Shea. "Reconnaissance of Prehistoric Sites on the Red Sea Coast of Eritrea, NE Africa." Journal of Field Archaeology, vol. 32, no. 1, 2007, pp. 1–16. JSTOR, www.jstor.org/stable/40026040.

32. Stringer C, Coasting out of Africa; Nature 405(6782):24-5, 27 June 2000 DOI: 10.1038/35011166.

33. The Guardian, 12 September 2017, 'Total monster': fatberg blocks London sewage system

34. Bath SC, Rayman MP. Iodine deficiency in the U.K.: an overlooked cause of impaired neurodevelopment? Proc Nutr Soc. 2013 May;72(2):226-35. doi: 10.1017/

S0029665113001006. PMID: 23570907.

35. Mail Online Sunday, May 12 2013. *Is man descended from the king of the swimmers? Forget about swinging in trees. Experts now say our earliest ancestors were apes who loved to monkey around in the water.* John Naish.

36. Rhys-Evans P.H and Cameron, M Surfer's Ear Provides Hard Evidence of Man's Aquatic Past, Human Evolution 2014, Vol. 29 Issue 1-3, p75-90.

37. Quoted in Tobias' article *Revisiting Water and Hominin Evolution,* published in "Was Man More Aquatic in the Past? Fifty Years After Alister Hardy Waterside Hypotheses of Human Evolution", ed. Mario Vaneechoutte, Algis Kuliukas, Marc Verhaegen (Bentham , 2011)

# Chapter 9

1. Recounted in The Smithsonian Magazine article, *Reagan and Gorbachev Agreed to Pause the Cold War in Case of an Alien Invasion*, by Danny Lewis, 25 Nov 2015 https://www.smithsonianmag.com/smart-news/reagan-and-gorbachev-agreed-pause-cold-war-case-alien-invasion-180957402/

2. Attenborough David, in Foreword to "Earth in Danger", by Ian Breach and Michael Crawford, 1076, Aldus Books, SBN 385 11345 5.

3. http://webarchive.nationalarchives.gov.uk/+/http://www.bis.gov.uk/foresight/our-work/projects/current-projects/global-food-and-farming-futures/reports-and-publications

4. Ogundipe E, Johnson M, Wang Y, Crawford MA (2016) Peri- conception maternal lipid profiles predict pregnancy outcomes, PLEFA, 114, 35–43. DOI: http://dx.doi.org/10.1016/j. plefa.2016.08.012

5. Rees G Doyle W, Srivastava A, Brooke ZM, Crawford MA, Costeloe KL (2005) The nutrient intakes of mothers of low

birth weight babies – a comparison of ethnic groups in East London, UK, Maternal and Child Nutrition, 1(2), 91–99.

6. Colombo SM, Rodgers TFM, Diamond ML, Bazinet RP, Arts MT (2020) Projected declines in global DHA availability for human consumption as a result of global warming. Ambio. 2020 Apr;49(4):865-880. doi: 10.1007/s13280-019-01234-6. PMID: 31512173

7. At the time of writing UNICEF's latest report on the subject was The State of the World's Children 2019 – Children, food and nutrition: Growing well in a changing world, October 2019
https://www.unicef.org/reports/state-of-worlds- children-2019

8. Elia and Smith 2009 - Improving nutritional care and treatment
Perspectives and Recommendations from Population Groups, Patients and Carers, produced for BAPEN (British Association for Parenteral and Enteral Nutrition)
https://www.bapen.org.uk/pdfs/improv_nut_care_report.pdf

9. See for example Global nutrition group issues first-ever consensus criteria for diagnosing malnutrition, University of Vermont, 11 September 2018, https://onlinelibrary. wiley. com/doi/full/10.1002/jpen.1440; and Kim et al. 2019, Microglial UCP2 Mediates Inflammation and Obesity Induced by High-Fat Feeding, Cell Metab. 2019 Aug. pii: S1550-4131(19)30439-5. doi: 10.1016/j.cmet.2019.08.010

10. See Stephen Hawking Says Humans Have 100 Years to Move to Another Planet, by Julia Zorthian, Time, 4 May 2017

11. Stephen Hawking, This is the most dangerous time for our planet, The Guardian 1 December 2016

12. The IUCN Red List of Threatened Species, established in 1964, and the leading authority on extinctions. https:// www. iucnredlist.org/

13. Thomas D. (2997) The mineral depletion of foods available to us as a nation (1940-2002) – a review of the 6th Edition

of McCance and Widdowson. Nutr Health. ; 19(1-2):21-55. PMID: 18309763

14. Spratt DJ and Dunlop I, Existential climate-related security risk: A scenario approach, Breakthrough - National Centre for Climate Restoration, Melbourne, May 2019, https://www. academia.edu/40017142/

15. Trends in International Arms Transfers, 2017, Pieter D Wezeman, Aude Fleurant, Alexandra Kuimova, Nan Tian, and Siemon T Wezeman.

16. UK reclaims place as world's second largest arms exporter, The Guardian, 30 July 2019

17. Wang Y, Lehane C, Ghebremeskel K, Crawford MA. (2009) Modern organic and broiler chickens sold for human consumption provide more energy from fat than protein. Public Health Nutr; 4:1-9.

18. Crawford, M.A. (1991) Fat animals - fat humans. in World Health, WHO, Geneva, July-August: 23 - 25

19. Doyle, W., Crawford, M.A. and Laurance, B.M. (1982) Dietary survey during pregnancy in a low socio-economic group. J. Hum. Nutr. 36A: 95-106

20. Doyle, W., Crawford, M.A., Wynn, A.H.A. and Wynn, S.W. (1989) Maternal Nutrient Intake and Birth Weight. J. Hum. Nutr. and Diet. 2: 407 - 414.

21. The Disadvantaged Child (1970) Harcourt, Brace & World, Inc, NY,ISBN 0-125725-6 Library of Congress 78-102443,USA.

22. Wynn, S.W., Wynn, A.H.A., Doyle, W. and Crawford, M.A. (1994) The association of maternal social class with maternal diet and the dimensions of babies in a population of London Women. Nutr. Health 9: 303-315.

23. Crawford, M.A., Doyle, W., Craft, I.L. and Laurance, B.M. (1986) A comparison of food intake during pregnancy and birthweight in high and low socioeconomic groups. Prog. Lipid Res. 25: 249-254.

24. Rees G Doyle W, Srivastava A, Brooke ZM, Crawford MA,

Costeloe KL (2005) The nutrient intakes of mothers of low birth weight babies – a comparison of ethnicgroups in East London, UK, Maternal and Child Nutrition, 1(2), 91–99.

25. Louise Brough, Gail A Rees, Michael A Crawford, R. Hugh Morton and Edgar K Dorman (2010) Effect of multiple-micronutrient supplementation on maternal nutrient status and infant birth weight and gestational age at birth in a low income, multi-ethnic population. Br J Nutr, Apr 23:1-9. doi: 10.1017/S0007114510000747. PMID: 20412605.

26. Taha AY, Cheon Y, Faurot KF, Macintosh B, Majchrzak- Hong SF, Mann JD, Hibbeln JR, Ringel A, Ramsden CE. (2014) Dietary omega-6 fatty acid lowering increases bioavailability of omega-3 polyunsaturated fatty acids in human plasma lipid pools. Prostaglandins Leukot Essent Fatty Acids. 2014 May;90(5):151-7. doi: 10.1016/j.plefa.2014.02.003. PMID: 24675168

27. Fiennes, R.N.T.-W., Sinclair, A.J. and Crawford, M.A. (1973) Essential fatty acid studies in primates: linolenic acid requirements of Capuchins. J. Med. Prim. 2: 155-169.. PMID: 4203709

28. Taha AY, Cheon Y, Faurot KF, Macintosh B, Majchrzak- Hong SF, Mann JD, Hibbeln JR, Ringel A, Ramsden CE. (2014) Dietary omega-6 fatty acid lowering increases bioavailability of omega-3 polyunsaturated fatty acids in human plasma lipid pools. Prostaglandins Leukot Essent Fatty Acids. 2014 May;90(5):151-7. doi: 10.1016/j.plefa.2014.02.003. PMID: 24675168

29. Nyuar KB, Min Y, Ghebremeskel K, Khalil AK, Elbashir MI, Crawford MA.(2010) Milk of northern Sudanese mothers whose traditional diet is high in carbohydrate contains low docosahexaenoic acid. Acta Paediatr.c;99(12):1824-7.

30. Nyuar KB, Khalil AK, Crawford MA. Dietary intake of Sudanese women: a comparative assessment of nutrient intake of displaced and non-displaced women. Nutr Health. 2012 Apr;21(2):131-44. doi: 10.1177/0260106012467244.

PMID: 23275454

31. Izzeldin SH, Crawford MA, Ghebremeskel K. (2009) Salt fortification with iodine: Sudan situation analysis. Nutr Health; 20(1):21-30.

32. Wang Y, Lehane C, Ghebremeskel K, Crawford MA. (2009) Modern organic and broiler chickens sold for human consumption provide more energy from fat than protein. Public Health Nutr; 4:1-9.

33. Leigh Broadhurst C., Cunnane. S.C. and Crawford M.A. (1998) Rift Valley lake fish and shellfish provided brain specific nutrition for early Homo. Br J. Nutr. 79: 3-21.

## Chapter 10

1. Geist, Helmut (2005). The causes and progression of desertification. Antony Rowe Ltd. Ashgate publishing limited. ISBN 9780754643234.

2. K. Wright, David; Rull, Valenti; Roberts, Richard; Marchant, Rob; Gil-Romera, Graciela (26 January 2017). "Humans as Agents in the Termination of the African Humid Period". Frontiers of Earth Science. 5 (Quaternary Science, Geomorfology and Paleoenvironment). :

3. http://www.fao.org/dryland-forestry/en/ Drylandrestorationinitiative.

4. Hansen HS, Jensen B. (1965) Essential function of linoleic acid esterified in acylglucosylceramide and acylceramide in maintaining the epidermal water permeability barrier. Evidence from feeding studies with oleate, linoleate, arachidonate, columbinate and alpha-linolenate.Biochim Biophys Acta. 17;834(3):357-63. PMID: 3922424

5. Crawford, M.A., Gale, M.M. and Woodford, M.H. (1969) Linoleic acid and linolenic acid elongation products in muscle tissue of Syncerus caffer and other ruminant species. Biochem. J. 115: 25-27.

6. Crawford, M.A., Gale, M.M., Woodford, M.H. and Casperd,

N.M. (1970) Comparative studies on fatty acid composition of wild and domestic meats. Int. J. Biochem. 1: 295-305

7.  Williams, G. and Crawford, M.A. (1987) Comparison of the fatty acid component in structural lipids from dolphins, zebra and giraffe: possible evolutionary implications. J. Zool. Lond. 213: 673 - 684.

8.  Elagizi A, Lavie CJ, O'Keefe E, Marshall K, O'Keefe JH, Milani RV. An Update on Omega-3 Polyunsaturated Fatty Acids and Cardiovascular Health. Nutrients. 2021 Jan 12;13(1):204. doi: 10.3390/nu13010204. PMID: 33445534; PMCID: PMC7827286.

9.  Clapp LH, Gurung R (2015) The mechanistic basis of prostacyclin and its stable analogues in pulmonary arterial hypertension: Role of membrane versus nuclear receptors. Prostaglandins Other Lipid Mediat;120:56-71. Doi doi: 10.1016/j. prostaglandins.2015.04.007 PMID: 25917921

10. Colussi G1, Catena C, Dialti V, Pezzutto F, Mos L, Sechi LA. (2014) Fish meal supplementation and ambulatory blood pressure in patients with hypertension: relevance of baseline membrane fatty acid composition Am J Hypertens.:471-81. doi: 10.1093/ajh/hpt231.. PMID: 24390292

11. Guo XF, Li KL, Li JM, Li D.(2019) Effects of EPA and DHA on blood pressure and inflammatory factors: a meta-analysis of randomized controlled trials. Crit Rev Food Sci Nutr.:1-14. doi: 10.1080/10408398.2018.1492901. PMID: 29993265

12. Djuricic I, Calder PC. Beneficial Outcomes of Omega-6 and Omega-3 Polyunsaturated Fatty Acids on Human Health: An Update for 2021. Nutrients. 2021 Jul 15;13(7):2421. doi: 10.3390/nu13072421. PMID: 34371930; PMCID: PMC8308533.

13. Williams, G. and Crawford, M.A. (1987) Comparison of the fatty acid component in structural lipids from dolphins, zebra and giraffe: possible evolutionary implications. J. Zool. Lond. 213: 673 - 684.

14. Taylor Merrow: https://504collaborationoption.

weebly. com/natural-selection-in-giraffes.html

15. Schmidt-Nielsen, K. Desert animals: Physiological problems of heat and water (Oxford, Clarendon Press, 1964)

16. Taylor C.E. (1968) The minimum water requirements of some African bovids. in "The comparative nutrition of wild animals", (1968) Symposium no 21 of the Zoological Society of London, pp195-206. ed M A Crawford, Academic Press, Library of Congress no. 68-17679

17. Wright DK (2017) Humans as Agents in the Termination of the African Humid Period Earth Sci., https://doi.org/10.3389/feart.2017.00004

18. https://en.wikipedia.org/wiki/Gobi_Desert

19. Treus V and Kravchenko D (1968). Methods of rearing and economic utilization of eland in the Askaniya-Nova Zoological Park, *Symp. Zool. Soc. London*, 21, pp.395-411

20. Crawford, M.A. (1968) Possible use of wild animals as future resources of food in Africa. Vet. Rec. 82: 305-314.

21. Origin of Species 1859 facsimile.djvu/53

## Chapter 11

1. http://www.oecd.org/greengrowth/fisheries/45692295.pdf

2. https://www.nationalgeographic.co.uk/environment-and conservation-/2020/03/greta-wasnt-first-demand-climate-action-meet-more-young

3. https://www.youtube.com/watch?v=KAJsdgTPJpU

4. For a transcript of Greta Thunberg's "How dare you" speech to world leaders at the United Nations in NYC, December 2019, see:https://eu.usatoday.com/story/news/2019/09/23/greta-thunberg-tells-un-summit-youth-not-forgive-climate- inaction/2421335001/

5. The quote is from Vice Admiral Richard Carmona, who was the seventeenth Surgeon General of the United States,

appointed by President George W. Bush in 2002. He made this remark and repeated it during a military conference in Washington DC, 2014 (published in Military Medicine, 2014, volume 179) discussing mental health. These words referred to the need to deal with the rise in mental ill health.

6. https://www.mirror.co.uk/news/world-news/shocking-true-extent-climate-change-23257939

7. https://climate.nasa.gov/vital-signs/arctic-sea-ice/.See also Stroeve J and Notz D (2018), Changing state of Arctic sea ice across all seasons, *Environ. Res. Lett.* 13 103001, https://iopscience.iop.org/article/10.1088/1748-9326/aade56

8. https://www.iea.org/articles/global-co2-emissions-in-2019#reference-1

9. https://www.iea.org/articles/global-co2-emissions-in-2019

10. https://blueplanetsociety.org/2020/01/the-hidden-dolphin-massacre-in-eu-waters/

11. https://www.express.co.uk/news/politics/1370316/eu-supertrawlers-brexit-news-eu-boris-johnson-cfp-greenpeace

12. https://www.medpagetoday.com/primarycare/obesity/90142

13. https://www.gov.scot/publications/scottish-health-survey-2018-volume-1-main-report/pages/62/

14. Wang Y, Lehane C, Ghebremeskel K, Crawford MA. (2009) Modern organic and broiler chickens sold for human consumption provide more energy from fat than protein. Public Health Nutr; 4:1-9.

15. Ghebremeskel, K., Crawford, M.A. (1994) Nutrition and health in relation to food production and processing. Nutr. Health 9: 237-253.

16. Malnutrition and obesity now a global problem, say experts; The Guardian 16 December 2019, https://www.theguardian.com/global-development/2019/dec/16/

malnutrition-and-obesity-now-a-global-problem-say-experts

17. https://en.wikipedia.org/wiki/Dr._Strangelove

18. See for example *America shaken after pro-Trump mob storms US Capitol building*, The Guardian, 7 January 2021, https://www.theguardian.com/us-news/2021/jan/06/trump-mob- capitol-clash-police-washington

19. https://www.express.co.uk/news/world/1379510/russia-news-latest-nuclear-war-icbm-missile-hypersonic-sarmat- putin-world-war-3

20. Julia Zorthian, *Stephen Hawking Says Humans Have 100 Years to Move to Another Planet,* Time, 4 May 2017, https://time.com/4767595/stephen-hawking-100-years-new-planet/

21. It was made into a film in 1975, directed by Miloš Forman and starring Jack Nicholson, and became the second film ever to win five major Academy Awards.

22. Dr Jo Nurse, National Lead for Public Mental Health and Well-Being, Department of Health Westminster Health Forum Keynote Seminar – Mental Health – New Horizons, the National Service Framework 17th July 2008 © Westminster Health Forum Important: note conditions Page 10 -13 Public Mental Health in the UK

23. Tronson, Natalie C. *How COVID-19 might increase risk of memory loss and cognitive decline*, The Conversation, How COVID-19 might increase risk of memory loss and cognitive decline 7 August 2020

24. Crawford MA, Schmidt WF, Broadhurst Leigh C, Wang Y. Lipids in the origin of intracellular detail and speciation in the Cambrian epoch and the significance of the last double bond of docosahexaenoic acid in cell signaling. (2021). Prostaglandins, Leukotrienes and Essential Fatty Acids 166 (2021) 102230. https://doi.org/10.1016/j.plefa.2020.102230

25. Strating JRPM and van Kuppeveld FJM (2017) Viral rewiring of cellular lipid metabolism to create membranous

replication compartments, Current Opinion in Cell Biology, v 47, pp. 24-33 https://doi.org/10.1016/j.ceb.2017.02.005

26. See https://www.bmj.com/content/372/bmj.n544/rapid-responses

27. Bermano et al., (2020) Selenium and viral infection: are there lessons for COVID-19?, Br J Nutr. 2020 Aug 6: 1–10. doi: 10.1017/S0007114520003128

28. Hamer et al., (2020), Lifestyle risk factors, inflammatory mechanisms, and COVID-19 hospitalization: A community-based cohort study of 387,109 adults in UK, Brain Behav Immun. 2020 Jul; 87: 184–187. doi: 10.1016/j.bbi.2020.05.059

29. Phiri P et al., (2021), COVID-19 and Black, Asian, and Minority Ethnic Communities: A Complex Relationship Without Just Cause, JMIR Public Health Surveill 2021;7(2):e22581, doi:10.2196/22581

30. The phrase was first used in McCarrison's Cantor Lectures of 1936. See https://mccarrison.com/free-libraries-2/mccarrison-library/nutrition-and-national-health-the-cantor-lectures-sir-robert-mccarrison-c-i-e-m-a-m-d-d-sc-ll- d-f-r-c-p-major-general-i-m-s-retd/for a full transcript.

31. UK Government Office https://assets.publishing.service.gov.uk/government/uploads/system/uploads/attachment_data/file/288329/11-546-future-of-food-and-farming-report.pdf

32. Omega-3 Fatty Acids: Nutritional Armor for the Warfighter and Historical Trends Behind Optimal Warrior Performance Richard H. Carmona, MD, MPH, FACS. Military Medicine, Volume 179, Issue suppl_11, November 2014, Pages 176–180, https://doi.org/10.7205/MILMED-D-14-00208, Published: 01 November 2014

33. https://ourworldindata.org/wp-content/uploads/2013/05/ourworldindata_u5_deaths_by_cause_2013_lancet_data.png

34. https://data.unicef.org/topic/nutrition/malnutrition/.

35. Smylie, M (2011) *Herring A History of the Silver Darlings*

(History Press, ISBN-13 : 978-0752459516)

36. Kurlansky, M (1998) Cod: A Biography of the Fish That Changed the World (Penguin, ISBN-13 : 978-0140275018)

37. http://www.bbc.co.uk/news/science-environment-18353964

38. Hamilton, L; Butler, M J. (2001). Outport Adaptations: Social Indicators through Newfoundland's Cod Crisis. Human Ecology Review. 8 (2): 1–11.

39. U.S. Declares a Disaster for Fishery in Northeast, Jess Bidgood and Kirk Johnson, New York Times, 13/09/2012 https://www.nytimes.com/2012/09/14/us/commerce-dept- declares-northeast-fishery-a-disaster.html

40. For a transcript of Greta Thunberg's "How dare you" speech to world leaders at the United Nations in NYC, December 2019, see:https://eu.usatoday.com/story/news/2019/09/23/greta-thunberg-tells-un-summit-youth-not-forgive-climate- inaction/2421335001/

41. https://www.vitalchoice.com

## Chapter 12

1. The opening pages of "What We Eat Today", by Michael and Sheilagh Crawford (Neville Spearman, 1972) describes the classical puzzle which can only be solved by thinking outside the box; so, on this occasion, coining this now overused phrase is justified!

2. See Tanaka T, Introducing a successful Japanese Marine Ranching Project: Shiraishijima Island's Marine Ranching Project in Okayama, in The Proceedings of the FRA-SEAFDEC Joint International Workshop on Artificial Reefs for Fisheries Resource Recovery, 2011 http://nrife.fra.affrc.go.jp/reprint/ gyosyou%20ws.pdf

3. Pacella SR, Brown CA, Waldbusser GG, Labiosa RG, Hales B (2018) Seagrass habitat metabolism increases short-term extremes and long-term offset of $CO_2$ under future

ocean acidification. Proc Natl Acad Sci USA. 2018 Apr 10;115(15):3870-3875. doi: 10.1073/pnas.1703445115.

4. See for example Elizabeth Preston, "Dolphins that work with humans to catch fish have unique accent", The New Scientist 2/10/2017, https://www.newscientist.com/article/2149139-dolphins-that-work-with-humans-to-catch- fish-have-unique-accent/

5. Boyages S. UK survey finds that 69% of a sample of teenage schoolgirls have some degree of iodine deficiency. Evid Based Nurs. 2012;15(2):47-8.

6. Nyuar KB, Min Y, Ghebremeskel K, Khalil AK, Elbashir MI, Cawford MA.(2010) Milk of northern Sudanese mothers whose traditional diet is high in carbohydrate contains low docosahexaenoic acid. Acta Paediatr.c;99(12):1824-7.

7. Drury, P.J. and Crawford, M. A. (1990) Essential fatty acids in human milk. in Clinical Nutrition of the Young Child. Raven Press, New York. 302 - 312.

8. Stephen Cunnane,(2005) The Survival of the Fattest, World Scientific Publishing Co. Pyc Ltd. ISBN 981-256-191-9

9. In What We Eat Today by Michael and Sheilagh Crawford the prediction is crystallised in a review by Graham Rose in the Sunday Times, 5th November 1972. Somewhat expressively he wrote that unless something is done, we "will become a race of morons". He got the message!

10. Aquaculture is the cage-farming of fish such as salmon and trout – not to be confused with the sustainable sea agriculture we are talking about here. The level of DHA in farmed salmon fell by 50% from 2010–2020.

11. Dr Takehiro Tanaka, Director of Fisheries Division, Department of Agriculture, Forest and Fisheries Okayama Prefectural Government. The kelp farm photo was taken from a National Geographic magazine 2000,

12. The Sahara is the largest of these deserts. Since 1900 it has expanded by 250 km to the south over a stretch of land from west to east 6,000 km long. The reasons for the continued

march south and proposals for its reversal have been discussed, but little if anything is being done to address the situation.

13. Fewer beaches get quality rating, BBC News, 22/05/2009, http://news.bbc.co.uk/2/hi/uk_news/8061242.stm

14. See *SAS's year that was 2009*, 22/2009, https://www.sas.org. uk/news/campaigns/sass-year-that-was-2009/

15. Earth in Danger by Ian Breach and Michael Crawford, 1976, Doubleday and Company Inc., Garden City, New York, USA, SBN 385 11345-5.

16. Hibbeln J 2007, From homicide to happiness - a commentary on omega-3 fatty acids in human society. Cleave Award. Nutrition and health 19:9-19, DOI: 10.1177/02601060070190020

17. https://www.bing.com/videos/ search?q=josette+sheeran+ted+talk&docid=60801836375 1533732&mid=D8914FA777C3B0BDD383D8914FA777C3 B0BDD383&view=details&FORM=VIRE

18. *The Sixth Extinction* by Elizabeth Kolbert, Henry Holt, 2014.

19. Paul R. Ehrlich, The Population Time Bomb (Sierra Club Balantine Books, 1968)

20. http://www.unicef.org/mdg/childmortality.html

21. http://www.fao.org/publications/sofi/en/

22. Improving Child Nutrition,UNICEF

23. http://www.fao.org/docrep/013/i2050e/i2050e00.htm

24. https://news.un.org/en/story/2019/08/1043921

25. http://www.theguardian.com/global-development/2013/ jun/06/malnutrition-3-million-deaths-children.

26. The Sixth Extinction: An Unnatural History, a 2014 book by Elizabeth Kolbert about the Holocene extinction, Bloomsberry Publishing,. NY and London, UK.

27. *https://phys.org/news/2011-06-farming-blame-size-brains. html*
https://www.bbc.com/future/article/20220503-why-human-brains-were-bigger-3000-years-ago.

In addition health audits in the EU 2005, 2010, and in the UK 2007, 2010, (DoH) 2013 (Wellcome Trust) all put the cost of brain disorders at the top and increasing with time. With the pile of scientific evidence from the 1970s, and 3 FAO/WHO joint reports on the essentiality of specific fatty acids for the brain in short supply and deficiency leading to cognitive and learning loss, you would have thought someone would have done something about that. BUT NO! Why? Who is responsible? We hear Greta Thunberg "How dare you". Lack of action is and will damage present and future children.

28. https://www.prb.org/stunting-among-children/

29. Ludmila Belayev and 14 ithers. DHA modulates MANF and TREM2 abundance, enhances neurogenesis, reduces infarct size, and improves neurological function after experimental ischemic stroke.

    CNS Neuroscience and Therapeutics.26,:9, 2020. https://doi.org/10.1111/cns.13444.

30. Bazan NG. Docosanoids and elovanoids from omega-3 fatty acids are pro-homeostatic modulators of inflammatory responses, cell damage and neuroprotection. Mol Aspects Med. 2018;64:18-33. doi:10.1016/j.mam.2018.09.003.

31. Pharoah PO, Platt MJ, Cooke T.(1996) The changing epidemiology of cerebral palsy. Arch Dis Child Fetal Neonatal Ed. 1996 Nov;75(3):F169-73. PMID: 8976681.

32. Nelson KB. (1986) Cerebral palsy: what is known regarding cause? Ann N Y Acad Sci.477:22-6. PMID: 3545016

33. Stanley FJ, Watson L (1992) Trends in perinatal mortality and cerebral palsy in Western Australia, 1967 to 1985 BMJ; 304(6843):1658-63, PMID: 1633518

34. Ogundipe E, Johnson M, Wang Y, Crawford MA (2016) Peri- conception maternal lipid profiles predict pregnancy outcomes, PLEFA, 114, 35–43. DOI: http://dx.doi.org/10.1016/j. plefa.2016.08.012

35. https://www.who.int/whr/1998/media_centre/executive_summary6/en/

36. https://news.sky.com/story/uk-and-ireland-among-five-nations-most-likely-to-survive-a-collapse-of-global-civilisation-study-suggests-12366136

37. Although hard evidence on dementia is currently lacking, it is most likely linked to long-term, adverse nutrition for the health of the brain exacerbated by genetic susceptibility.

38. White, Tim D.; Asfaw, B.; DeGusta, D.; Gilbert, H.; Richards, G. D.; Suwa, G.; Howell, F. C. (2003), "Pleistocene Homo sapiensfrom Middle Awash, Ethiopia", Nature, 423 (6491): 742–747, Bibcode:2003Natur.423..742W, doi:10.1038/nature01669, PMID 12802332.

39. In the image of the skull the size of the brain is given as 1.5L

40. See Darwin's Origin of Species, Chapter 6, last paragraph, all editions.

41. Ambio. 2018 Nov 19. doi: 10.1007/s13280-018-1115-y. Global challenges for seagrass conservation Unsworth RKF1,2, McKenzie LJ3, Collier CJ3, Cullen-Unsworth LC4,5, Duarte CM6, Eklöf JS7, Jarvis JC8, Jones BL4,5, Nordlund LM9

42. Sutherland WJ1, Butchart SHM2, and 23 others Trends Ecol Evol. 2018 (1):47-58. doi: 10.1016/j. tree.2017.11.006. Epub 2017 Dec 4. A 2018 Horizon Scan of Emerging Issues for Global Conservation and Biological Diversity.

43. Ecology. Rapid domestication of marine species.Duarte CM, Marbá N, Holmer M.Science. 2007 316(5823):382-3. PMID: 17446380

44. For more on Tubby Isaacs and his successors, see https://spitalfieldslife.com/2013/06/13/so-long-tubby-isaacs-jellied-eel-stall.

45. https://en.wikipedia.org/wiki/Wye_College.

46. Cooksey report recommends central coordinating body for research. BMJ 2006; 333 doi: https://doi.org/10.1136/bmj.39059.559213.DB (Published 14 December 2006) Cite this as: BMJ 2006;333:1239. A review of UK health research funding - Full Text: Ref: ISBN 0118404881

47. M.A. Crawford, Y. Wang, D. E. Marsh, M. R. Johnson, E. Ogundipe, A. Ibrahim, H. Rajkumar, S. Kowsalya, K.S.D. Kothapalli, J.T. Brenna, Neurodevelopment, nutrition and genetics. A contemporary retrospective on neurocognitive health on the occasion of the 100th anniversary of the National Institute of Nutrition, Hyderabad, India, Prostaglandins, Leukotrienes and Essential Fatty Acids, 180, (2022). 102427, ISSN 0952-3278, https://doi.org/10.1016/j.plefa.2022.102427.

# AFTERWORD
# DARWIN'S VOICE IS HEARD AGAIN

In this book, after 150 years, Darwin's voice can ring out again with his complete thesis, no longer silenced by self-interested curtailment. We explained in chapters 2 and 3 how Darwin stated that all species, both animal and plant, were influenced by the environment, and that those "best fitted" to it would survive. He called this the "conditions of existence', or 'conditions of life".

In 1890 Weismann cut off the tails of many generations of mice, and because they did not start begetting tailless mice, claimed he had proved that the conditions of existence - the environment - was irrelevant. This was crass and mind- blowingly unscientific, with broad implications: it was clearly mutilation, not environmentally induced modification. Yet, astonishingly, it was accepted by English speaking (not French) academics, and very extensive deductions were made from this simple result. From that day until now, abetted by UK PHILOSOPHER Herbert Spencer's distortion of Darwin's phrase 'best fitted' to 'fittest' (in 1864) the environment has been abused, because humans dominate the planet, they have regarded themselves as the fittest to do so. This distortion has led to the rape of the planet, leading to the potential of wholesale destruction of life itself.

The discovery of DNA as the information chemistry of genetics in the 1950's re-affirmed the genome as the centre for scientific, commercial and popular thought. Any suggestion that the environment could influence the gene was ridiculed. Despite the undeniable importance of the DNA, we have challenged this dogma as the sole arbiter of life. After 150 years Darwin's voice can again be heard. British embryologist C. H. Waddington, a medical researcher, came up with the term epigenetics in 1942 when he described environmental influences on the genome. His views were countered by evolutionary biologists including Theodosius Dobzhansky and Ernst Mayr as too Lamarkian. Resistance to his ideas were fierce but as Professor of Human Genetics at Edinburgh University he persevered. He died in 1975 (REF 83).

The evidence accumulated leading to the publication of 'The Handbook of Epigenetics' in 2010. This gave birth to a new paradigm, that of epigenetics, which has proved that the heritable somatoplasm (body cells, phenotype) can and indeed does change through environmental influence, without altering the genotype (germ-plasm - DNA) and can be reversible. Epigenetics shows Weismann's thesis to be false absolutely. Nature is far more nuanced than the simplistic Weismannian / Spencerism would have us believe.

This in turn vindicates Darwin's original, undistorted, thesis that the 'conditions of life' - the environment - influences what is 'best fitted' to survive therein, so we need urgently to ensure that the planet, our environment, remains 'best fitted' for life, ours included (see Darwin's Origin of Species, Chapter 6, last paragraph, all editions).

# APPENDIX for chapter 3

## Human Genome Map and the Encyclopaedia of DNA elements -ENCODE

The major international effort was launched in 2004 to provide a more biologically informative representation of the human genome by using high-throughput methods to identify and catalogue the functional elements it encodes. In its pilot phase, 35 groups provided more than 200 experimental and computational datasets that examined in unprecedented detail a targeted 29.998 Mb of the human genome.

In their report of the pilot phase of the project the authors said "To our surprise, many functional elements are seemingly unconstrained across mammalian evolution. This suggests the possibility of a large pool of neutral elements that are biologically active but provide no specific benefit to the organism. This pool may serve as a 'warehouse' for natural selection, potentially acting as the source of lineage-specific elements and functionally conserved but non-orthologous elements between species."

Further in their analysis of control of DNA transcription it emerged that an extremely large number of interacting elements are involved, including non-protein coding transcripts and the pervasive effect of histone modification of DNA controlling the state of transcriptional activity. In other words epigenetics effects are dominant in regulating the whole genome. Since epigenetic effects are environmentally influenced **and** do not involve actual mutation of chromosomal DNA **and** are transmitted vertically, we must now accept that there is a mechanism for an evolutionary process that does not depend of selection of random mutations on the basis of fitness. This is opposite to the orthodox neo-darwinian understanding of natural selection. It gives back to the conditions of existence that Darwin repeatedly referred to as a mechanism of influencing inheritance directly.

The main conclusions obtained during the 4 years of the pilot ENCODE project are listed below [#]:

1. The transcription occurs in almost the whole genome such that most of its bases are committed with at least one primary transcript. Many transcripts link distal loci segments to protein-coding regions.
2. Various novel non protein coding transcripts were identified. Many of these transcripts originate from overlapping protein-coding loci and from regions previously considered transcriptionally silent.
3. Many transcription start sites were identified. Many of them present chromatin structure and protein-binding specific sequences similar to the well-known promoters.
4. The regulatory sequences that surround the transcription start sites are symmetrically distributed, with no bias towards upstream regions.
5. The accessibility to chromatin and histone modification patterns are highly predictive of both the presence and the activity of transcription start sites.
6. The DNA replication timing is related to the chromatin structure.
7. A total of 5% of the bases in the genome can be considered under evolutionary restriction in mammals. For 60% of these bases, there is evidence for function based on results of experimental tests accomplished to date.
8. A general overlapping between the genomic regions identified as functional by experimental tests and those

under evolutionary restriction was not observed. One of the most surprising conclusions from this first phase concerns the remarkable excess of experimentally identified functional elements which lack evolutionary constraint. This means that apparently many functional elements are not restricted to mammal evolution. The consortium suggested the existence of a large pool of neutral elements that are biochemically active, but that do not provide a particular benefit to the organism. This pool may serve as a storage to natural selection, potentially acting as a source of lineage specific elements.

As concluded by the consortium, this surprise suggests that we take a more "neutral" view of many of the functions conferred by the genome [#]."

What we can take all this to mean is that so called purifying selection is not supported by the data from the genomic analysis. Something else is going on and that something has to be epigenetics setting: in other words the influence of the environment is paramount as over against the survival of an elite set of favourable genes which individually confer selfish advantage. How could an individual gene gain an advantage anyway, as if a haemoglobin molecule could exist on its own? What is preserved in the struggle for existence is a set of environmentally shaped preferred settings of a common genome... thus highlighting the importance of Darwin's original phrase - namely "the survival of those **best fitted** to their conditions".

Occasionally alleles are selected by a population bottleneck that occurs as a result of a pandemic. Those who survive due to a minor variant of a gene that prevents infection by a particular pathogen repopulate the earth.

These alleles are not found to go to fixation as pandemics peter out due to reduction in number of susceptible subjects before complete elimination of the population lacking the resistance allele. It remains the case that more shaping of phenotype is done epigenetically than selectively.

# The Encode Project Consortium (2007) Identification and analysis of functional elements in 1% of the human genome by the ENCODE pilot project. Nature 447 (7146), 779–816. doi: 10.1038/nature05874. See also:
Fernanda Moraes and Andrea Goes (2016) A decade of human genome project conclusion: Scientific diffusion about our genome knowledge. Biochem Mol Biol Educ. 2016 May 6;44(3):215-23. doi: 10.1002/bmb.20952. Epub 2016 Mar 7. PMID: 26952518.
E-mail: acgoes@uerj.br

# INDEX

Milton Keynes UK
Ingram Content Group UK Ltd.
UKHW020719120624
443704UK00007B/82